fP

YOU

On a Diet

The Owner's Manual for Waist Management
Revised and Updated

MICHAEL F. ROIZEN, MD,
and MEHMET C. OZ, MD

With Ted Spiker, Lisa Oz, and Craig Wynett

Illustrations by Gary Hallgren

Free Press

New York   London   Toronto   Sydney

*f*P

FREE PRESS
A Division of Simon & Schuster, Inc.
1230 Avenue of the Americas
New York, NY 10020

FREE PRESS and colophon are trademarks
of Simon & Schuster, Inc.

Designed by Ruth Lee Mui

For information regarding special discounts for bulk purchases,
please contact Simon & Schuster Special Sales at 1-866-506-1946
or business@simonandschuster.com

The Simon & Schuster Speakers Bureau can bring authors to your live event.
For more information or to book an event, contact the Simon & Schuster Speakers
Bureau at 1-866-248-3049 or visit our website at www.simonspeakers.com.

Manufactured in the United States of America

3   5   7   9   10   8   6   4

Library of Congress Cataloging-in-Publication Data

Roizen, Michael F.
You, on a diet : the owner's manual for waist management /
Michael F. Roizen and Mehmet C. Oz ; with Ted Spiker, Lisa Oz, and Craig Wynett ;
illustrations by Gary Hallgren. — Rev. and expanded.
p.   cm.
Includes bibliographical references and index.
1. Low-fat diet.   2. Low-fat diet—Recipes.   3. Weight loss.   I. Oz, Mehmet.   II. Title.

RM237.5.R65 2009
613.2'5—dc22   2009045040

ISBN 978-1-4391-6496-9
ISBN 978-0-7432-9896-4 (ebook)

Disclaimer

This publication contains the opinions and ideas of its authors. It is intended to provide helpful and informative material on the subjects addressed in the publication. It is sold with the understanding that the authors and publisher are not engaged in rendering medical, health, or any other kind of personal professional services in the book. The reader should consult his or her medical, health, or other competent professional before adopting any of the suggestions in this book or drawing inferences from it.

The authors and publisher specifically disclaim all responsibility for any liability, loss, or risk, personal or otherwise, which is incurred as a consequence, directly or indirectly, of the use and application of any of the contents of this book.

To the millions who have dieted hard,
so they can learn to diet smart

Contents

Part 3:
The Science of the Mind

Appendices:
The Medical Options

Part 1

What a Waist!

How Your Body Is Supposed to Look—and Work

Introduction
YOU: On a Diet

Work Smarter, Not Harder

Most diets promise commonsense solutions to tight-pants problems: Eat less, and you'll weigh less. Keep your mouth closed, and you'll keep the pounds off. Sweat like a sauna-dwelling sumo wrestler, and you'll wind up skinnier than a sheet of paper. Straightforward enough. But if it really worked that way, our bodies wouldn't be large enough to be spotted by Google Earth. If it really worked that way, then most diets wouldn't fail. If it really worked that way, then we all must be a bunch of rebellious hellions with mayo-covered lips and belt-busting bellies who don't feel like following a few simple instructions.

Or it could be that most diets have it all wrong.

We believe it's the latter.

You know why? Because most diets instruct you to take on the corn chips, meatball specials, and dessert trays with brute force. It's you versus food in a lifetime heavyweight fight. But in that scenario, the fight is always fixed—and not in your favor. That's because the battle against extra pounds isn't won with force, with sweat, with *trying* to diet. It's won with elegance, with smarts, and with healthy choices that become as automatic as a Simon Cowell barb.

When it comes to dieting, trying to whip fat with our weapon of willpower is the food equivalent of holding your breath underwater. You can do it for a while, but no matter how psyched up you get, at some point your body—your biology—forces you to the surface gasping for air. And with most diets, your body forces you to gasp (or gulp) for food. No matter how hard you try not to eat, some hidden force deep inside is always prying your mouth back open, making it impossible for willpower to win. Instead of sparring with your waistline, it's time you made your body an ally in the fight against fat.

Our process is to look at our overweight bodies the way scientists would: Identify the underlying biology of the problem, then find the cures. Why? Because we're lucky enough to be in the right place at the right time—a time when the scientific world has just now started to unlock the biological mysteries that have caused us to store fat and gain weight. For the first time in our history, the scientific community is uncovering the medical evidence about food, appetite, and satiety that will allow you to tackle weight problems with the real weapon against fat: knowledge. By making this knowledge simple and accessible, we're going to give you tools and actions to crack the code of true and lifelong waist management. In fact, our plan will help you avoid the dangerous yo-yo cycle of weight gain and weight loss. We're going to help you reprogram your body so that you can keep off the weight you lose forever.

Through the years, many of us have been led to believe that our weight problem is about two things: calorie counting and mental toughness. While some of us may say that the weight problem is too much of the twelve-cheese lasagna, the real problem is that most of us have as much of a clue about how our bodies work as we have about how our cars do. Sure, we know the major parts and generally what they're supposed to do. The real danger of thinking we have most of the answers is that we stop asking the questions. If we look under our hood, do we really understand the systems that make our bodies accelerate to a life of fat and the ones that slam the brakes on the dangerous cookie-and-cake collisions that take place every day? Probably not, and that's what we're here to help you learn.

Above all, we're going to teach you that when it comes to dieting, you need to work smart, not hard.

Following our plan, you can expect to drop up to two inches from your waist (or a dress size) within two weeks and see results steadily after that. While the end goal is what many of us look for, we believe that the path you choose to get there is what really dictates whether you make it or not. Our path looks like this:

Part 1: What a Waist! Starting here, we'll talk about our major principles for how the body is designed to work and how our program is geared toward those functions. And we'll also give you the biological ideals of the human body—how our bodies originally looked and functioned. We'll also give you some self-assessment tools for figuring out your own body's ideals. Once you know where you're going, you'll have a better idea of how to get there.

Part 2: The Biology of Fat. Here you'll follow morsels of food from the pantry to the porcelain bowl and everywhere in between. We'll start by exploring the physiology of appetite, and then we'll dive into the science of fat—how we store it, how we burn it, how we fight it. Obesity is really only a twenty-year-old problem (not for you but for society). Since 1990, we've gone from 1 percent of North Americans with the dangerous disease of inflammation from fat in the liver to 35 percent who have it now. You'll learn what a truly amazing system your body is when you steer it in the right direction through wise nutritional and activity choices.

Part 3: The Science of the Mind. When it comes to overeating, most of us put more emphasis on what we're noshing than on what we're thinking. But you can't discuss weight issues without exploring the scientific and chemical (and even spiritual) reasons why your brain hormones and your emotions drive you to the eight-enchilada special. You'll learn why some foods are addictive. More important, we'll show you the strategies for making your emotions and the chemicals that drive them work for, not against, your waistline.

Part 4: The YOU Diet and Activity Plan. After you read and learn about the intricacies of your body, you'll find the eating and activity plan that will teach your body to eat and work smart. Your body will become your gym as you gain sleek strength in your body's foundation muscles—all without using weights. And you'll learn to make the right decisions in the supermarket aisle and at the fast-food window. The fourteen-day plan outlines recipes, exercises, and actions you can take to live leaner and healthier.

(In our appendices, we'll explore the medical options for dealing with weight issues—for times when you may plateau, and for those people whose weight problems have led to major medical problems.)

Now, with all the diet information that's circulating today, sometimes it's hard to know what's right, and sometimes it's hard to remember what to do even if it is. That's why we feel that while the program is important, how you learn it—how you ingrain it as part of your lifestyle—is just as vital. As we travel through the four parts of the book, you'll notice various ways you'll learn about your body and how to change it. These are the five main elements we'll use along the way:

YOU-reka Imp

YOU-reka Moments! Like Einstein suddenly realizing that $E = mc^2$ you'll develop deep insights that challenge your preconceptions about diets, about fat, and about your body. In the margin, you'll see our **YOU-reka** imp— the signal that we're about to come upon a moment of enlightenment by busting a myth or explaining something to you about diets that may seem 180 degrees from what you believe is true.

YOUR Body: In Parts 2 and 3, as we explore the biology of your body, we'll start each chapter by giving quick biology lessons about what really happens inside your body. We ask that you put on your metaphorical scrubs and gloves as you whiz through your arteries, travel through your intestines, and hang out in your stomach. We'll get up close to your fat so we can see how your body handles it and how it manipulates your body. We believe that by learning about how the inside of your body works, you'll develop the smarts you need to change how the outside looks.

YOU Tests. Through interactive quizzes and measurements, you'll establish baselines for such vital statistics as your ideal body size and your eating personality. And you'll also be able to test for the secret things that could be contributing to a weight problem (get a load of our tongue test on page 76). You can start in a few pages by taking the Fat Facts Test on page 18.

YOU Tips: After we explore the biology of your body to show you what bad things can happen if you make the wrong choice or have cross-wired genetics, we'll immediately give you actions that can help turn your body around. At the end of each chapter, we'll outline intelligent strategies—big and small—for living, eating, and moving in a more healthful way.

The YOU Diet and Activity Plan: In Part 4 (on page 217) we'll detail the specific and simple strategies, recipes, and exercises that will lead you to the body you want—for the rest of your life. The fourteen-day YOU Diet (it's actually so easy that we crafted a seven-day plan that you do twice) and the no-weights-required YOU Workout provide all the tools and instructions you'll need. Best of all, they don't take a lot of time, and they're so easy that you can incorporate them into your life today. You'll be rewarded for the time you spend planning, exercising, shopping, and cooking with more energy and a better mood—and you'll enjoy looking in the mirror more!

So where do we start? With our first **YOU-reka!** moment: Your body naturally wants to take you to your optimum weight, as long as you don't get in its way.

That's right. For almost everyone, no matter what your genetics, the systems, organs, and processes of your body all want you to function at an ideal weight and size. With the following few principles that we'll develop throughout the book, we're going to teach you how you can make that happen without having to bludgeon yourself in frustration with a butter knife. These are our major principles for achieving your very best and very healthiest body.

YOU Will Choose Elegance over Force

Most dieters try to defeat their Oreo/Cheeze Doodle/custard pie infatuations with will, with deprivation, with sweat, with a "my-brain-is-stronger-than-your-crust" attitude. But trying to beat your body with mind power alone may be more painful than passing a melon-size kidney stone. Instead, you have to learn about the systems and actions that influence hunger, satiety, fat storing, and fat burning to fine-tune your corporeal vehicle so it runs on autopilot and takes you to your ultimate destination: a healthy, ideal body. (For those who want to skip ahead, you've probably already peeked at Part 4; however, getting to know the nuances of your body is what will help you achieve and maintain a truly healthy-size body.)

YOU Will Learn How Your Body Thinks

True body improvement is about science. It's about making the leap from witchcraft to hard data, from alchemy to chemistry, from speculation about what works for your body to explanations of how your body actually works. The only way you'll understand the way calories and fat travel from that 2,000-calorie onion loaf to the back of your arm is by bringing alive the physiology of hormones, blood, organs, and muscles—by explaining the processes of digestion, starvation, fat storage, and muscle movements. When you understand the magic of physiology and the fun of biology, you'll know what actions to take—and why you're taking them—to reboot your body back to where it wants to be. Just as when you're trying to help a tantruming toddler or kick-start a frozen computer, you can't fix it unless you know what's wrong. Know the *why*, and it's much easier to handle the *how*—when you need to. Let's face it, we're not going to be sitting next to you at 10:30 p.m. when you're pilfering a Pop-Tart. So you need to be equipped with knowledge of how your body works and reacts to that Pop-Tart so that you can defend against the little sugar-coated bugger.

YOU Will Challenge Your Beliefs about Diets

Throughout our lives, we've been conditioned to believe that if one thing is good for us, then more of it must be better. If you eliminate 100 calories from your daily diet, then eliminating 400 must qualify you for size 2. If you walk to lose weight, then running a marathon must nuke the fat right off your body. Well, neither idea is true. Worse, not only aren't they true, but many of the diet myths perpetuated today actually *hurt* our bodies. Food deprivation, for example, drops your metabolism and makes your body want to *store* fat. Many of the rules, ideas, and principles you may believe about dieting—that you assume work when dieting—simply aren't true and can very well contribute to weight issues because they keep the vicious cycle of fat loss and fat gain revolving faster than Lance Armstrong's front wheel.

Throughout the book, you'll learn all about this perfect storm of factors that contribute to our ability to gain so much weight—and our inability to lose it. You'll see that some of these reasons are biological, some are environmental, and some are psychological, and only when you learn how to navigate these tricky waters will you find true success when it comes to achieving and maintaining a healthy size.

One of the reasons why most so-called diets fail is because of a psychological and behavioral flaw that many dieters have. We desperately want to believe the simple, comforting promises that diets make—that

> **FACTOID**
>
> In men, the supplement L-carnitine—at a dose of 3 grams a day—helps muscles use carbohydrates, but it is also good for blood vessel function in both men and women.

doing A always gets us B. Because once we see that A (eating wheat germ 24-7) doesn't always equal B (the cover of *Vogue*), then we get frustrated and angry, and give in to the gods of cream-filled baked goods.

Unfortunately, your body and your fat do not have a linear, two-step relationship. Instead, think of your body as an orchestra. All of its systems, organs, muscles, cells, fluids, hormones, and chemicals play different instruments, make different sounds (your intestines have dibs on first-chair tuba), and produce different results depending on how you use them. They work independently, but only when they're played together can you appreciate the magnificent symphony of your own biology. As the conductor of your biological orchestra, you control how the instruments interact and what the final result will be.

YOU Will Make Dieting Automatic

While we want you to "not think" about eating good foods, we also know that "not thinking" may be how you got into this pants-stretching mess in the first place. When you don't think about the consequences of ordering football-size calzones, you wind up with such pleasantries as high LDL (lousy) cholesterol, low HDL (healthy type of) cholesterol, a fat-filled liver, inflammation in your arteries, and a higher risk of aging arteries that cause memory loss, heart disease, even wrinkles, as well as a steady stream of coupon offers from the large men's department. We want your body to guide you to the *right* choices—without thinking about them—so that they'll lead to the results you want. It will take some effort at the start to retrain your habits, palate, and muscles, but this program will serve as a lifelong eating, activity, and behavior plan that will become as routine as going to the bathroom before bed.

Unless you're the rare kind of person who responds to dietary drill sergeants, you won't find long-term solutions using traditional weight-loss methods: willpower, deprivation, fads, phases, or dead-bolting the lid of the butter pecan. Instead, using this plan, you will train yourself to *never* think about how much you're eating, *never* think about getting on a diet or worry about coming off one, and *never* have to figure out formulas, zones, or, for the love of (fill in the deity of your choice), place a chicken breast on a food scale.

YOU Will Focus on Waist Management

Our society seems almost as obsessed with pounds as it is with celebrity breakups, but it's time to shift your thinking: Studies have shown that waist circumference, not overall weight, is the most important indicator of mortality related to being overweight. Of course you'll lose pounds on this plan, but we want you to switch your focus from a number that measures your *weight* to one that measures your *waist*. Because of its proximity to your organs, your belly fat is the most dangerous fat you can carry.

In addition to helping you shrink your waist through diet, we'll also teach you the exercises that will help you achieve and maintain a healthy waist size. Now, we don't want you to think that exercise must involve sweating like a waterfall and panting like an obscene caller, because it doesn't. But you do need to start thinking about your body as a dartboard: It's all about what's in the center. You'll be focusing on the physical activities that will help control your waist size—specifically walking and foundation-muscle training of your entire body (without growing igloo-size muscles). We'll teach you simple moves that will develop all of your foundation muscles, and we'll teach you how to tighten your belly, improve your posture, and develop the muscles that will make you fit into your clothes better. That translates into a shapelier waist, which, studies (and pick-up line frequency charts) show, makes you more attractive to others.

But let's not overlook the management part of the waist management equa-

Take Out the Tape

Some people haven't stepped on a scale since *Laverne & Shirley* played in prime time. And that's a good thing. For our purposes, you don't need to know how much you weigh (but if you want to check your progress on this program, then go ahead and peek). All you need is a tape measure. Measure the circumference of your waist at the point of your belly button (suck in; you will anyway), and record the score here. (Depending on how your weight is distributed, you may need to make an adjustment to where you place the tape. If you're overweight, keep the tape measure parallel to the floor during measurement.)

YOUR SIZE: _____

For optimum health, the ideal waist size for women is 32½ inches; once you hit 37 inches, the dangers to your health increase. For men, the ideal is 35 inches, and the dangers to your health increase once you hit 40 inches.

While we're going to emphasize waist over weight in this book, we also know that many of you won't be able to resist the siren of the scale. When it comes to actual weight, you do need to stop thinking about one specific number. ("I want to get down to one hundred thirty.") All of us have an ideal playing weight—not a weight for running marathons or making All Pro linebacker or posing for an airbrushed-anyway centerfold. This ideal playing weight is a *range* in which you live lean and healthy, and one in which you significantly reduce the risks of aging diseases associated with being overweight (more on all of this in Part 2).

tion. We all know how good managers work: They plan ahead and create systems that play to people's strengths, they set realistic goals, they measure progress, and they don't force their employees down roads that are designed to give them a pack-your-things meeting with HR. You need to train yourself to be a good waist manager by following a plan that's designed to help you become the CEO of your body.

You Will Focus on YOU, but Not Rely on YOU

It doesn't matter whether you look at presidents (Lincoln or Taft), musicians (Usher or Heavy D), or tennis players (Sharapova or Serena), it's clear that we all have different builds, just as we all have different genetics, metabolic rates, and chemical interactions. Still, there are some fundamental biological facts that are true whether you're built like a branch or a stump. As a species, we're programmed to gain and preserve the right amount of weight. That's simply what our bodies are designed to do (more on that coming up). The trick is to figure out your factory settings. Then, we'll give you the all-important lock-setting tools that will help you to reboot those factory settings so that your body maintains its ideal size and shape.

While this is a very individual challenge, it doesn't have to be a lonely one. Life is a team game; you've got sports teams and surgical teams, restaurant staffs and office staffs, hip-hop clubs and calculator clubs. And of course you have the ultimate team: your family. The most successful teams all work the same way: Everybody plays a different role and contributes in his or her own way. You may have a Shaq, Kobe, or LeBron on your team, but the team can't win the title unless everybody, not just the stars, works for the team goal.

Somehow, though, when it comes to weight control, you believe that you're solely responsible for dropping your excess pounds and changing your habits. To make it worse, when you're gaining weight, even the fans are chipping in on your side; the world around us wants us to gain weight in the form of big portions, drive-throughs, and family dinners that could feed a small municipality. Then when you're trying to lose weight, it's as if everyone's against you; they bring junk food into the home, suggest that everyone go out for ice cream, and feast on pork fat while you're trying to gnaw on cauliflower. You can think of this as being green at the same time. What's good for the outside environment (more plant food, less four-legged food) is good for your environment too.

You have to stop thinking that this game is you versus a stadium full of rib-loving opponents. Sure, you need to be the quarterback of your waist control team, but you won't achieve success without a team that can block for you, high-five you when you're doing well, and give you an encouraging smack on the butt when you're not. Your starting lineup should include your doctor, maybe a nutritionist, maybe a personal trainer, and certainly scads and scads of fans like your family and friends (online or in person) who can push you, support you, and yank the bowl of candy corn away from you. But you shouldn't be the only one relying on other people; you should use this opportunity to find a support partner who needs you as much as you need her. After all, the best kinds of satisfaction shouldn't come from the sixth spoonful of cake batter, but from sharing knowledge and support, and helping others lose inches.

YOU Will Stop Blaming Yourself

The classic psychology of fat is this: If you're thin, then you believe that fat people must be doing something wrong to make them fat. But if you're fat, then you blame the environment, or your genetics, or anything else. Well, we're going to try to eliminate that blame and use medical insights to explain the epic saga of weight-related problems. We want to move dieting past a guilt-driven and blame-ridden system, and make it a science-based system.

Of course not everyone can look like a Beyoncé or a Brad Pitt. To get an idea of what your healthy weight, waist, and shape should be, you'll need to take into account such things as bone structure, muscle mass, genetics, and risk factors associated with your weight. Here's a fact that goes virtually unmentioned: There are clinically obese people who live with no risk of health problems, and there are CD-thin people whose risk of dying prematurely is more than a chuteless sky-diver's. Our goal is to get you to the point where you strip away inches, you strip away the risks of being overweight, and you strip away the guilt associated with the process of always trying to do so.

YOU Will Never Be Hungry

We know exactly how you've felt when you've dieted in the past. Hungry. Famished. Three seconds away from steamrolling through a triple-dip cone with sprinkles. That recipe for dieting is one you can tear up. In fact, the only place hunger ever got you was a pair of pants that could double as curtains. To eat and work smart, your goal is *never* to be hungry and *never* to be in a state of dietary angst, where your only salvation is the 99¢ menu at the drive-through window. By keeping your hunger (and internal chemicals) in check, you'll avoid the impetuous behaviors that send fat on an express ride to your belly.

YOU Will Make Mistakes

Look, we don't care how motivated you are, how willing you are, how inspired you are by Eva Longoria's body. Someday, and someday soon, a volleyball-size muffin is going to get the best of you and nudge, bribe, or cajole its way into your stomach. That's OK. Hear that? That's *OK*. You're going to have moments when your eyes, body, and curious fingers won't be able to turn their radar lock off of the queso dip. You have to get past the concept that diets have *side effects*—that is, unexpected negative consequences. Instead, realize that eating plans have *effects*—offshoot actions, behaviors, and emotions that are simply part of everyday living. One of those effects is that you will occasionally eat things that are nutritional cigarettes; though one may not hurt you forever, it can get you addicted to some bad behaviors. Because of that, waist management is about developing contingency plans—plans that allow you to make mistakes and then get back on the right road. We're going to teach you how to make a YOU-Turn when you do make mistakes with Twinkies or Tootsie Rolls or any bad-for-your-waist foods. That way, your dietary fender benders won't turn into hundred-car Autobahn pileups.

YOU Will Be Flexible—and Have Fun

Most of us want our diets to be a little like having the remote control; we want the power to make lots of choices, depending on everything from our mood to the time of day. It's clear from research that the most successful eating plans are low-maintenance: You can follow them with your family, and you won't feel overwhelmed by cravings. If you can do that, you'll get results. But try to stay on a diet where you feel more isolated than a Yankees fan at Fenway Park, then chances are that the result will feel like the box-office numbers of a B-level horror flick—a miserable failure.

Eating right shouldn't be about feeling bad. It should be about feeling strong, increasing energy, living better, feeling healthier, and having more fun than a front-row rock fan. It should be about eating without thinking and without obsessing about every forkful. Of course, we all have reasons for overeating or eating the wrong kinds of food (stress, boredom, comfort, five-cent wing specials). But our goal isn't just for you to make by-the-book food substitutions or come to grips with your Devil Dog demons. You should be grinning—not grimacing, grunting, and growling—as the inches melt away from your waist, and laughing as your lipid profile improves. You'll understand how, after we show you how the mind-stomach connection works by explaining how brain and belly chemicals control what the mind thinks, how the fork acts in your bodily orchestra, and how this relationship can become a cacophony in the wrong hands.

So now that we're about to begin, you're probably asking, What are we going to do, and how are we going to do it? Well, we're going to give you everything you need to make a body change—through a series of elegant and effective changes based on hard science—that will stick with you for your life. Simply, this book will serve as your lifelong waist management, body-changing plan.

Best of all, when you put it all together and integrate automatic actions into your life, you'll live by the principles you'll need to stay fit and healthy, so that you can achieve and maintain exactly what you're striving for:

Your ideal body.

The Fat Facts Test

What Do You Really Know about Fat, Diets, and Other Weight-loss Solutions?

To help you determine your level of dietary knowledge, take this Fat Facts Test. In less time than it takes to listen to an *American Idol* off-key clunker, you may just learn more about your body and belly than you've ever known before.

1. ***What is the first historical event that we can point to as contributing to the rise in excess pounds?***
   a. The development of agriculture.
   b. The development of whipped cream in coffee.
   c. The development of more office jobs.
   d. The development of fast food.

2. ***What is the reason most diets fail?***
   a. They're designed so that they're impossible to stick to long-term.
   b. They're so complicated that you need a math degree to follow them.
   c. There are only so many carrot sticks and celery stalks a person can take.
   d. Mozzarella sticks. Mmm!

3. **Which of the following strategies is most recommended for people trying to lose weight?**

   a. Weighing yourself once a week.

   b. Eating two to three small meals a day.

   c. Eating nuts every day.

   d. Ex-Lax smoothies for everyone!

4. **What's the most important number for determining whether an increased waist size is putting you at risk for health problems?**

   a. Bra size.

   b. Blood pressure.

   c. Cholesterol.

   d. Heart rate.

5. **What is ghrelin?**

   a. The name of a *Harry Potter* character.

   b. A hormone that makes you want to eat more.

   c. The name of fat cells in your belly.

   d. The chemical in your brain that makes you feel good.

6. **What is leptin?**

   a. The name of the dude on the Lucky Charms cereal box.

   b. The muscle-building protein that helps burn fat.

   c. The nutrient in fruit that works in conjunction with fiber.

   d. A chemical from fat that tells your brain you are full.

7. **Which spice has been shown to be helpful for controlling weight?**

   a. Cinnamon.

   b. Thyme.

   c. Oregano.

   d. The one married to David Beckham; Posh, is it?

8. **Which one does not stimulate eating high-calorie food?**

   a. Too little sleep.

   b. Too little sex.

   c. Too little water.

   d. Too much work.

9. **What does your body most want to do in periods of extreme stress?**

   a. Stay away from food.

   b. Gorge on food.

   c. Seek crunchy foods.

   d. Crumple up into a pile of jelly and retreat to a warm bath.

10. **An ideal buddy is:**

    a. Tall, dark, and handsome.

    b. Someone who has more fat than you to lose.

    c. Someone who loves to celebrate with molten chocolate cake.

    d. Someone who is on the same journey as you.

11. **Of the following choices, which is least dangerous to a long-term waist management strategy?**

    a. A 1,000-calorie-a-day diet.

    b. Higher than usual colonics to remove all fat.

    c. Training for a marathon.

    d. Playing video games.

12. **Which organ is most responsible for metabolism?**

    a. Heart.

    b. Stomach.

    c. Liver.

    d. Kidneys.

13. The perfect storm for waist gain means:

  a. You eat more because corner stores and fast-food restaurants that serve high-calorie foods are everywhere.

  b. That high-fructose corn syrup can overwhelm an already fatty liver, producing a storm of inflammatory compounds and making the liver fatter. And you want to eat more and find a corner store that offers half price on anything with corn syrup in it.

  c. You get too much sleep, so your metabolic rate slows; high-calorie food is easy to get, so you make up for oversleeping with overeating.

  d. You can float more easily during a storm surge.

14. Calorie for calorie, what fills you up for the longest amount of time?

  a. Fat.

  b. Fiber.

  c. Fructose.

  d. French fries.

15. At least how much must you walk daily for optimum waist control?

  a. Thirty minutes.

  b. Two hours.

  c. Any time you can spare.

  d. Any, as long as it's not traveling to and from the fridge.

16. What is the main purpose of liposuction?

  a. To help people lose weight.

  b. To target problem body parts.

  c. To keep some Hollywood docs in business.

  d. To ensure another season of successful reality TV.

17. What is your omentum?

  a. A badly misspelled word.

  b. The part of your brain that's stimulated to store fat.

  c. A chemical that controls hunger.

  d. A fat-storing tissue that becomes metabolically active.

18. Health-wise, what is the optimal waist size for a woman?

a. As little as possible.

b. 32½ inches.

c. Under 35 inches.

d. Whatever slides into that little black dress, honey.

19. Which part of your body that plays a role in weight gain works most like your brain?

a. Your stomach.

b. Your heart.

c. Your small intestine.

d. Your unmentionables.

20. What is CCK?

a. The former Soviet Union.

b. A hormone that regulates insulin levels by changing your blood sugar level.

c. Colonic Creations by Katherine.

d. Cholecystokinin, a chemical that tells your brain to stop eating the waffle.

21. Of the following items, what contributes most to weight gain?

a. Periods of low levels of willpower.

b. Short periods of high-intensity stress.

c. Long periods of low-intensity stress.

d. Periods of high-intensity dessert trays.

22. The difference between an allergy to and intolerance of gluten is:

a. Five trips to your doc.

b. Whether milk is eaten with gluten.

c. The degree of T-cell involvement in your gut.

d. Whether you have a deficiency of an enzyme or too great an immune response to gluten chemicals.

23. Which of the following can be an effective medical option for weight loss?

    a. Aspirin.

    b. Beta-blockers.

    c. Statins.

    d. Antidepressants.

24. Which activity is most helpful for waist control?

    a. Crunches.

    b. Cardiovascular training like running.

    c. Resistance training like weight lifting.

    d. Naked salsa dancing every other Tuesday.

25. What's the worst side effect of losing weight?

    a. Increased risk of chocolate withdrawal.

    b. Increased risk of muscular and joint aches.

    c. Increased risk of yo-yo dieting.

    d. Increased risk of astronomical tailor bill.

Answers

1. a. The development of agriculture meant that we could now have foods we wanted, not needed. And that's what provided the foundation for indulgence.

2. a. Most diets don't reprogram you to think and eat automatically, so that eventually you'll go *off* the diet just as surely as you went *on* it.

3. c. Eating a handful of nuts has been shown to help you stay full, while skipping meals can be detrimental because your body will go into a fat-storing, starvation mode when it doesn't have enough calories.

4. b. Of these risks, blood pressure is the greatest indicator of health risks associated with being overweight.

5. b. Ghrelin makes you want to eat more.

6. d. Leptin keeps you full.

7. a. Cinnamon increases insulin sensitivity, which helps enhance the satiety center in your brain (and also reduces blood sugar levels as well as cholesterol levels).

8. d. All four satiety centers (for food, sleep, thirst, and sex) are collated in your brain; too little sleep or sex or too much thirst makes you crave sugary foods. Work will increase calorie intake only if you are stressed out and cope through eating.

9. a. Extreme stress (as in the case of a car accident, or even exercise) turns off your hunger. Chronic stress (like a long line of looming deadlines or family problems) can make you crave feel-good carbohydrates.

10. d. You and your buddy adopt each other's habits (and looks, to a degree).

11. d. Playing video games works because it keeps your hands busy, so you can't eat. (Training for a marathon is actually destructive to your body because of the risk to your joints, and for most people, 1,000 calories is a dangerously low daily caloric intake. Do we really need to explain colonics?)

12. c. Your liver is responsible for most metabolic functions.

13. b. Your body has a biochemical perfect storm. Too much fructose presented to a fatty liver makes the liver process it differently from fructose delivered slowly, as it does in whole fruit. The rapid delivery is believed to cause your liver to produce an inflammatory chemical that damages your liver, arteries, and immune system. We've gone from consuming 0 pounds per person of high-fructose corn syrup in 1960 to 63 pounds now.

14. b. Fiber fills you. A cup of oatmeal in the morning has been shown to prevent you from afternoon gorging.

15. a. Walk at least thirty minutes—at once or in intervals—every day.

16. b. Liposuction should be used to sculpt problem areas, not to remove a lot of fat.

17. d. Located next to your stomach, your omentum is fat that can cause damage to surrounding organs.

18. b. While 32½ inches or less is ideal, 37 inches is when women start seeing a greatly increased risk of weight-related disorders.

19. c. Your small intestine—with 100 million neurons—has anatomy similar to your brain.

20. d. CCK is a chemical that directly and indirectly sends a message to your brain from your guts that you're full.

21. c. Chronic stress makes your body store more fat.

22. d. An intolerance is caused by a deficiency of the enzyme that metabolizes gluten; an allergy provokes a too-great immune response to a gluten antigen or protein.

23. d. Bupropion, an antidepressant, has been shown to help control cravings and lead to about a 7 percent weight loss. Other antidepressants, such as tricyclic antidepressants or selective serotonin reuptake inhibitors (SSRIs), can often be associated with weight gain.

24. c. Adding a little muscle through resistance training helps your body burn more fat throughout the day.

25. c. Yo-yo dieting not only has physiological effects, because you end up gaining more weight after you've lost it, but it also has psychological effects.

Scoring

You get one point for each correct answer.

20 and above: Congratulations, doc. You're an anatomical expert.

11–19: You're average, but then again, the average person is overweight, so maybe this isn't so good. Maybe you'd better read on.

10 and below: Don't worry, you're about to enroll in the ultimate course in the biology, history, and anatomy of fat—which is the best way to change your body.

Chapter 1

The Ideal Body

What Your Body Is Supposed to Look Like

Diet Myths

- ❖ Your body doesn't need any fat.
- ❖ Fast food is responsible for most of our fat problems.
- ❖ Dieting has to be hard.

The most common question heard among overweight people isn't "Can I have more sour cream?" It's "Why can't I lose weight?" While you may think you know the answer (severe pancake addiction), the real reason is biological:

We're actually hardwired to store some fat.

Our bodies have more systems that allow us to gain weight than to lose it. Historically, as we'll see in a moment, that served us well. Today, though, we've poisoned the systems that help us lose weight and empowered the ones that allow us to gain it—botching up our anatomy and turning our bodies into fat-storing machines. One of your goals will be to reprogram your body so that your internal systems can work the way they did when the greatest enemy we faced was a charging wildebeest, not a cheese-drowned pork roll.

Our ancestors survived by gaining and storing weight to survive periodic famines. That has left our bodies prone to storing fat and gaining weight, tendencies that willpower alone can rarely overcome. To see how our bodies have morphed from rock-hard to sponge-soft, let's look inside the bodies of early man and woman. They looked like stereotypical superheroes: strong, lean, muscular, able to jump snorting mammals in a single bound.

As we evolved, we created systems and behaviors to survive when droughts and poor eyesight made picking and hunting less than successful. We learned to thrive, and we learned to eat. In early times, our diets consisted of fruits, nuts, vegetables, tubers, and wild meat—foods that were, for the most part, low in calories. That's not to say our ancestors didn't enjoy their foods. They consumed their sugars through fruit, and they even splurged when they came across the Paleolithic Cinnabon—a honeycomb. The difference between their splurges and ours? They came across the sweet treats only rarely; it's not as if they popped in for a 900-calorie sugar bomb every time they went shopping for a new buffalo hide. Add that to the fact that their definition of "searching for

The Heavyweight Fight: Genetics Versus Environment

It's easy to argue that lifestyle choices and lack of willpower are responsible for weight problems (it's the argument that lean people tend to make). But it doesn't explain the 95 percent failure rate after two years of people who have lost fifty pounds or more; they had plenty of willpower to lose but regained the weight nonetheless. Researchers argue that obesity is more genetically linked than any other trait except height—and at least 50 percent of obesity cases clearly have genetic components. Our take: The waist control game requires two players—environment and genetics. Even if your genes have made you predestined for a life of taking up two seats, that doesn't mean you should abdicate control over your body. When you make the right environmental, behavioral, and biological changes that we outline, you'll be able to stay healthy and avoid the bad side effects of excess weight, like diabetes, high blood pressure (hypertension), and arterial inflammation. While 10 percent of the obese population has genetic challenges that may make a supermodel contract impossible, the bigger risk with these genes is not in the weight itself but in the predisposition to risks associated with obesity. For example, genetic problems associated with being overweight are called leptin resistance and leptin deficiency (leptin is a hormone associated with satiety, which we'll discuss in the next chapter). Folks who either don't produce leptin or block its signals usually become morbidly obese, and the problem is surely genetic.

While some people have these abnormalities, they tend to be the minority of the population. If you need to worry about losing twenty-five, thirty-five, even fifty pounds, your problem is not likely to be genetic. Only when your excess weight exceeds one hundred pounds would most doctors consider testing for genetic abnormalities. Still, the example of leptin is only the tip of the scientific iceberg as far as genetics and obesity are concerned. As the fight against obesity continues, we'll see more and more drug companies target genetic reasons for weight gain—that is, drugs that attack the genetic biochemical problems that may be contributing to your weight problem. That said, the onus of waist management still falls on you, to improve your environment and your behaviors so that your genetics can work for you, not against you.

food" included walking, stalking, and chasing, not sliding the milk carton out of the way to find the pudding pack. It was a lot of work to get food, so they naturally burned many of the calories they consumed through the physical activity of hunting and gathering.

Because salt and sugar were scarce, our ancestors mostly feasted on grains, vegetables, and meats—for good reason. The meat provided the protein, vitamins, minerals, and fatty acids that helped them grow taller and develop larger brains, while the other foods gave them nutrients such as glucose, a simple sugar found in fruit and the complex carbohydrates of plants, that they needed to grow and develop, and for energy to move. And, of course, food was always fresh, as there was no canning or refrigeration to store up food for Super Bowl parties, or to sneak in an 11 p.m. bowl of sugar-coated oats.

Another difference was that the meat our ancestors ate wasn't like the meat we know today. Theirs was low in fat and high in protein; ours often comes in the form of corn-fed cows pumped up to make fattier, tastier cuts. Even today's buffalo burger is corn-fed. Truly wild game has about 4 percent fat, while now most commercially available beef has nine times that amount. (The theory behind protein-heavy diets such as Atkins is that protein reduces overall food intake and could reduce calorie intake as well. The flaw is that eating proteins dripping in saturated fat, such as bacon, isn't exactly the same as eating the leaner, healthier forms of protein, such as chicken and fish.)

The result: Your tribal forefathers and foremothers could eat anytime they could harvest or catch something, and still not put on excess weight.

The lesson: Our ancestors never thought about a diet in the way we do—and their bodies had the approximate density of granite. Us? We obsess about diet more than red-carpet reporters obsess about designer dresses, and our bodies have the consistency of yogurt.

Still, we can't blame the advent of fast food and waffle cones for all of our weight issues. The downfall started in the pre-G.A. (pre–Golden Arches) era—over 10,000 years or so ago, when agriculture first appeared. Agriculture allowed us to make more advances than a seventeen-year-old boy in a movie theater, but we paid a price for

Myth Buster

them. Besides sparing the lives of countless mammoths, the rise of agriculture ensured that we'd always have a steady supply of food—an advantage during times of famine, a disadvantage at the $6.99 Mama's Kitchen Eat-Everything Buffet. With a constant source of food, people became less nomadic, and communities grew closer together. While the average life span increased (thanks to the elimination of the extreme sport of tiger chasing, with, perhaps, some help from sanitation and immunization), agriculture also brought its share of downsides: more bacterial infections, shorter stature, and rotting teeth that come from eating refined sugar and less nutritious farm-raised food (overused soil cannot produce nutrient-rich food). Our ancestors' diets shifted from vegetables and meat to grains from the farms, essentially hindering them from getting the diverse mix of protein and micronutrients needed for brain development.

The advent of agriculture started the sociological shift that altered the way we live—and the way we eat—up until this day. We could now produce food, so we could now produce what we wanted, not necessarily what we needed. Instead of making foods that could both complement our bodies and appeal to our taste buds, we started making ones that were kinder to our tongues and pocketbooks than they were to our waists.

We're not in the business of trying to make you live like cavemen, or help you score a blue-jeans billboard, or help you become thin enough to escape between two jail bars. What we should acknowledge is that we live in a world with free will, with temptations, and with more eating options than the stores at Mall of America. Biologically, our bodies want us to eat right. But in today's society (cavemen didn't have bad bosses or deadlines for annual reports), our biological drive to be the right weight and to eat right can be overcome by stress or temptation. And that has shifted many dietary decisions from biological necessities to psychological reactions. What we're going to do is teach you how to reprogram your body to work the way it's supposed to work—so that you eat to satisfy and to fuel rather than to console or excite. Controlling your fat isn't about being banished with a life sentence of broccoli florets (although four servings per week does decrease breast and prostate cancer risks considerably). It's about teaching your body a little bit about the way our ancestors ate. Naturally and automatically.

YOU TIPS!

Automate Your Eating. If your waist management plan is going to work—as in, really work, for your whole life—then eating right has to become as automatic as it was for our ancestors. That's not as insurmountable as it seems. Just look at one study from the *Journal of the American Medical Association*. Two groups were assigned two different diets. One went on a diet rich with good-for-you foods like whole grains, fruits, vegetables, nuts, and olive oil, foods found in the typical Mediterranean diet. The other group was not given any specific direction in terms of foods to eat but was instructed to consume specific percentages of fat, carbohydrates, and protein daily. In short, they had to think a lot about preparing foods and dividing amounts, while the first group only had general guidelines about foods to eat.

Myth Buster

The groups weren't given guidelines about how much to eat; they let their hunger levels dictate their hunger patterns. And when they did that, what happened? Without trying, the first group ate fewer calories, lost inches, and dropped pounds.

YOU-reka! The point: The people in the good-foods group ate the foods that naturally kept them satiated so their bodies could seek their playing weights.

❖ The "good-for-YOU-foods group" ate significantly more fiber than the control group (32 grams versus 17 grams).

❖ The "good-for-YOU-foods group" ate higher amounts of good-for-you omega-3 and omega-9 fats in the form of olives, fish, and nuts (especially walnuts). Those fats help increase the level of chemicals that make you feel satiated.

❖ The "good-for-YOU-foods group" more than doubled their consumption of fruits and vegetables.

The "good-for-YOU-foods-group" ate the foods we recommend in this YOU Diet, didn't obsess about calories, and enabled their bodies to do what they're supposed to do: regulate the chemicals that are responsible for hunger and for satiety (more on this in Chapter 2).

Don't Undereat. When our ancestors couldn't find food and went for long periods of time without it, their bodies acted like a life preserver, storing fat in anticipation of the inevitable periods of famine. The same system works today. **YOU-reka!** When you try to "diet" by going for long periods of time without eating or by eating way too few calories, your brain senses the starvation and sends an SOS signal through your body to store fat because famine is on its way. That's why people who go on extreme fasts and extremely low-calorie diets don't lose the expected weight. They store fat as a natural protective mechanism. To lose weight, you have to keep your body from switching into starvation mode. The only way to do it: Eat often, in the form of frequent healthy meals, and snacks.

Plan Your Meals. Start every day knowing when and what you're going to eat. That way, you'll avert the 180-degree shift between starving and gorging that occurs when you skip meals. Our fourteen-day diet (in Chapter 13) will show you how to plan your meals so that you feed your body regularly to avoid extreme periods of overeating and undereating that can lead to a gain in weight and inches.

YOU Test

Remember Your Ancestry

Some people say their family has big bones or big cells. Some say their family has big appetites. Some say their family just has big beer coolers. If you gained weight as an adult, you can get a relatively accurate picture of what your ideal size should be by thinking about what you looked like when you were eighteen (for women) or twenty-one (for men); a time when you were at your metabolically most efficient and when you weren't stapled to an office chair for sixty hours a week. Most people gain their weight between the ages of twenty-one and sixty, so by looking at your size at eighteen or twenty-one, you'll have a good, though not quite scientific, idea of your factory settings. (If you're over forty, with today's adolescent obesity, such comparisons may not work in the future.) It's not perfect, but it's a thumbnail sketch of where you want to be. You can record your waist size (or closest guess) from when you were eighteen, but, more important, think about your shape. Ask your parents about their body sizes—or find pictures of them— when they were eighteen, to help give you a good idea of what you're supposed to look like.

Stand in Front of the Mirror. Naked.
Without Sucking in Your Belly.

For some of you, this assignment may feel natural, but for most, the exercise is as uncomfortable as a coach-class airline seat. We're having you do this not to benefit the neighborhood peepers, but for two other reasons. First, we want you to realize that we're emphasizing healthy weight. Not fashion-magazine weight, not featherweight, but *healthy* weight. And we think that means you have to start getting comfortable with the fact that every woman isn't as light as a kite, and every man won't have the body of Matthew McConaughey. Where you want to be may not be *exactly* where your body wants you to be. We're not saying you need to accept a belly that looks like four gallons of melted ice cream, but we want you to get closer to your ideal health—and that means physically and emotionally.

Second, we want you to look at your body. Now draw an outline of your body shape (both from the side and front views). Ask a partner or close friend to look at the shape you drew and tell you—honestly—if that's approximately what your body looks like. (Your clothes can be back on at this point.) This is just a quality-control check to make sure you have an accurate self body image. (Those with eating disorders have very distorted body images, making it an obstacle for getting back to a healthy weight.) This might be the first time you've ever had to articulate things about what your body looks like—and that's good. In *YOU: Being Beautiful,* we help you evaluate your feelings about your shape with a YOU-Q Test.

Part 2

The Biology of Fat

Food, from Start to Finish—Why Our Bodies Want It,
How We Store It, and How We Burn It

Chapter 2

Can't Get No Satisfaction

The Science of Appetite

Diet Myths

- Hunger is primarily dictated by what's happening in your stomach.

- The biggest battle in dieting involves willpower.

- As long as a food is low-fat, it's not going to make you fat.

As much as an iPod bud in the ear, fat has become a regular part of our landscape. We see it *everywhere.* We see it tethered to a hunk of prime rib. We see it masquerading as a Nutter Butter. We see it crammed into evening gowns or cascading over belt buckles. We've seen paparazzi-haunted celebrities gain it and lose it, lose it and gain it. And, if we can bear a confidence-crushing six seconds of nudity in front of a mirror, most of us have seen our own share of flesh that droops, sags, or jiggles. So reason would tell you that we should know as much about fat as we know about Angelina Jolie's private life. But we don't.

Sure, we know what it looks like, what it feels like, and that it can be as bad for our health as a steak knife lodged in our hand. But few of us really know how fat works biologically—how the Twinkie morphs from a wonderfully yellow spongy cake to the flab that conjoins our inner thighs, or how our skinny-as-a-straw friend can wolf down a meat-lover's supreme while we feel bloated if we as much as sniff four carrots.

Starting in this chapter and continuing throughout the rest of Part 2, we'll show you the way that food travels—from the time your body wants you to eat it, to the time it exercises squatter's rights on your hips, to the time you fry it into oblivion. The best place to start? With your appetite. Appetite really comes in two forms: physiological signals that make you hungry and emotional coaxes that lure you to food.

In this chapter, we'll explore those physiological signals, because understanding and controlling your hunger and satiety signals will help you adopt a healthy eating plan. (We'll explore the psychological and emotional aspects in Part 3.) Once you know that those mechanisms have much more powerful control over how you eat than do your taste buds, then you can make the environmental, behavioral, attitudinal, and biological adjustments you need to live at your healthy weight.

Above all, there's one sign that will clue you in to whether you've become an effective processor of food. It's the sign that you, not a bag of gummy bears, are in control of your weight. It's the sign that you, without having to work at it, have been pro-

Myth Buster

Fat's Bad Rap

Sure, nobody likes body fat, especially when it beats you through the door by five or six seconds. But despite potentially serious consequences, fat, by nature, is good. (That's not a typo.) Besides helping Santa hopefuls land December jobs, it also helps your cells function and provides insulation. Most of your fat is stored in a reservoir throughout your body. You have drums and drums of it, sitting passively, just waiting to be burned. But you have another kind of fat too. It's called brown fat and is usually found on the back of your neck and around your arteries (and has absolutely nothing to do with how much chocolate you eat). This increases in outdoor workers during cold spells to protect them from the weather; it insulates our vital organs. Though you have a fairly small percentage of brown fat as an adult, about one-third of fat in babies is brown fat, and it's used primarily to keep them warm. What makes brown fat different? **YOU-reka!** Brown fat is *alive.* It has nerve fibers, like any organ, and it also has leptin receptors. When the level of this hormone goes up, it turns on energy consumption in the brown fat and burns it. This is important because it shows that the right leptin levels can signal you to immediately get rid of this fat. And it's also symbolic of the inherent goodness of body fat—when it's found in the right amounts. Perhaps what's most interesting is that we also have the ability to get brown fat going—to burn calories. Typically, fat that isn't burned to produce body heat is stored on our hips, thighs, stomach, and so on (the body-heat process is called thermogenesis). A change in internal or external temperature can trigger the fat-burning processes—a move into colder temps (like 55 to 65 degrees) can trigger brown fat to go into action. But we're also seeing that brown fat can be induced by other things, such as exercise.

moted to captain of your waist management vessel. And it's the sign that you've ultimately reprogrammed your biology so that your body uses food as a medicine to make you stay healthier so that you live long enough to see how *Lost* ends.

That sign? Satisfaction.

As you change from *always* thinking about diet to *never* thinking about it, you will be reprogramming your body so that it's not your eyes, tongue, or overzealous utensils that will guide you.

YOU-reka! Instead, it will be the chemicals in your brain and body.

By tuning in to your body's signals, you'll allow your anatomy to work the way it's supposed to: so that you'll never be famished, you'll never pop a button at the table, and you'll never bounce between hunger extremes. Instead, you'll get a little hungry, you'll eat, you'll stop. Satisfied.

The Anatomy of Appetite

You'd think that the first place we'd start to talk about how appetite influences fat would be the spot that's covered by an XXXXL shirt.

But to understand appetite, you have to navigate farther north—to the place that may hold the least "storage" or excess fat. In your brain, you'll find the hypothalamus, a key command center for your body. Among the biological functions it controls are your temperature, your metabolism, and your sex drive. Located in the center of your brain, the hypothalamus (see Figure 2.1) also coordinates your behaviors that involve appetite—not just for food but also for thirst, sleep, and even for sex. So while it may appear that call-to-duty signals come from your stomach growling or your loins tingling like a static shock, it's actually your brain that's sending out the signals that you crave either a quiche or a quickie. (At least one person we know helped curb an eating problem by having regular, monogamous, healthy sex. When the appetite function for sex was satisfied, the appetite function for food was diverted.) It's also one reason inadequate sleep or sex translates to more hunger for food.

Hidden in your hypothalamus, you have a satiety center that regulates your appetite. It is controlled by two counterbalancing chemicals that are located side by side (see Figure 2.2).

FACTOID

As you get older, you have fewer leptin receptors in your hypothalamus—meaning that you have fewer satiety signals, which makes you more prone to gaining weight.

FACTOID

Your brain is actually about 60 percent fat; you really are a fat head. But the fat is largely part of the membrane around your nerve cells or other support cells. In fact, more than 50 percent of all brain fat should be omega-3 DHA. Thus, you use fat in your brain as a structural element, rather than as a storage depot.

❖ The satiety chemicals led by CART (the *C* stands for cocaine and the *A* for amphetamine, since these drugs put this chemical into overdrive). CART stimulates the surrounding hypothalamus to

Figure 2.2 **Chemical Reaction** If we look closely at the hypothalamus, we see that a small nucleus at the bottom houses NPY and CART, which fight the yin-yang battle to control the brain biochemistry of hunger. Each chemical readily travels to other nuclei in the hypothalamus. NPY causes our temperature to drop and our metabolism to decrease as we feel hungry. CART stimulates the opposite influence. The nearby mammillary body (literally shaped like a nipple) is part of our limbic system, where we store memories and emotions—just the right combination to create a craving for a favorite food. The thalamus is the body's relay station and rapidly transmits orders throughout the brain based on the desires of the eating center.

increase metabolism, reduce appetite, and increase insulin to deliver energy to muscle cells rather than be stored as fat.

❖ The eating chemicals driven by NPY (a protein called neuropeptide Y). NPY has the opposite effect on the hypothalamus; it decreases metabolism and increases appetite.

Think of these two command chemicals as any game or sport that involves offense and defense, like soccer, checkers, or even dating. The offense is always trying to make advances, trying to score points, and trying to attack, while the defense protects its territory.

Your eating chemicals play offense. They want as many points as possible, so they fire off those signals for your body to score: eat, eat, eat, calories, calories, calories, chimichanga, chimichanga, chimichanga. The biological message: Prevent starvation by eating. Meanwhile, your satiety chemicals play defense, like a goalkeeper, the back row of checkers, or a protective parent. They send the messages to your brain that you're full, to shield you from steadily pumping bacon-wrapped scallops down your gullet. How do we know these centers work this way? For one, by looking at extremes and seeing what happens when the feeding system is turned completely on or off. When we study animal models, we see that if a rat's eating center is destroyed, for instance, it forever forgets to eat. The resulting severe anorexia starves the body of all energy and nutrients so that it withers away to the approximate width of an envelope. In rats whose eating center is overstimulated, though, food is always on the radar screen. And those rats eat themselves to death—literally—by increasing their fat-induced diseases such as diabetes, hypertension, and arthritis.

In a perfect system, your offense and defense complement each other; you get the foods you need and stop when you've had enough. Unfortunately for everyone except elastic-waistband manufacturers, a lot of things can mess up those systems (many of which we'll discuss in a moment). But these obstacles aren't insurmountable. You can take comfort (and find motivation) in the fact that your body wants you to reach your goals. Your body doesn't want to be bigger than it should be. Your body doesn't want lots of excess fat. Take the case of rats made obese by force-feeding. When they're allowed to eat freely, they go back to their control weight. *They eat what they should eat, without thinking.* Same goes for starving rats. When allowed to eat again, they don't gorge. They naturally go back to their control weight. And we know from years and years of research that what rats do is a pretty fair indication of what humans will do under the same circumstances. (Humans, of course, will do what rats do when they're motivated only by biology. A rat isn't upset by stress at home or work, which is why controlling the emotional aspect of eating plays such a big role in effective waist management, as we'll discuss in Part 3.)

YOU-reka! If you can allow your body and brain to subconsciously do the work of controlling your eating, you'll naturally gravitate toward your ideal playing weight. You do it by developing a well-trained defense that naturally balances the offense. When you do, you'll win the diet game every time, whether you have willpower or not.

Though it may not always be the case in football or Scrabble, when you pit offense against defense in your body, the offense in your body typically attacks more aggressively. It's simply easier to scoop up bean dip than it is to leave it for others.

The Hunger On and Off Switches

Duct tape over your mouth isn't how your body regulates food intake. Your body does it naturally through the communication of substances controlled by your brain. Although there are many hunger- and obesity-related hormones waiting to be discovered, there's enough evidence to suggest that two hormones have as much influence for dictating our hunger and satiety levels as a head coach does on offense and defense—hour to hour and year to year.

Lovin' Leptin: The Hormone of Satisfaction

In sumo champions, a little extra fat can produce good results. But we also think that fat has an unfair knock against it. Fat is treated a little like an accused suspect; it sometimes gets a bum rap. Fat produces a chemical signal in your blood that tells you to stop eating. Left to its own devices, fat is self-regulating; the problem occurs when we override our internal monitoring system and continue to stuff ourselves long after we're no longer hungry. Your body knows when it's had enough, and it prevents you from wanting any more food on top of that. How does fat curb appetite? Through one of the most important chemicals in the weight-reduction process: leptin, a protein secreted by stored fat. In fact, if leptin is working the way it should, it gives you a double whammy in the fight against fat. The stimulation of leptin (the word comes from the Greek word for "thin") shuts off your hunger *and* stimulates you to burn more calories—by stimulating CART.

But our bodies aren't always perfect, and leptin doesn't always work the way it's supposed to. In some research, when leptin was given to mice, their appetites decreased, as expected. When it was given to people, they initially got thin, but then something

> **FACTOID**
>
> Neuropeptide Y is a stress hormone that increases with severe or prolonged stress. This may be why some people in chronically stressful situations tend to gain weight. Testosterone, the male sex hormone, seems to stimulate NPY secretion, while the female sex hormone, estrogen, seems to have a varying effect depending on the stage of a woman's cycle.

strange happened: They overcame the surge of leptin and stopped losing weight. This indicates that our bodies have the ability to override leptin's message that our tank is full. How? When leptin tells your defense—the satiety chemicals—to kick in and protect you against stray bonbons, the pleasure center in your brain says, "Uh, yeah, three more this-a-way." That surge from the pleasure center, which we'll discuss in more detail in Part 3, can overrule leptin's messages that you're full. That's called leptin resistance (there's another form of leptin resistance as well, which happens when cells stop accepting leptin's messages, called leptin-receptor resistance). Most obese people, by the way, have high leptin levels; it's just that their bodies have the second form of leptin resistance—they don't receive and respond to leptin signals.

That doesn't mean leptin is always on the losing end of this chemical battle. **YOU-reka!** The challenge is to let leptin do its job so that the brain demands less food. One way to do it: Walk thirty minutes a day and build a little muscle (that's part of our activity plan in Part 4). When you lose some weight, your cells become more sensitive and responsive to leptin.

Ghrelin Is the Gremlin: The Hormone of Hunger

Your stomach and intestines do more than hold food and produce Richter-worthy belches. When your stomach's empty, they release a feisty little chemical called ghrelin. When your stomach's growling, it's this gremlin of a hormone that's controlling your body's offense; it sends desperate messages that you need more points, you need to score, you need to FedEx the chili dogs to the GI tract immediately. Ghrelin makes you want to eat—by stimulating NPY. **YOU-reka!** To make things worse, when you diet through deprivation, the increased ghrelin secretion sends even more signals to eat, overriding your willpower and causing chemical reactions that give you little choice but to line your tongue with bits of beef jerky.

Ghrelin also promotes eating by increasing the secretion of growth hormone (*ghre* is the Indo-European root word for "growth"). So when you increase ghrelin levels, you stimulate that growth hormone to kick in, and growth hormone builds you not only up but out as well.

Your stomach secretes ghrelin in pulses every half hour, sending subtle chemical impulses to your brain—almost like subliminal biological messages (carrot cake, carrot cake, carrot cake). When you're really hungry or dieting, those messages come fast—every twenty minutes or so—and they're also amplified. So you get more signals and stronger signals that your body wants food.

After long periods, your body can't ignore those messages. That's why sugar cookies usually trump willpower, and that's why deprivation dieting can never work: **YOU-reka!** It's impossible to fight the biology of your body. The chemical vicious cycle stops when you eat; when your stomach fills is when you reduce your ghrelin levels, thus reducing your appetite. So if you think your job is to resist biology, you're going to lose that battle time after time. But if you can reprogram your body so that you keep those ghrelin gremlins from making too much noise, then you've got a chance to keep your tank feeling like it's always topped off.

Food Fight: The Ghrelin Versus Leptin Grudge Match

So now let's get back to that offense and defense. The natural state is for you to have a give-and-take relationship between your eating and satiety chemicals—between your ghrelin and leptin levels—to influence NPY and CART, respectively. It's the relationship between the impulse that says, "I'll take a large pepperoni with extra cheese," and the one that says, "No more passengers, this belly is full."

This battle over eating isn't between your willpower and the Belgian waffles; it's between your brain chemicals. The NPY is the villain—encouraging you to buffets, driving you to the pantry, pointing its chemical finger to the convenience foods, while CART is your dietary guardian angel, which encourages a cascade of allies to keep you full and satisfied and in no way interested in creamed anything. Think of the two substances—NPY and CART—competing for the same parking space, the one that will ultimately determine whether or not you eat (see Figure 2.3). They both arrive at the same time and want that space. Either more NPY or more CART sneaks into the spot, thus sending the all-important go or stop signal to your brain to influence the hormones that make you feel full or hungry.

Here's how they all work together: Ghrelin works in the short term, sending out those hunger signals twice an hour. Leptin, on the other hand, works in the long term, so if you can get your leptin signals high, you'll have a greater ability to keep your hunger and appetite in check. Isn't that great? Leptin can outrank ghrelin—to keep you from feeling like feasting on anything short of fingernails every few minutes. If you focus on ways to influence your leptin levels, and, more important, leptin effects (through leptin sensitivity), your brain (through CART) will help control your hunger.

Sometimes, it may seem like we don't have much control over the chemical reactions taking place within our arteries or inside our brains. But just as you can control things like cholesterol and blood pressure by changing the foods you eat or altering your behaviors, you can also control the satiety center of your brain. How? Through your choice of foods.

At least as far as your body is concerned, foods are drugs; they're foreign substances that come in and switch around all those natural chemical processes going about their business within your body. When your body receives foods, different chemical reactions take place, and messages get sent throughout your system—turning on some things, turning off others. While your body internally gives orders, you set the tone and direction of those orders through the food you're

Figure 2.3 **In a Jam** The satiety center is waiting to be turned off by NPY or stimulated by CART. Whichever fills up the receptor docks first is what controls whether you want to eat more or not. In turn, these two proteins are influenced by lack of water, sleep, and even sex. They're also influenced by ghrelin coming from your stomach, which stimulates NPY so you get hungry, and leptin from your fat, which is further stimulated by a chemical called CCK, released from your intestines after a meal.

feeding it. Eat the right foods (like nuts), and your hormones will keep you feeling satisfied. But eat the wrong foods (like simple sugars), and you'll cause your body to go haywire hormonally and become addicted to these harmful foods. And that ends up with one result: the next notch in your belt.

A major gang leader against your body is fructose, found in high-fructose corn syrup (HFCS), a sweetener in many processed foods. Here's how it works: **YOU-reka!** When you eat calories from healthy sources, they turn off your desire to eat by inhibiting production of NPY or by producing more CART. But fructose in the HFCS, which sweetens our soft drinks and salad dressings, isn't seen by your brain as a regular food.

Because your brain doesn't see any of the fructose in the thousands of HFCS-containing foods as excess calories or as NPY suppressants, your body wants you to keep eating (which means that even low-fat foods can have extremely bad consequences, calorie- and appetite-wise). Americans have gone from eating no pounds of this stuff per person in 1960 to eating more than sixty-three pounds of it every year (that's 128,000 calories). That's a contributor to weight gain, since the fructose in HFCS doesn't turn off your hunger signals. Foods with fructose—which may in fact be labeled as low-fat—make you both hungry and unable to shut off your appetite. They are also rich sources of calories: the perfect storm of weight gain. So you constantly get the signal that you're hungry, even after you've jammed your gut with two baskets of calorie-laden, fructose-loaded biscuits. That HFCS causes another perfect storm (we talk about the environmental one in Chapter 10). HFCS can cause your liver to be overwhelmed by fructose, which in turn causes inflammation. See, your liver can handle a small amount of fructose, as it would if you ate a piece of fruit every hour. But large amounts of it quickly overwhelm your liver. Your liver can't fully handle it, so it processes it by an alternate pathway that produces inflammatory substances that damage your liver, arteries, and immune system, promoting heart disease and cancer.

YOU TIPS!

Get Over Sticker Shock. You should read food labels as actively as you read the stock ticker or the horoscopes. We have a *YOU: On a Diet* "Rule of 5s." If any food has any one of the five ingredients below as any one of the first five ingredients on the label, don't let it near your mouth.

❖ Simple sugars
❖ Enriched, bleached, or refined flour (this means it's stripped of its nutrients)
❖ HFCS (high-fructose corn syrup—a four-letter word)
❖ Saturated fat (four-legged animal fat or palm or coconut oil)
❖ Trans fat (partially hydrogenated vegetable oil)

Putting them into your body is like dunking your cell phone in a glass of water. It'll cause your system to short out your hormones and send your body confusing messages about eating. Today's yearly per capita consumption of sugar is 150 pounds, compared to 7.5 pounds consumed on average in the year 1700. That's twenty times as much! When typical slightly overweight people eat sugar, they on average store 5 percent as ready energy to use later, metabolize 60 percent, and store a whopping 35 percent as fat that can be converted to energy later. Any guess as to where 50 percent of the sugar we consume comes from? HFCS in fat-free foods like salad dressings and regular soft drinks.

Choose Unsaturated over Saturated. Meals high in saturated fat (that's one of the aging fats) produce lower levels of leptin than low-fat meals with the exact same calories. That indicates you can increase your satiety and decrease hunger levels by avoiding saturated fats found in such sources as high-fat meats (like sausage), baked goods, and whole-milk dairy products.

Don't Confuse Thirst with Hunger. The reason some people eat is because their satiety centers are begging for attention. But sometimes, those appetite centers want things to quench thirst, not to fill the stomach. Thirst could be caused by hormones in the gut, or it could be a chemical response to eating; eating food increases the thickness of your blood, and your body senses the need to dilute it. A great way to counteract your hormonal reaction to food is to make sure that your response to thirst activation doesn't contain unnecessary, empty calories—like the ones in soft drinks or alcohol. Your thirst center doesn't care whether it's getting zero-calorie water or a megacalorie frap. **YOU-reka!** When you feel hungry, drink a glass or two of water first, to see if that's really what your body wants.

Avoid the Alcohol Binge. For weight loss, avoid drinking excessive alcohol—not solely because of its own calories, but also because of the calories it inspires you to consume later. Alcohol lowers your inhibition, so you end up feeling like you can eat anything and everything you see. Limiting yourself to one alcoholic drink a day has a protective effect on your arteries but could still cost you pounds, since it inhibits leptin.

Watch Your Carbs. Eating a super-high-carb diet increases NPY, which makes you hungry, so you should ensure that less than 50 percent of your diet comes from carbohydrates. Make sure that most of your carbs are complex, such as whole grains and vegetables.

Stay—Va-Va-Va-Voom—Satisfied. In any waist management plan, you can stay satisfied. Not in the form of a dripping double cheeseburger but in the form of safe, healthy, monogamous sex. Sex and hunger are regulated through the brain chemical NPY. Some have observed that having healthy sex could help you control your food intake; by satisfying one appetite center, you seem to satisfy the other.

Manage Your Hormonal Surges. There will be times when you can't always control your hormone levels; when ghrelin outslugs your leptin, and you feel hungrier than a lion on a bug-only diet. Develop a list of emergency foods to satisfy you when cravings get the best of you—things like V8 juice, a handful of nuts, pieces of fruit, cut-up vegetables, or even a little guacamole.

Chapter 3

Eater's Digest

How Food Travels through Your Body

Diet Myths

- ❖ Fat turns to fat, protein turns to muscle, and carbs turn to energy.
- ❖ The fullness of your stomach is what tells you to stop eating.
- ❖ Sugar gives you an instant high to help combat hunger.

Once your brain tells you to eat, that's exactly what you do. You eat. Maybe you gorge. Maybe you nibble. And then maybe you forget about that hefty portion of mac 'n' cheese until it winds up on the back of your thighs. But in between mouth and thighs, there's an amazing system of digestion that takes place—a system that determines whether that food gets burned, stored, or expelled faster than a delinquent high schooler.

Now that you know the biochemical reasons why you shuttle food to your mouth, it's time to start exploring the biology of what happens to food once it's in there. In this chapter, we'll discuss what happens in the early part of your digestive system, and in the next chapter, we'll discuss the effects of food as it interacts with the rest of your digestive organs.

Your Digestive Highway: The On-ramp

On your gastrointestinal interstate, everything enters via your physiological toll booth: your mouth. The nutritious powerhouses slide through the express toll to give you the power, energy, stamina, and strength to live your life. Toxic (though sometimes tasty) foods can enter too, but you'll pay a heavier toll later for the damage they do along the way and after. Throughout its journey, your food and all of its nutrients (and toxins) will pull over at various organs, slow down on winding roads, speed up, merge with other nutrients, and even get pulled over by the bowel brigade for nutritional violations. (See Figure 3.1.)

During every trip, your food hits a symbolic three-pronged fork in the road:

❖ Either it will be broken down and picked up by your bloodstream and liver to be used as energy.

❖ Or it will be broken down and stored as fat.

❖ Or it will be processed as waste and directed to nature's recycling pot: the porcelain junkyard.

Figure 3.1 Gutting It Out Food pulls over at various spots in the intestinal track, so disease of these areas can cause nutritional deficiencies even if two people are eating identical foods. Not all of the nutrients that come from food and supplements get absorbed in the same place; they're absorbed throughout your GI tract. Here are the rest stations where nutrients are absorbed:

Stomach: alcohol

Duodenum (first part of the small intestine; takes off from the stomach): calcium, magnesium, iron, fat-soluble vitamins A and D, glucose

Jejunum (middle part of the small intestine): fat, sucrose, lactose, glucose, proteins, amino acids, fat-soluble vitamins A and D, water-soluble vitamins like folic acid

Ileum (last part of the small intestine; leads to large bowel): proteins, amino acids, water-soluble vitamins like folic acid, vitamin B12

Colon (also known as the large bowel): water, potassium, sodium chloride

Here's how the system starts: Before a morsel even reaches the tollbooth, your body has a radar gun to let you know that food is coming—powered by such physiological cues as sight, smell, and the fact that you've been drooling like an overheated Saint Bernard at the thought of a fried-cheese appetizer special. In response to that sensory information, glands in your mouth start to secrete enzymes to help break down your food; then your stomach quickly constructs its version of a roadside welcome center by pumping out stomach acid to help prepare your body for the digestion process.

Now, don't underestimate your stamp licker as a player in this digestion process. Back in the day of buffalo-hide cocktail dresses, people relied on their tongues (and their noses) for survival; if it tasted good, then it was safe, and if it tasted like dinosaur dung, then it could be poisonous or toxic.

We do the same things, but in slightly different ways. Since our bodies use our senses to process information, we rely on our tongue for information about food. The information we acquire sends messages to the brain, and then the brain sends messages to our forks: keep eating or stop eating. That message largely comes from our five tastes (sweet, sour, salty, bitter, and unami, which recognizes the inherent deliciousness in foods like juicy filet mignon), but it also comes from what we smell. Some researchers say that three-quarters of how we "taste" certain foods actually comes from how we smell it. What's this have to do with your waist growing? For one, there's the obvious: the more you like a bad-for-you food, the more likely you are to keep eating it. But the genetics of taste and taste buds may play an even more subtle and fascinating role. As you'll see in the box on page 74 ("Are You a Supertaster?"), the physiological makeup of your tongue could make you more or less disposed to eating good or bad foods.

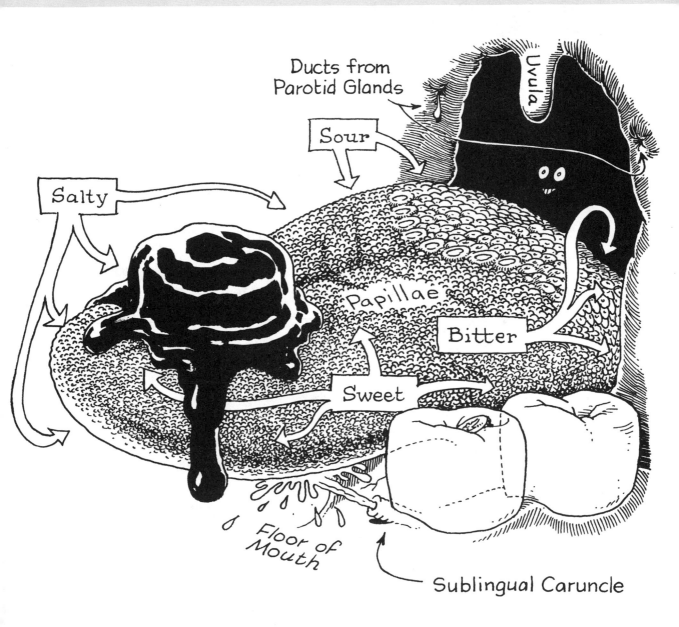

Figure 3.3 **Chewing the Fat** One of the reasons we can gain weight so readily is the efficiency of our teeth, which fit perfectly with one another to ensure that every morsel of food is crushed completely. Salivary glands near the lower teeth and at the back of the mouth secrete enzymes to hasten digestion before swallowing. The sight and smell of food warn these systems of what's to come.

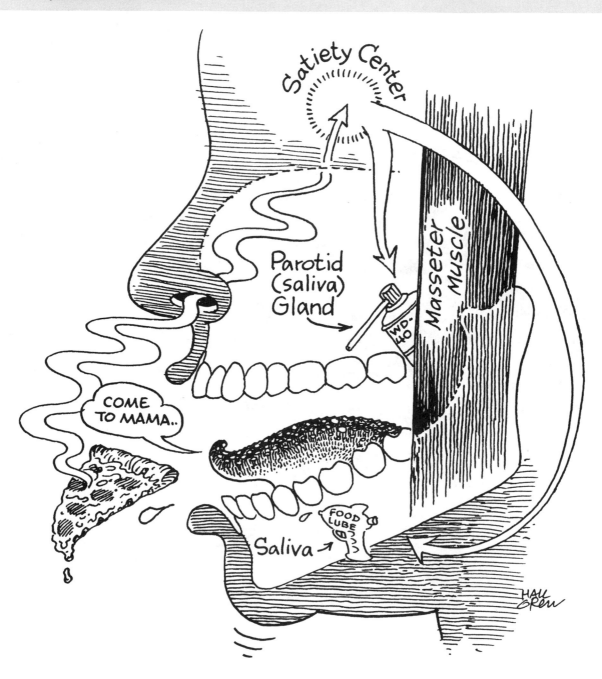

Unlike other animals, we waste very little energy eating because of our highly efficient perfectly opposing molars (see Figure 3.3). The powerful crushing motion helps us extract every possible calorie from the prime rib deluxe. Other animals waste or burn a lot of calories while they eat because their teeth do not efficiently mush the food when they move prey to belly. In humans, once that food actually does breeze past the tollbooth, it accelerates onto the on-ramp of the esophagus—that's the tube that links your mouth to the interstate that is your GI system.

After your Double Whopper slides down the on-ramp, it has to make a tricky merge in the form of a sharp turn to enter the stomach. That angle—the gastroesophageal junction—is what keeps stomach acid from spilling back into your esophagus and making your chest feel like an arson victim. (When you have extra fat in your belly, that angle is pried open, allowing acid to spill upward and cause heartburn. See "The Word on GERD," page 68.) Once your Whopper chunks have entered your stomach, serious digestion begins. The food is held in your stomach until your body directs it to the small intestine, where most of the nutrients are absorbed and passed along to the rest of your body through your bloodstream (to the liver, which is the next stop for absorbed nutrients), or to the large intestine on the way to evacuation.

Food Processor:
How Your Body Breaks Down Nutrients

In terms of weight and waist gain, a calorie is a calorie is a calorie. Calories not used immediately by your body for energy are either eliminated as waste or stored as fat. **YOU-reka!** But that doesn't mean that all calories are treated equally by your body.

Myth Buster

Oh, the Gall

Your gallbladder may seem as unnecessary as bad goatees, but one of its functions is to help store bile—that digestive juice that helps your body absorb nutrients. Obese people have a greater than 50 percent chance of developing gallstones. Why? An overworked liver caused by being overweight makes bile, which is more like sludge than liquid, and predisposes them to developing stones. It's also more likely that you'll develop stones when you lose weight fast, like after weight-loss surgery—because the gallbladder doesn't empty enough when it doesn't see any fat. So it's not uncommon for a surgeon to remove the gallbladder during a gastric bypass procedure. The risk factors for developing the painful stones are easy to remember, because they sound like an R & B group. They're the 4 Fs: female, fertile, fat, and forty. (We don't mean this to be a gender issue, but the fact is that women are more likely to have gallstone symptoms than men.)

For example, protein and fiber with high water content have a great effect on satiety, and simple carbohydrates have the least effect on satiety. (Fat, by the way, has an effect on satiety similar to that of protein and fiber, which is why low-fat diets leave people hungry all the time.) When it comes to converting calories, your body processes fat most efficiently—meaning that you actually keep more of it, because your body doesn't need to expend as many calories trying to store it. On the flip side, your body works hard to process protein, to make it highly flammable to your body's metabolic furnace.

Contrary to popular belief, not all ingested protein becomes muscle, and not all the fat in your food gets stored on your hips. Everything has the potential to turn into fat if it's not used by your body for energy at the exact time it is absorbed through your intestines. And energy is energy is energy (see Figures 3.4a and 3.4b). Here's how the different nutrients are processed:

Simple sugars (as in a cola): When sugar, which is quickly absorbed and sent to the liver, meets the liver in the digestion process, the liver tells your body to turn that sugar into a fat if it can't be used immediately for energy.

Complex carbohydrates (as in whole grain foods): They take longer to digest, so there's a slower release of the carbohydrates that have been converted in your bowel to sugar to become sugar in your bloodstream. That means your diges-

Figure 3.4a **Department of Energy** The three major types of energy are contained in carbohydrates, proteins, and fats, which can come from healthy or waist-busting forms. Complex carbs enter the blood slowly, so we do not tax our hormones. Amino acids are converted inefficiently to sugars, and fats cannot be converted at all. Fats come in forms our bodies recognize (like nuts) and naturally less common forms that poison us (like trans fats). Most foods, like meat, are a combination of energy sources; as the food digests (or sometimes rots) in your intestines, nutrients are absorbed in different places. By the way, even though the liver is the symbolic center of the metabolic universe, the intestines, as evidenced by your bathroom time, aren't really a closed loop.

Figure 3.4b **Food Use** Simple sugars from carbohydrates are the most versatile energy source, so they're preferentially used by our organs, especially the finicky brain, which refuses to tolerate any other source. Fats are a backup system to supply muscle with energy; this is why actually using muscles is needed to selectively lose fat, and why exercise works so well. Amino acids from proteins are crucial for building the body, but are used only as a last resource for exercise energy.

tive system is not stressed as much. Still, if your body can't use this slower sugar when it's released, it gets converted to fat.

Protein (as in meat): It gets broken down into small amino acids, which then go to the liver. If the liver can't send them to your muscles (say, if you're not exercising and don't need them for muscle growth or maintenance), then, yep, they get converted to glucose, which then gets converted to fat if you can't use it for energy.

Fat (as in funnel cake): It gets broken into smaller particles of fat and gets absorbed as fat. Good fats (like those found in nuts and fish) decrease your body's inflammatory response, and bad fats increase it. That inflammatory response, which we'll explain in the next chapter, is a contributing factor to obesity and its complications. If you're exercising and have used up all readily available carbohydrates (sugar), your muscles can use fat for energy, which is a great way to erode your love handles.

Your Digestive Highway: The Main Drag

At the bottom of your stomach and top of your intestines, your food hits an important traffic signal: It's the red light that tells your brain you're full and don't need another large order of onion rings (or the cheese sauce for dipping or the beer to wash it down). That red light is delivered by the vagus nerve, which is a large nerve that comes from the brain and stimulates the contraction of the stomach (see Figure 3.5). The vagus nerve is also the main cable controlling the parasympathetic system, which is the relaxation section of your nervous system. **YOU-reka!** The key messenger switching the vagus on is a peptide produced in your gastrointestinal track called CCK, which is released when your bowel senses fat. Technically, it stands for

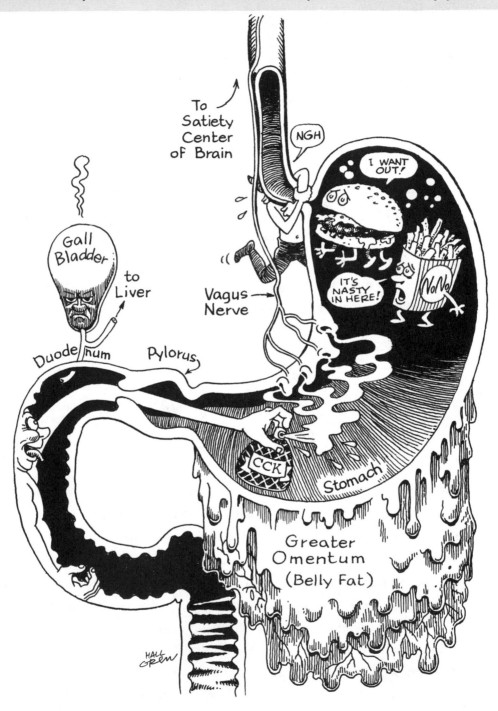

cholecystokinin, but for our purposes, let's think of it as the Crucial Craving Killer because its main purpose is to tell your brain via the vagus nerve that your stomach feels fuller than a *Baywatch* bathing suit.

Myth Buster Without having to go through the chemical pathways of your body (your bloodstream), CCK acts as a very direct message and indicator of your fullness. (Remember, leptin is more of a long-term indicator of your satiety; CCK provides a very short-term, intense message.)

After the food spends some time in your stomach, it will slowly leave that reservoir and go into the small intestine via the duodenum, the first part of your intestines that comes right after the stomach. That's when CCK puts up a digestive detour sign, in a very clear physical signal that makes you feel full. It causes the pylorus—the opening at the end of the stomach—to slam shut; that keeps food from moving into the small bowel. That's how your stomach gets full physically and how you feel full mentally. One interesting note: High-saturated-fat diets lead to less CCK sensitivity, so you do not feel as full as you should after eating a steak.

After the stomach, your food enters the small intestine and has a head-on collision with bile. Bile is the thick green digestive fluid that's secreted by the liver, stored in the gallbladder, and released into the small intestine. (CCK also has a third effect: It's what causes the gallbladder to contract.) After fat is broken down into smaller particles by substances called lipases, which are released by the pancreas, these tiny particles interact with bile to form a compound that is easily absorbed by the cells of your body. Bile surrounds the **Myth Buster** fat in our meal like soap surrounds grease on our hands so it can be scrubbed from the intestinal wall and better digested and absorbed.

Once it reaches the bloodstream, food continues to influence how hungry you may feel. Elevated blood sugar sends your brain the message that it's time to take your plate to the sink and hit the couch. When your blood sugar is low, that's what stimulates hunger and causes you to feed like a rat in the Kraft aisle.

Many of us get into trouble when we eat foods with simple sugars (think

The Word on GERD

Fat doesn't just pose problems for your belly and subway turnstiles; it also can mess with your throat. About half of obese people have the chest-burning condition called GERD (gastroesophageal reflux disease). The thinking is that extra fat in the belly, hanging off your stomach, pulls down on your stomach, thereby opening the angle of the GE junction and pushing it toward the chest. (Remember, it's at an acute angle to keep food from going back up your throat every time you eat.) The pried-open angle makes it easier for acid and food to be pushed back up. Plus, the extra fat in the belly puts pressure on the contents of your bowel. More pressure, more GERD. What's the big deal? Besides the unpleasant sensation of tasting your food on the way *up,* GERD also burns your esophagus—in the same way that the sun burns your skin. After a burn, it takes a couple days to heal, but if the burning happens over and over, it means you're burning the tissues and are more likely to develop cancer there, just like repeated sunburns increase your risk of skin cancer. Taking half a full aspirin or two baby aspirin (you want 162 mg) with a glass of water decreases this risk by about 35 percent. By the way, alcohol, coffee, pepper, acidic foods like tomatoes and OJ, and, to a lesser degree, chocolate increase GERD symptoms. The best way to manage symptoms until you lose weight is to avoid meals within three hours of bedtime and to put blocks under the head posts of your bed so that you sleep at a slight tilt. (Pillows usually don't work, since your head will typically roll off the pillow.)

soft drinks, jelly, cake). Simple sugars create a rebounding effect. You're feeling blah, so you eat a 3 Musketeers. That sugar surge works like an electrical jolt, and you instantly feel more energy. But less than two hours later, that energy surge (in the form of elevated blood sugar levels) plummets, and then you feel blah again. Your conclusion? You must need another Musketeer. That rebound effect (combined with the desire for the taste that's stimulated by the pleasure center in your brain) can put your body in biological turmoil, where you eat to feel better, though what you're eating is actually making you feel sluggish, so you swirl and swirl around, always feeling like you need to eat.

YOU-reka! At the bottom end of your small intestine (before it joins your large intestine), food hits the ileal brake—another signal that you're full. At this juncture there's a traffic signal that slows the passage of the slurry of intestinal contents from the small intestine to the large

Figure 3.6 **Acid Trip** Fat presses on the gastroesophageal junction and unkinks this connection, which makes acid and reflux move up toward the throat. Pressure on the stomach from intra-abdominal fat increases the backwash.

intestine. It's called the ileocecal valve. The squeezing required to overcome this traffic signal valve is reduced naturally by some foods, since your body feels that you're still digesting and not ready to evacuate those foods yet. Very little absorption of nutrients occurs in the colon (except by your bacteria, which gorge on it), so once the food passes the ileocecal valve, not much more happens except that you reabsorb water while consolidating the waste you've formed. The result: You have a traffic backup in your gut, and if you try to send more cars down the road, the problem's only going to turn into a fuller feeling. It's one of the reasons why fiber kills cravings, because fiber slows down the transit of food from your small intestine to your large intestine, keeping that full feeling. In the next chapter, we'll pick up the rest of the digestive journey in the intestines, where some of the key fat-storing processes take place.

The System of Satisfaction

Though it may seem that we have endless reasons to eat—to celebrate holidays, to beat stress, to pass time between Super Bowl commercials—there's only one real reason why we need food: for energy. That energy allows our organs to function, our muscles to move, and our bodies to keep warm. And to a large extent, our brains help control how we convert food to energy. To help understand the process that your body goes through to use energy, we'll break down the metabolic path into two phases.

Digestive Phase: Your hypothalamus orchestrates this phase of metabolism by receiving signals from throughout your body about whether you're hungry or not, so that your body can use energy to power itself. Here's how: Your body has a short-term reservoir for energy in the form of glycogen, a carbohydrate primarily stored in your liver and muscles. After eating, when you have glucose (sugar) and insulin (the hormone produced in the pancreas to transport glucose), your body uses all of the glucose it needs for immediate fuel but takes the rest and stores it as glycogen. If your blood glucose level falls, your pancreas stops releasing insulin—and then releases another G substance, glucagon, which converts the stored energy (glycogen) to sugar (glucose). So the effect is that when your intestinal gas tank empties of sugar (in other words, when our ancestors were fasting between bison hunts), your body is still able to supply crucial energy to your central nervous system by converting glycogen to glucose.

Fasting Phase: When you're sleeping or go long periods without eating, your body needs to have a supply of energy to keep your organs functioning. Once you use up all of your available glucose during the digestive phase of metabolism (your body stores only about 300 calories in the short-term glycogen reservoir), it taps a long-term reservoir: fatty tissue in the form of triglycerides (molecules that include a carbohydrate-containing glycerol). This keeps you going until you break the fast with breakfast.

Figure 3.7 **First-degree Burning** Feasting allows our livers to store excess sugar as glycogen, so we can access energy without eating for hours. Once glycogen stores are full, we save the excess energy from an ice cream sundae as fat. To break down fat, we first have to use up glycogen, which can take a half hour of exercise. That's when the body automatically begins burning up fat.

Storing Energy

Using Energy

YOU TIPS!

Slow the Process. Especially before your meal. If you have a little of the right kinds of fat just before you eat, you can trick your hormonal system by sending the signal to your brain that you're full. If you eat a little fat twenty-five minutes before your meal (70 calories or so of fat in the form of six walnut halves, twelve almonds, or twenty peanuts), you'll stimulate production of CCK, which will both communicate with your brain and slow your stomach from emptying to keep you feeling full. (CCK release and ghrelin reduction take about twenty-five minutes to kick in and take about 65 calories of fat to stimulate.) That way, you'll be able to sit down for a meal and eat for pleasure, not for hunger—which is one way to ensure you'll eat less. The average person is finished eating well before his satiety signals kick in, thus counteracting any possibility that his hormones can help him. For the same reason, you should eat slowly. If you down your food faster than a MiniVac, you won't allow your satiety hormones time to kick in.

Set the Early Fiber Alarm. Many of us may associate fiber with better health and increased toilet time, but fiber is the speed bump of your GI interstate. It slows everything way down. Technically, it works by slowing the transit of food across the ileocecal valve, keeping your stomach fuller for longer. The result: a greater feeling of satiety and an increase of appetite-suppressing CCK-like signals. While you should aim for around 30 grams of fiber a day, the key is bulking up in the morning. Studies show that consuming fiber in the morning (at breakfast) makes you less hungry in late afternoon—a notorious candy-sucking, diet-busting time of day. Great sources of breakfast fiber include steel-cut oatmeal, 100 percent whole grain cereal, whole grains, and fruit. (You'll note that every breakfast in the YOU Diet—see Part 4—has a lot of fiber in it, whether it's the cereal or the vegetables in an egg-white omelet or the whole wheat bread. And morning snacks, like an apple, also have fiber.)

Besides controlling blood sugar levels and decreasing insulin levels, fiber also reduces calorie intake for up to eighteen hours a day. Start with 1 to 2 grams of dietary fiber before meals and at bedtime and slowly increase to 5 grams. (If you add it all at once, you'll produce more gas than a Saudi oil field.) The supplement konjac root also seems to have a fiber-related effect. One study showed a nearly six-pound weight loss in eight weeks for those who ate 1 gram of it an hour before their meals.

Step Down to the Plate. Monstrous portion sizes are one of our stomach's biggest enemies: Studies show that when you're served bad foods in large containers, you'll eat up to one-third more than if you were served in smaller containers. By getting served in larger popcorn boxes, bigger dishes, and taller cups, we've automatically been tricked into thinking that availability should dictate how much we eat, rather than physical hunger. You don't have to go through drastic changes to make small ones. For starters, change your serving plates to the nine-inch variety to give yourself the visual and psychological cue that you're full when your physical appetite has been sated. That's important, because studies show visual cues help determine how full you are, in that you may not feel satisfied until your plate is clean, no matter how large the plate is. That's also reason never to eat directly out of a box or carton and always to remember that one serving size of a food is often about the size of a fist.

Slow Down. Stomach growling stimulates appetite, but growling doesn't really tell you how hungry you are. It tells you to eat, but not how much to eat. That's why meal size is so important. You're hardwired to eat, but you're not hardwired to eat a lot. Having a big meal quickly won't stop you from wanting to eat a few hours later. So slow down and let your CCK act; it takes about twenty-five minutes after the nuts to decrease your desire to eat.

Add Pepper. Red pepper, when eaten early in the day, decreases food intake later in the day. Some credit the ingredient capsaicin for being the catalyst for decreasing overall calorie intake and for increasing metabolism. It also appears to work by inhibiting sensory information from the intestines from reaching the brain, which is particularly effective in reducing appetite in low-fat diets. Capsaicin works by killing—or at least stunning—the messages that you're hungry. So add red pepper to your egg-white omelet.

Are You a Supertaster?

We all know that foods we like may send others seeking gas masks. But your tongue-related genetics may play an even bigger role in waist management. It could mean that you're either not getting the right foods, or more prone to downing an after-dinner pie before the check arrives.

If you're classified as a "supertaster," you tend not to eat fruits and vegetables because they may taste very bitter, thereby putting yourself at a higher risk of certain diseases and colon polyps because you're not getting the nutrients from fruits and vegetables. You should supplement your diet with half a multivitamin morning and night to ensure you're getting the right nutrients, as well as use fruits and veggies to enliven other things—as in salads and desserts and as moisturizers on breads (tomato sauce works great here). And if you're an "undertaster," you may be more prone to eating (and overeating) sweets because it takes more of a taste to satiate you. By the way, researchers say about 25 percent of us are supertasters and 25 percent are undertasters, while the rest of us are regular tasters.

Which taster are you?

The Saccharin Test: Mix one pack of saccharin (Sweet'N Low) into two-thirds of a cup of water; that's about the size of a tennis ball. Now taste the water. You'll probably taste a mix of both bitter and sweet, but see which taste is stronger. If sweet is dominant, then it means you're probably an undertaster, and if bitter is dominant, it means you're probably a supertaster. If it's a tie, you are like half the population, so don't sweat it. To be sure, you may have to do the test more than once to tease out differences.

The Blue Tongue Test: Wipe a swab of blue food dye on your tongue and see the small circles of pink-colored tissue that polka-dot the newly painted blue canvas. Those are your papillae. Then put a piece of paper—with a four-millimeter hole, or the size of a hole punch in three-ring paper—over your tongue. Using a magnifying glass, count the little pink dots you see in the hole. If you have fewer then five dots, it means you're an undertaster, while more than thirty indicate you're probably a supertaster.

Chapter 4

Gut Check

The Dangerous Battles of Inflammation in Your Belly

Diet Myths

- ❖ Your stomach is the place where you store your belly fat.
- ❖ Diets are mostly about calorie control.
- ❖ Your brain is the only part of your body that reacts emotionally to food.

We all know about the daily skirmishes that play out in the battle against obesity. You versus the ranch dressing, you versus the dessert tray, and in the title fight, your butt versus your college jeans. But it would be a mistake to think that every weight-loss war happens at the table or in the privacy of your own closet. In fact, millions of little firefights break out inside your gut every time you eat or drink—and these are the most influential battles in your personal crusade against excess weight. Deep inside your éclair-encrusted gut, you have cells and chemicals that react and respond to food in two ways: as an ally or as an enemy.

As we move along in our digestive journey to the second half of our digestive system, we'll explore these battles and how they influence your waistline. Here, your body doesn't just form allies or fight enemies according to how many calories a particular food has, or how greasy it is, or whether its mascot is a red-haired clown. When interrogating nutrients as they pass through your digestive system, your body classifies them by what kind of inflammatory effect they have; the enemies contribute to inflammation, and the allies quiet it.

We're not just talking about the inflammation that happens when your belly balloons to the size of a convention center, or the inflammation that happens to your joints if you have arthritis. We're talking about the chemical reaction of inflammation that happens within your cells and is an underlying cause of weight gain. This process is like the rusting of our bodies. Just like metal rusts when exposed to oxygen, inflammation is caused when oxygen free radicals (no political affiliation) attack innocent bystanders in our bodies.

Inflammation happens on many different levels and through several different mechanisms, many of them having to do with food. Not only can you get inflammation through allergies to food, but you can also get inflammation in the rest of your body—through the way your liver responds to saturated and trans fats, and through the way your body and belly fat respond to such toxins as cigarettes and stress. In turn, these inflammatory responses can cause things like hypertension, high lousy (LDL) cholesterol, and insulin resistance—and *those* inflammatory responses influence the total-body mother of all inflammation in your arteries, which leads to heart disease. (We'll discuss these at length in the next chapter.)

How Tolerant Are You?

With more than 100 million neurons in your intestines, gastrointestinal (GI) pain is immediate, but the level of GI discomfort you feel depends on your genetics; specifically on your tolerance of or allergies to certain foods and your genetic disposition for feeling the effects of those GI land mines. While there are certainly pharmaceutical solutions for dealing with the digestive explosions, there are also foods that produce an anti-inflammatory effect and can come in and put out the fire (see YOU Tips). During these inflammatory firefights, your intestines are contracting too much, or are being dilated—a painful process that works through the vagus nerve. Too much stimulation or distension of the bowel is what causes the pain. Some of us are less sensitive to those internal motions, so we may not always be getting the clue from our gut. These are some of the more common GI firestorms involving food intolerance:

❖ *Enzyme deficiencies:* When your intestines lack enzymes to metabolize specific foods like milk or grains or beans, the food remains undigested, so you start feeding your intestines' ravenous bacteria. The result: lots of intestinal dilation and more gas than a Hummer fuel tank. The most common of these is lactose intolerance (the lack of GI agreement with dairy products), and a close second is an allergy to the protein gluten from wheat (and rye and barley; nutritional good guys). As an example, when you lack the enzyme lactase (which happens more as you get older), the sugar lactose in the milk reaching your intestine is not metabolized, so it's presented to your intestinal bacteria, which metabolize the lactose in your intestines, producing a lot of gas. You don't feel so good either. The cure: avoiding lactose (milk and milk products) and/or gluten (see more on page 100).

❖ *General GI disorders:* Problems like irritable bowel syndrome, which causes gut-related symptoms like diarrhea and abdominal pain, are caused by sensitive nerves and result in inflammation in the intestinal walls. For example, we usually all pass the same amount of gas a day (about fourteen times, or 1 liter total), but some of us sense discomfort from that gas more than others do.

❖ *Psychological responses:* Food aversions can develop if, say, a person had a bad vomit-inducing shrimp dinner one night. The response would be to associate the shrimp dinner with the painful aftereffects and avoid it.

Of course, there are a number of extreme-end GI problems like infections, parasites (worms are the world's most successful weight-loss technique—but we don't recommend the *Fear Factor* diet), and violent and even lethal allergic reactions to food. The point is that we all may have degrees of intolerance in ways we may not even recognize. And we need to start listening to what our small intestine is trying to tell us about what we eat. Once you recognize that the general sense of "feeling off" can be caused by the foods you eat, you can identify—and work to eliminate, reduce, or substitute—the substance that makes your gut twist like an animal balloon.

Here, we'll look at how inflammation happens at the gut level, and then, in the next chapter, how that can lead to inflammation at the total-body level.

Inflamed Gut: The Intestinal Firefights

At the intestinal level, foods can cause inflammation of your intestinal wall through such things as allergies, bacteria, or other toxins. When food incites inflammatory responses in your gut, it's as if a grenade has been launched throughout your digestive system (see Figure 4.1 on page 85). Then in response to this already damaging grenade, your body tosses more grenades to create an apocalyptic digestive War of the Worlds. The effect is that the more inflammation we have in our intestines, the more toxins can enter our bloodstream.

During this firefight along the digestive border, your body perceives a foreign intruder and assigns its special forces—mast cells and macrophages—to eliminate the culprit. These are the cells that start an immune-response process throughout your body by ingesting foreign elements and alerting the rest of your body's protecting cells that intruders have entered the area. Foods that don't agree with your body's sensibilities are seen as foreign invaders, so the macrophages attack these foods and tell everyone that this war is going on. This causes your whole body to start firing away at these foods and at innocent bystanders— and thus causes inflammation in your bloodstream. In that way, eating unhealthy food is really like having a chronic infection that triggers an immune response, which then causes inflammation.

One of your body's goals is to get glucose into your brain cells—to feed those brain cells so that they can function. But inflammation in your body prevents sugar from getting to those cells, so you end up wanting more glucose and eating more sugary foods, which then increase inflammation and start the whole cycle again.

While we should be concerned about decreasing our body fat, we should also concentrate on decreasing our body's inflammatory response so we become more efficient in managing potential complications of our waist size. There's some genetic component to inflammation (some of us have more than others, and smokers tend to have higher levels of inflammation than nonsmokers). Most important, the process of gaining weight is often a process of inflammation. **YOU-reka!** When you decrease your body's inflammatory response, you will decrease your weight and waist as well.

The more inflammation you have, the less efficiently you use your food calories, and the worse you feel. The worse you feel, the more bad foods you eat to try to make yourself feel better. The more bad food you eat, the less well you can respond to the normal stresses of life, and the more inflammation you experience. And the more inflammation you have, the higher your risk of developing:

❖ diabetes and its cousin, metabolic syndrome
❖ high blood pressure
❖ high bad cholesterol numbers
❖ and all of the other conditions that contribute to your increase in size and your decrease in health

Plain and simple: Inflammation ages your body by making your arteries less elastic and by increasing atherosclerosis (the rusting of blood vessels). Inflammation also makes it more likely that your DNA will be damaged, and a cell will

FACTOID

Probiotics like *Lactobacilli* GG, *Bacillus coagulans,* or *Bifidus regularis* repopulate your small intestine's bacteria with healthful bacteria, especially after a course of antibiotics. The good bacteria calm down the dangerous ones—meaning that they can help you have less GI irritation, less gas, and less risk of an inflammatory uncivil war breaking out. Furthermore, some of the bacteria in your gut produce a poop that has proteins in it that you can absorb. And some of those proteins seem, in emerging research, to cause depression or high blood pressure. So we like bacteria whose poop does you no damage.

become cancerous. And it increases your risk of infections. If the inflammatory mediators are fighting in the arteries, they can't be defending elsewhere, and this situation increases the risk that your body will turn on itself, causing an autoimmune disease in which you attack your own tissues (for example, some forms of rheumatoid arthritis and thyroid disease).

Inflammation stresses your body.

Inflammation fattens your body.

Obesity isn't just a disease of doughnuts and baked ziti. Obesity is a disease of inflammation. As we travel through the rest of our digestive journey, we'll be stopping at three digestive landmarks to see how foods influence inflammation and how inflammation influences fat:

Your Major Interstate of Food: Your Small Intestine. This approximately twenty-foot-long organ (it's about three times your height) serves as your second brain, deciding which foods agree with your body and which foods cause your body to rebel like sixth graders with a substitute teacher.

Your Parking Lot of Fat: Your Omentum. The omentum, which is located next to your stomach, serves as your primary storage facility of fat, where you park some or (in really bad cases) all the

Abdominal Pain Is a Pain in the Neck

Your abdominal discomfort may be caused not by what's happening inside your belly but by what's happening outside. According to one researcher, there's such a thing as Tight Pants Syndrome, which is abdominal pain lasting two to three hours after a meal. Its cause? Yup: pants that are too tight. (The researcher says there's as much as a three-inch difference between waist size and waistband.) Funny, but the same thing happens with men and shirt size. Two-thirds of men purchase shirts with a neck size that's too small, so they get headaches, changes in vision, and even changes in blood flow to and from the brain.

excess foods you eat. Ideally, the garage is empty. But as we gain weight, some of our bellies are housing four stories of Winnebago-worthy fat. Most important, the omentum serves as our body's ultimate stress gauge: **YOU-reka!** As we'll explain in a moment, bigger bellies indicate higher levels of inadequately managed chronic stress—which causes chronic levels of inflammation.

Your Post Office Processing Facility: Your Liver. Your liver is the second-heaviest organ in your body (the largest, your skin, is actually twice as heavy) and is your body's metabolic machine. Your liver works a lot like an urban postal center, taking in all the incoming mail (in terms of nutrients and toxins), sorting it, detoxifying it, and then shipping it off to different destinations for your body to use as energy.

While the three organs all play different roles, the upshot of their relationship is this: The small intestine initially processes your food, and your omentum helps store it. Inflammation occurs in your small intestine and omentum, but the big battle happens in your liver, where the mother of all inflammatory responses takes place. That's the one that makes you store fat—and experience the unhealthy effects of it. And certain foods increase inflammation produced by your liver (see more on page 52).

FACTOID

Fat is a storage tissue, except when it's in your middle, when it becomes like an organ. Omentum fat has more blood supply than any other kind of fat and is quickest to mobilize itself to feed the liver. And it produces inflammatory substances.

Yes, we know that in-your-gut physiology isn't always pretty, but we want you to keep in mind our main gut goal: By understanding how food travels through this leg of your digestive system, you'll be able to identify the foods that will help you reduce harmful and weight-related inflammation. When you do that, you'll have signed a digestive peace treaty that can end the war on your waist.

Gathering Intelligence

They say that a woman thinks with her heart, and a man thinks with his personal periscope, but when it comes to sheer anatomy, the organ closest to your brain isn't the one that flutters over a midnight serenade or the one that tingles over a lingerie catalog. It's the one that coils through your gut like a sleeping python.

From a purely physiological standpoint, your small intestine functions as your second brain. It contains more neurons than any organ but your brain (and as many as your spinal cord), and the physical structure of the small bowel most resembles that of the brain. In addition, after your brain, your small intestine experiences the greatest range of emotions—in this case, your feelings manifest themselves in the form of gastrointestinal distress. In your brain, you react to actions: You feel love when your spouse holds your hand, mad when he forgets an anniversary, humiliated when he takes off his shirt at the Bears game and thumps his densely forested chest for a shot at

Myth Buster

being on *SportsCenter*. Your small intestine does the same thing. It reacts to foods that enter its pathway, depending on their anti- or pro-inflammatory effect. Your foods dictate whether your small intestine feels mild annoyance (a little bloating), anger (gas), stubbornness (constipation), or all-out temper tantrums (a thar-she-blows case of diarrhea).

Why Some People Stall

We'd like to think that our bodies work like cars—press the accelerator to go faster, tap the brakes to slow down. But our body's metabolic switches don't quite work that way: We may not gain or lose weight at the rate in which we expect to. When we have inflammation, our bodies are less efficient, meaning that we burn more calories—as a way to protect you, even as you gain weight. As we lose weight and decrease inflammation, our bodies go back to being efficient, and we may not burn calories at the proportional rate in which we gained them. So when we eat the right foods and more efficiently metabolize them, weight also may stall temporarily—meaning you still may be heavy, but might not have as many health risks associated with the weight.

Of course, you're the one who decides what foods you'll eat, but your small intestine works like an undercover agent—gathering information about all the nutrients and toxins that enter your body.

Your small intestine feels. Your intestine thinks. And your intestine performs a critical job during digestion: It helps guide you in all of the decisions *you* make about eating, because it tells you which foods agree with your body and which ones don't. How does it do that? Through the absorption of those foods. Your small intestine has an absorptive surface area that's 1,000 times larger than its start-to-end length because of all of the accordion-like nooks, crannies, and folds within it. Those spaces are where your body actually absorbs nutrients. So your intestinal absorption area isn't just 20 feet long; it's the equivalent of 20,000 feet long. No wonder you absorb so much of what you eat. When you have inflammation in the wall of your small intestine (through a food allergy or intolerance), it dramatically cuts down on that absorptive surface area—from about 2 million square centimeters to 2,000 square centimeters—because of swelling and poisoning of the functional surface cells. And if the intestine can't absorb nutrients, you experience an upset stomach and diarrhea.

While we're all familiar with those overt, emergency intestinal crises, our intestinal emotions also influence us in ways we don't normally associate with food. The reason we may feel groggy or have less energy than a drained nine-volt

You may hear that celebrities get colonics because they seem like some sort of miracle weight-loss cure. Here's how they work: You get a tube pushed up into your lower intestines (via your back end). You're infused with a solution, and you roll around to wash out your colon, then the fluid gets sucked out (you're given coffee, to help you go to the bathroom quickly). The purpose is to cleanse out the toxins and "reboot" your intestines. You'll produce a lot of waste after a colonic, but the main waste here is of money. Your colon only absorbs water, so there's no weight-loss benefit from colonics. In fact, you can get the same colon-cleansing and toxin-eliminating effect with a twenty-four-hour fast, coffee, and water.

could be because our intestines are trying to tell us we're choosing the wrong foods. If you pulled out the small intestines of your entire family and laid them on the back deck to compare them (latex gloves, please), you'd see that they all look alike; they're the classic, wormy tubes that wind throughout your gut. In terms of basic physiology, we all have the same intestines, just as we all have the same basic brain structure. But just as all of our brains don't function the same way even though we have the same parts, our intestines don't function the same way either. **YOU-reka!** Our intestines are as different as our smiles, as our laughs, as our political views, as our fetishes. A particular food can make one person feel energized and make another person feel as lethargic as a rag doll.

Anatomically, your intestinal wall is Clint Eastwood tough. With more than a trillion bacteria living in your intestines at any given time (most of them helpful, but at least 500 species of which are potentially lethal), your body protects itself with a fortified infrastructure to keep the bacteria out of your bloodstream. But

Figure 4.1 **Internal Conflict** Food and toxins continually line the frontier of our intestines. Good foods slip through to provide us nutrition, but combatants stimulate an aggressive response from local immune cells. The resulting inflammation causes swelling, gas, and belly cramps.

your body—though it relies on that Fort Knox–like wall—has to have a way to give clearance to authorized visitors. That is, it needs to allow nutrients to get through the wall to your bloodstream so you can use food as energy to keep your organs functioning, to go to work, to pry the kid's fingers from the panicked frog's leg. (One of the ways this penetration system works is through bile, which tricks the wall's security so fats can get through to the bloodstream.) This selection of what stays in your intestines and what can cross the line is one of the least understood anatomical processes, but it's part of the inflammatory battle that plays out daily in your body. When your intestinal wall is inflamed, some unauthorized visitors get in.

Essentially, alien bacteria are living in your intestines, trying to get into your bloodstream to multiply (which is their goal) and cause havoc, but they're being fought at the intestinal wall by those who guard it. (Your gastrointestinal tract, but especially your intestines, is one of three places where your body interacts with the external world; your skin and lungs being the other two.) In your small intestine, your mast cells and macrophages, which are part of your immune system, serve as the bowel brigade, fighting alien invaders.

When foods enter the small intestine and are transported across the intestinal wall, they're met by this bowel brigade border patrol, which screens the nutrients. The bowel brigade lets the food through because it has an authorized ID card—it's food, and your body wants it. But if it's the wrong

Milking It

If you suffer from a milk allergy, it can make your gut feel like a washing machine in the rinse cycle. Here are some ways you can help manage it:

❖ Milk's one of the easiest ingredients to substitute in baking and cooking by using an equal amount of either water, fruit juice, or soy or rice milk.

❖ Watch out for hidden sources of dairy. For example, some brands of canned tuna fish and other nondairy products contain casein, a milk protein. The U.S. Food and Drug Administration (FDA) is currently working on requiring products to eliminate the term nondairy if they contain milk derivatives. If any of the eight most common allergic foods (peanuts, milk, wheat, soy, tree nuts, fish, shellfish, and eggs) are in a product, they're supposed to be clearly identified on the label.

❖ In restaurants, tell your server about your allergy. Many restaurants put butter (which comes from milk) on steaks and other food after they've been grilled or prepared to add extra flavor, but you can't see it after it melts.

❖ Some ingredients seem to contain milk products or derivatives but actually don't. These are safe to eat if you have a lactose allergy: cocoa butter, cream of tartar, and calcium lactate.

By the way, there's a higher ethnic predominance of lactose intolerance in those of non-European origin. It's just another example of how genes—not willpower—mix with your environment to help dictate what you can and cannot eat.

kind of food, if it contains some toxins, or if you are allergic to it, your bowel brigade responds by calling in more mast cells and setting off time-released bombs throughout your intestines. This is where the inflammation firefight starts. The result? Pain, gas, nausea, or general GI discomfort.

Why is this crucial? Not just because of the initial inflammatory reactions, but for the role it plays in your eating emotions (your small bowel is your second brain, and 95 percent of your body's serotonin, which is a feel-good hormone, is in your gut). How you feel influences how you eat, and how you eat influences how you feel. When you eat food that makes you feel

FACTOID

About 2.5 percent of us suffer from milk allergies, making it the most prevalent of food allergies. While allergies to dairy products are generally outgrown, peanut allergies are not (and they're the most potentially lethal). By the way, it seems like some allergies are more prevalent the earlier in life we're exposed to the foods.

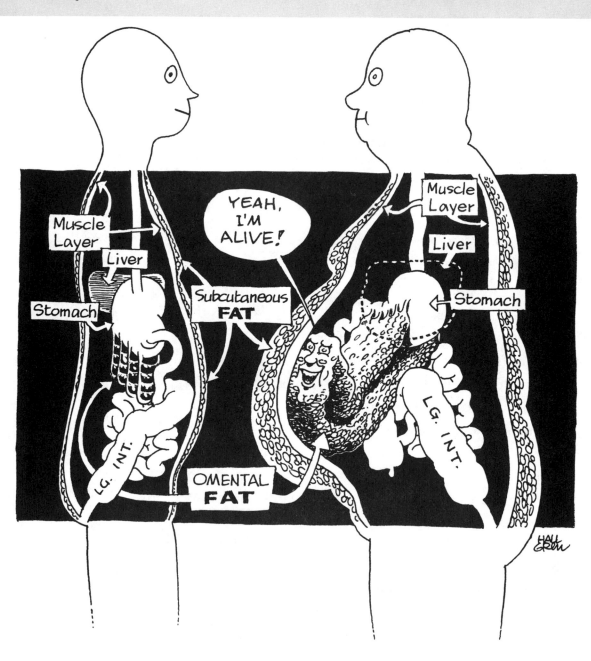

bad, you self-medicate with food that may make you feel good in the short term but will actually contribute to both inflammation and weight gain. Ultimately, when you're caught in a cycle of feeling bad and eating worse, you'll create a chemical stress response in your body—one that's handled by your parking lot of fat.

The Storage of Stress in Your Belly

The best way to tell how stressed you are: Take a look how much belly fat you have. The larger your waist, the higher your stress.

Along the intestinal freeway, the parking garage for fat that is your omentum looks like a stocking draped over a hanger (the stomach is the hanger), but changes depending on how many calories you're storing (see Figure 4.2). In a person with little omentum fat, your stomach looks as if it has nylons hanging off it—thin, permeable, with some webbing. But in a person with a lot of omentum fat, the hanger looks as if snow pants are hanging on it—the fat globules are so fat that there's no netting or webbing whatsoever. (While cells can convert to fat in the liver, getting fatter is more a case of your existing cells growing. When you add body fat, you don't get more fat cells, just more fat in each cell.)

Genetics certainly helps dictate whether you're going to have a big waist or a small one. But your lifestyle—in terms of stress—often plays a bigger role in deciding whether you'll have large amounts of belly fat or not. Here's how it works:

Historically, mankind has two types of stresses. The first kind is the immediate soil-your-loincloth stress (in other words, the dinner-seeking saber-toothed tiger is closing in fast). In that fight-or-flight scenario, your body produces the neurotransmitter norepinephrine to speed your heart rate, breathing, and 100-yard-dash time to the cave. When that happens, the last thing you're thinking about is grilling up some tubers on the campfire, so your hunger levels are squashed. That's because your body inhibits the peptide NPY during periods of acute stress (it's why exercise cuts appetite, because your body senses that you're in acute stress). So high levels of stress work in favor of your waist: They take away your appetite and speed up your metabolism.

The second kind of stress that early man faced is the chronic struggle brought on by drought and famine. In contrast to the thirty or forty seconds they sweated over tiger fangs, our ancestors worried about survival all the time, and their bodies had to deal with chronic stress. When they faced famine, they sought out as many calories as they could, and their metabolism downshifted to help them conserve energy. The modern-day version of this problem is chronic stress, which makes us seek out calories and then downshifts our metabolism. **YOU-reka!** Our bodies respond by storing the excess energy to call upon during periods where there may not be enough food. Those extra calories are stored in the omentum—our abdominal fat depot—to have on hand in case we are denied food. The liver, which is the relay station for energy circulation in the body, has immediate access to this omental fat, unlike the cellulose cluttering up the back of our thighs.

When people are under stress, their bodies release high amounts of steroids into their bloodstream in the form of the hormone cortisol. In acute cases (the tiger or a car accident), steroids stick around briefly. But when you're under chronic stress (the drought or the nagging task), your body needs to find a way to deal with those high levels of cortisol. So your omentum clears the cortisol steroids; it has receptors that bind to them and can suck them out of the bloodstream. (Unfortunately, this doesn't necessarily reduce

Figure 4.3 **Toxic Dump** All the nutrients we absorb through the intestines pass through the liver via the portal vein. Excess fat and inflammatory chemicals stored in the omentum can dump directly into the liver as well, which can start a cascade of toxic protein release into the body.

the stress level that you feel.) The steroids turbocharge the ability of omentum to store fat, so your belly fat (and subsequent waist size) becomes the best surrogate indicator of how well you are really coping with stress—despite what your brain might be claiming. That uptake of steroids throws your body into metabolic disarray by making your omentum resistant to insulin so that sugar floats around without being absorbed and used appropriately by needy cells. This:

- ❖ chronically raises your blood sugar, which damages your tissues;
- ❖ supercharges your omentum with inflammatory chemicals that destabilize the delicate equilibrium of your hormones;
- ❖ forces your omentum to pump high-octane fat directly into your liver—causing your liver to make even more inflammatory chemicals;
- ❖ causes NASH (nonalcoholic liver disease) or NAFL (nonalcoholic fatty liver) (more on page 99).

The Fight Against Inflammation

The liver—the organ that's responsible for your metabolism—receives its blood and nutrients from your gut. What it wants isn't the trans fat from the extra-large fries. It wants the other nutrients from the salmon slider: the protein from the fish, the carbohydrates from the 100 percent whole wheat bun, the lycopene from the tomato, the calcium from the spinach. The liver is always on the job, processing munchies after midnight, as well as 5 a.m. coffee. Your liver takes every chemical

FACTOID

Preliminary studies in animals show that the scent of grapefruit oil—yes, just the scent—has an effect of reducing appetite and body weight. Rats exposed to the scents for fifteen minutes three times a week enjoyed the effect. The cause? It's unclear, but it may work through grapefruit oil's effects on liver enzymes. Grapefruit oil is widely available through aromatherapy stores and websites. As a bonus, try to eat a couple of grapefruit while you're searching.

Infected and Inflated

While it's true that everything from your hair to that ankle tattoo technically belongs to you, the truth is that only 10 percent of the cells on and in your body are actually yours. The rest are microbes living on your skin and in your orifices (pleasant visual, eh?), and especially in your gut. Those gut-residing microbes provide the enzymes you need to digest the fiber in fruits and vegetables that would otherwise pass through your system without being absorbed (pleasant visual number two). That's right. Without the bacteria and viruses in your gut, the food-label warning about 100 calories per bite would be a gross exaggeration. Specifically, mice raised without exposure to any germs have 60 percent less body fat than ordinary mice, even though they eat 30 percent more food. More intriguingly, common gut bacteria inhibit proteins that normally prevent the body from depositing fat, so infected mice have more belly fat.

So what do a few blubbery mice have to do with obesity in humans? It turns out that people infected with a specific chicken virus in India carry an extra 33 pounds of fat compared with noninfected humans. More important, they have lower cholesterol and triglyceride levels—just the opposite of what we expect with weight gain. Why? Perhaps because the germs in the gut also digest cholesterol, so that less of it is absorbed. In an American study, the virus was found in 30 percent of obese subjects compared to only 11 percent of leaner people, and the folks who had the virus weighed significantly more than uninfected people. (And when twins with only one infected sibling are examined, the infected twin has 2 percent more body fat, despite having the same genes.)

Finally, we know that fat cells and our immune cells share lots of similarities. Fat cells can engulf bacteria and can secrete hormones that stimulate the immune system, possibly explaining why obesity causes an inflammatory response and leads to elevated C-reactive protein (a marker of inflammation). So how do you tell if you have a germ civil war inside you that's causing obesity? If your cholesterol and triglyceride levels are low and your C-reactive protein level is elevated, it might be worth testing yourself; Obetech (www.obesityvirus.com) makes a kit. This might reduce your guilt level, but since science is still gathering data and a cure is still lacking, you will still need to focus on other approaches. For now, anyway. This also may explain why probiotics are associated with weight loss; the healthy bacteria in your intestines from probiotics help keep unwanted viruses from setting up a permanent home in "their intestine."

in your body and processes it by binding it to a protein, transforming it into something the body can use.

So your poor overworked liver also gets the toxic trans fat directly from your intestines and from your omentum via that portal vein that feeds right into it. When your intestines send that convoy of fat pouring down into the vein, the liver sees it as a runaway train and tries to metabolize the foods. But in defending the body, additional inflammatory chemicals are released.

Help on the Horizon

"Fat free" can refer to marathoners and teen pop stars, but when you see it referring to food, you have to be skeptical. That's because either it tastes like a shoe box or it can be loaded with lots of sugar to compensate for fat—making that "fat-free" food more dangerous than a slowpoke in the passing lane. One goal for food manufacturers is to make foods that allow eaters to have the best of both worlds: great-tasting food that doesn't have waist-expanding ingredients. One such substance that may eventually change the way we eat is called Z-trim—it's a natural, zero-calorie fat substitute that's made from the fiber of such ingredients as oats, soy, rice, and barley. While there's no clinical data showing its effectiveness in weight loss, there's some evidence to suggest it can be used to cut the amount of fat usually used in a meal by 25 percent to 50 percent. The resulting food has all the "taste" benefits of fat (better taste, more creaminess, better mouth-feel) without the caloric load. Z-trim, which you can use with your own recipes, might also inhibit the hunger-inducing ghrelin because of its fiber content. The downside seems to be that by adding Z-trim, you also lose the benefit of the healthy oils in the food. Our tasters reported that foods with Z-trim had all the flavor of full-fat food, and that's enough to make us hopeful that nonfat won't always have to mean high-sugar or no taste.

In your liver, nutrients can be met by two substances. In our digestive town along our intestinal highway, let's think of one as the raucous frat house that stimulates inflammation, while the other is a nice, stately nonprofit group that quiets inflammation and performs good deeds throughout your body.

Eating foods that stimulate your liver to release the frat-house substance—which is called nuclear factor kappa B, or NF-kappa B—triggers a chain of events that causes the inflammation in your body and prevents the transport of glucose to your cells (and thus triggers hunger). Glucose (sugar) on the inside of cells stops hunger (in the specific satiety center of the brain). But you can also eat foods that stop the inflammation riot or foods that stimulate the release of the do-good substances that have an anti-inflammatory effect (see Figure 4.4). They're called PPARs (it stands for peroxisome proliferator-activated receptors, but we like to think of them as Perfectly Powerful Abdominal Regulators). The reason PPARs are so effective: Once they're activated, they decrease glucose and insulin levels, as well as cholesterol and inflammation. Though we all have different genetic dispositions for levels of PPARs, PPARs aren't self-starters; they need to be activated by foods to work.

Weird Causes of Obesity

Most people assume that being overweight means one of two things: that you eat too much or move too little. But some research suggests that overeating and inactivity shouldn't be the only things taking the blame for our moon-sized waist circumferences. Studies show that other explanations for obesity include things like—get this—what you stick under your armpits and the age of your mom when she gave birth. Here are some of the more unusual things theorized to be related to obesity:

Deodorants: Some deodorants contain chemicals that can disrupt your normal metabolism, making you more likely to gain weight. While we don't recommend ditching the deodorant and scaring off elevator mates, you should avoid deodorants that contain the ingredient aluminum or sprays with polychlorobiphenols.

The temperature: Air-conditioning in the summer and heating in the winter may make you less cranky, but they also may make you fatter. If you're in a cold room, for example, your body has to do more metabolic work to bring your temperature to normal (same for a warm room)—thus increasing your metabolism. You can increase your calorie-burning motors simply by lowering the temperature in your house during the winter (to 61 degrees Fahrenheit, where brown fat secretion kicks in) or raising it in the summer.

Stopping smoking: We recommend cigarettes about as much as we recommend DIY vasectomies, but nicotine can be a powerful weapon in the fight against fat. See our take on nicotine on page 462.

Your mom: Studies show that the older your mom was when she gave birth, the more likely you are to be fatter. While there's nothing you can do to change your family history, having a mom who was older at the time of your birth means you need to be more vigilant about watching your waist.

Your mate: Studies show that fatter people tend to choose fat mates, and that increases the odds that you'll produce an even fatter child. We're not in the matchmaking business, but it's worth noting that the best place to meet a mate isn't at the burger joint.

Some drugs: Some meds used to treat problems related to obesity, such as beta-blockers for high blood pressure, insulin for diabetes, and some antidepressants actually stimulate appetite, decrease metabolism, or have other effects that make weight gain more likely.

Now, if you look at PPAR and NF-kappa B at the cellular level, you can also see how they predispose us to obesity. Every human cell is run by DNA strands that carry blueprints for future growth. When the DNA mutates, it makes our cells less able to reproduce themselves rapidly and accurately, so our bodies age. What makes that DNA break down? Yes, inflammatory responses in your body cause oxidation (remember that this is your body's rusting process)—namely in

Figure 4.5 **Stress Mess** The cycle of stress affects weight by increasing hormones above normal levels, resulting in hunger and fat deposition, which causes inflammation, which causes more stress, and off we go.

Is There Such a Thing as a Bad Food?

Fast-food franchise owners aren't the only ones who may say that there's no such thing as good or bad food—that it's just the volume of food that you eat. There are plenty of dietitians, nutritionists, doctors, and food growers who believe the same thing. Our research leads us respectfully to disagree. Good, healthy foods satiate you, they decrease inflammation in your body, they turn down the activity of hazardous genes and turn up the production of beneficial proteins by good ones, they decrease the tendency to yo-yo, they're nutrient-dense, and they make you younger. Bad foods make you hungrier, increase inflammation in your body, turn up the production of proteins that foster heart disease and cancer by hazardous genes and turn down the activity of good ones, make you feel sluggish, make it more likely you'll yo-yo, have few nutrients, and make you older. After all, when you eat fries (no matter whether it's two fries or two bags), you're taking in calories that taste good but have as much nutrient value as plywood. In other words, bad foods add to your waste; good foods make waist management easier because they help keep you satisfied so that you never feel like gorging on nutrient-low and calorie-high foods. We call those good foods the YOU-th-FULL foods.

the form of increasing NF-kappa B with inadequate PPAR levels to put out the inflammatory fires. How do we stop that mutation, that oxidation, and that inflammation? By eating foods that increase your antioxidants or that have anti-inflammatory properties—foods that we'll cover in the waist management plan on page 255. These foods are particularly useful for those who are aging and unable either to exercise or to manage stress efficiently.

This is one of the primary battles you want to win—to quiet your inflammation and decrease your fat storage through the regulation of these two chemicals and their allies. To quash those hooligans living in the NF-kappa B house, you need to increase the effects of the noble PPARs throughout your body.

The Stress Response: Putting It All Together

Today, we don't experience droughts or famine, but we do have high levels of chronic stress, whether it comes in the form of workload, relationship troubles, or to-do lists that are longer than Route 66. And our bodies respond the same way

The Liver's Cheap Shot

When you think of damage to your liver, you typically think of one kind of shot—the kind that involves rocketing booze down your pipes. But when it comes to waist management, there's another kind of shot involved—the cheap shot. That cheap shot comes in the form of high-fructose corn syrup serving up a sucker punch to your liver.

Here's the story: When you're overweight, you typically have an increased food intake, an increase in the number of addictive foods that you eat, a decrease in physical activity, and some genetic component for storing belly fat. Bad enough, right?

Well, with that increase in belly fat, you also develop insulin resistance, which causes a lot of extra glucose to float around in your blood, as well as an increase in free fatty acids. Your liver goes into overdrive trying to process those fats, and you wind up with damaging inflammation.

When fructose is added to the mix—in the form of syrups (especially high-fructose corn syrup), not the natural kind found in fruits—things go from bad to worse. Fructose in syrups is absorbed into your body so fast it is thought it overwhelms your liver's ability to process it; instead, the excess goes down an alternative route of metabolism that causes release of toxins, and that's the sucker punch that results in liver damage that's not associated with alcohol (called NASH) or fatty liver (NAFL, nonalcoholic fatty liver). NAFL and NASH further limit your ability to handle fructose, producing more inflammatory substances, which further damage your liver, arteries, and immune system. Look at the *YOU: On a Diet* diet plan for the right way to throw a counterpunch.

as our ancestors' bodies did. But the difference is that we have plenty of food at our disposal. Chronic stress triggers an ancient response of calorie accumulation and fat storage, so we end up continually upgrading the size of our omentum storage unit. Here's where the cycle of fat spins out of control:

- ❖ When you have chronic stress, your body increases its production of steroids and insulin, which . . .
- ❖ Increases your appetite, which . . .
- ❖ Increases the chance you'll engage in hedonistic eating in the form of high-calorie sweets and fats, which . . .
- ❖ Makes you store more fat, especially in the omentum, which . . .
- ❖ Pumps more fat and inflammatory chemicals into the liver, which . . .

Go G-Free

These days, there's a whole lot of buzz surrounding the word "gluten" (and no, it has nothing to do with exercises to tone your butt muscles). It has to do with the issue of gluten intolerance, allergies, and diseases associated with the body's inability to handle gluten, the substance found in wheat, rye, and barley (it's the doughy stuff that holds it all together).

The difference, of course, between an allergy and intolerance is that an allergy can cause inflammatory reaction in the skin, mouth, and lungs, while an intolerance does not involve the immune system and manifests itself more in symptoms of discomfort such as gas, diarrhea, and abdominal pain. (Celiac disease, by the way, is permanent intolerance to the chemicals associated with wheat protein.) The problem with this host of problems is not only the symptoms that come along with them but also the fact that the changes in the intestines can make it difficult to absorb important vitamins and nutrients.

So if you're starting a waist management plan and suffer from one of these issues (gluten intolerance, for example, affects one in seven people), you need to know how to manage the nutritional limitations that may affect how and what you eat. Some tips for managing these problems:

Know Your Foods. You likely know the main foods that contain gluten: wheat, rye, barley, and all their derivatives, such as bran, couscous, and orzo. But you may not know some of the more stealthy foods that contain gluten, such as beer, artificial flavors, candy, lunch meats, Communion wafers, pasta, soy sauce, and lipstick. Luckily, some grains are gluten free. They include chia, buckwheat, flax, corn, quinoa, rice, and soy.

Label, Label, Label. Before you do your shopping, spend some time searching online for gluten-free products. It'll save you time in the supermarket until you get to know which brands are gluten free. Since online info isn't always accurate, check the labels of everything you drop into your cart. Under-the-radar, red-flag words include "modified," "hydrogenated," and "natural flavors."

* Creates a resistance to insulin, which . . .
* Makes your pancreas secrete more insulin to compensate, which . . .
* Makes you hungrier than a muzzled wolf, which . . .
* Continues the cycle of eating because you're stressed and being stressed because you're eating.

Don't Be Timid. Whether you're eating out or at a party, don't be shy about letting your host and server know about your allergy or intolerance. They may be able to accommodate you, but it's always best to plan ahead (by eating a little something beforehand or even bringing your own gluten-free snacks to a party). Either way, speak up—there's no sense in trying to hide it or fight it.

Sample Gluten-Free Shopping List

Fresh fruits	Peanut butter
Unflavored milk	Eggs
Canned salmon, tuna, and chicken	Popcorn
Dried beans, lentils, and peas	100% fruit juice
Most yogurts	Plain nuts and seeds
Fresh vegetables	Coffee and tea
Tofu	Cocoa
White or sweet potato	Jell-O
Corn	Spices and herbs
Plain brown rice	Pudding
Fresh pork and poultry	Canola and olive oil
Fresh fish or seafood	

To get an accurate diagnosis, you can have a celiac panel done to rule out celiac disease, an endoscopy and small-tissue biopsy (if the panel has shown that your risk is high), and a genetic testing (which can ID genes associated with celiac disease).

Interestingly, the more fat you store in your omentum, the more it reduces the effect of stress on your brain—it's your body's way of comforting you, assuring you that you'll be prepared during times of famine. It's why your omentum fat— the fat around your belly—isn't just an indicator of the size of your waist, it's also your own personal gauge of the size of your stress.

YOU TIPS!

Let Food Fight the Fight. Your best weapon against fat isn't a Tae-Bo video or a self-serve liposuction vacuum. It's food. Good food. Inflammation-reducing food. Food that turns on the factory of genes that make you younger and healthier. To reduce obesity-causing inflammation, you need to eat foods with nutrients that can do just that—either by having direct anti-inflammatory properties, or by stimulating the do-good PPARs or inhibiting the party-throwing pledges in the NF–kappa B frat house. Anti-inflammatory chemicals are often what gives a specific food its flavor, smell, and color. So eating more anti-inflammatory foods means eating more flavorful and brightly colored foods. (The foods you eat ought to be tasty; you can magnify a flavor by doubling up on it with two different food sources. For example, add sundried tomato bits to tomato sauce, or eat dried apples with sugar-free applesauce to bring out the flavor.)

Following is a list of nutrients that seem to have anti-inflammatory effects, and our recommended doses. Though they may not help you lose a ton of weight, they're known or thought to have anti-inflammatory effects, which will help you live healthier no matter what your weight.

Substances known to fight inflammation:

Omega-3 Fatty Acids: Omega-3 fatty acids—found in fish oils—seem to increase the number of PPARs, which will help reduce your inflammation. We recommend you get omega-3s in the form of three 4-ounce servings of salmon or trout per week or a 2-gram fish oil capsule each day or 600 milligrams of vegetarian DHA from algae (where the fish get their DHA) or an ounce of walnuts a day (twelve halves provide beneficial omega-3s too). Saturated fats, by the way, increase inflammatory properties, and trans fat undermines the effects of omega-3s.

Green Tea: The thinking is that catechins in green tea inhibit the breakdown of fats and also inhibit production of NF-kappa B. Studies have found that drinking three cups of green tea a day reduced body weight and waist circumference by 5 percent in three months. It also increased metabolism (all nonherbal teas contain substances that increase the metabolic rate).

Substances we think may fight inflammation:

Beer (in moderation, Tiger): The bitter compounds that come from beer derived from hops seem to activate PPARs in animal studies. But you have to get them in the form of only one drink a day. Consumption of twenty-one eight-ounce beers, twenty-one glasses of wine, or twenty-one shots of whiskey a week has a clear correlation with belly fat, independent of all other risk factors.

Turmeric: A gingerlike plant that has curcumin as its active ingredient, turmeric seems to activate more PPARs to reduce inflammation. Just add the right dose—a pinch (⅛ of a teaspoon) several times a day if you want. Add any more, and your food will taste like mustard. A teaspoon of inexpensive mustard has about the right amount of turmeric—the less expensive mustards use turmeric to cover the lack of mustard seeds. But that turmeric makes them a benefit.

Jojoba Beans (They are really seeds): They've been shown to tune up the system in the ways we want, like increasing good cholesterol levels and raising leptin levels to curb hunger. The supplement jojoba extract (the supplement simmondsin is also made from jojoba) seems to work by stimulating CCK. The dose is about 2.5 grams to 5 grams for most people (50 milligrams per kilogram of weight).

The Main Ingredients

Though the effects are not completely proven, there's some evidence that the following substances and ingredients have a meaningful anti-inflammatory effect:

Substance	Found In
Isoflavones	Soybeans, all soy products
Lignans	Flaxseed, flaxseed oil, whole grains such as rye
Polyphenols	Tea, fruits, vegetables
Glucosinolates	Cruciferous vegetables such as broccoli and cauliflower, plus kale
Carnosol	Rosemary
Resveratrol	Red wine, grapes, red or purple grape juice, or knotweed plants
Cocoa	Dark chocolate
Quercetin	Cabbage, spinach, garlic

Drink Java. Coffee is Americans' largest source of antioxidants (aside from caffeine, which has its own antioxidant properties). It is chock-full (pun intended) of polyphenols and is a great low-calorie fluid when you have cravings. You can drink decaffeinated versions to avoid the side effects. The second-biggest source of antioxidants? Bananas, which have seven times less than coffee.

Go through the Process of Elimination. To change the way you feel, the way you process food, and the way you store fat is to get at the root of the system: You need to figure out what foods may be causing you GI trouble, no matter how subtle your symptoms may be. The best way to do that is through the food-elimination test. What you'll do is completely eliminate certain groups of foods for at least three days in a row. (Sometimes, the elimination of a food takes two or more weeks to show its benefits in how you feel.) During that time, take notes about all the different ways you feel: your energy levels, fatigue, and how often you go to the bathroom. Take notes when you eliminate foods and when you reintroduce them—that way you'll really notice what changes make you feel worse or better.

Here's the order we suggest: wheat products (including rye, barley, and oats; see our G-Free Plan), dairy products, refined carbohydrates (especially sugar), saturated and trans fats, and artificial colors (which are tough to get rid of because they're in everything). While the experiment will help you ID your personal digestive destructors, it has an added benefit: Eliminating a group of foods for several days at a time will help train your body to eat smaller portions all the time.

Get Moving after a Big Meal. If you've made a mistake and gorged on a tub's worth of food, make your body work in your favor. Stay awake for a few hours and take a thirty-minute walk to help your body with the breakdown of nutrients and so that it uses the food for energy, rather than storing it as fat. Once the calories are in your stomach, don't try to vomit; vomiting can damage your stomach, burn your esophagus, and even discolor your teeth if you do it enough. Also, don't eat sweets after gorging, because sweets will increase insulin and help deposit excess calories in your belly.

Pick Your Poison. High amounts of sucrose (sugar) cause inflammation; you can reduce the effect by using alternative sweeteners. Besides causing sudden spikes in blood sugar, foods with high sugar content have high calorie content, and if not burned off or used as fuel, those calories will be stored as fat. Though some sweeteners are low- or no-calorie, there is a downside: Sweeteners found in diet soft drinks, in diet foods, and on restaurant tables next to the sugar packets go unrecognized by the brain. They're essentially invisible to your brain's satiety centers, so it doesn't count them as real food and still desires to be fulfilled by calories from somewhere else. There's no clear-cut proof of the effects of these sweeteners—on either a health level or on a weight-loss level—but we do know one thing: Prehistoric man wasn't putting Splenda in his water. Artificial sweeteners, while lacking calories, may have side effects such as intestinal problems and headaches. If you're having a hard time losing weight or don't feel well, these are some of the first things to cut out, even though they can be an alternative to high-calorie sugars. There's no clear-cut data on which sweeteners work most effectively, but here's how we rate them:

Sweetener	The Scoop	Here's the Skinny
Sucralose (Splenda)	Discovered in 1976 but not introduced for wide-spread use for many years. More than 500 times sweeter than sucrose, stored in body fats, suitable for baking, and does not affect levels of blood sugar.	The research is least complete on this one, but go ahead and keep it in the cupboard. Its widespread use is too new for us to know any of the long-term effects, but it appears the most promising—and it's the best one to use for cooking.
Aspartame (NutraSweet)	Entered the market in 1981. Several studies have found that it has adverse health effects, but those studies were very limited.	It's come under a lot of scrutiny and has basically stood the test of time. But it's the sweetener that hangs around the longest in your body, and it cannot be heated—it turns into formaldehyde (which could help you save on funeral expenses). It's also rumored to limit the brain's ability to use certain vitamins, antioxidants, and the mineral magnesium.
Saccharin	Has been around since the early 1900s, and while some studies found a health risk, those studies have significant limitations.	It appears to be one of the safest sweeteners and the only one with real long-term data, even if some of the data is not positive. (If you consume more than eighty twelve-ounce diet sodas a day, you're at an increased risk of bladder cancer—good luck!)
Agave nectar	Is a hypersweet natural substance.	Try it. Though it's very high in calories, you need only a fraction of the amount of sugar needed to gain the same level of sweetness. You can order through www.veganessentials.com or www.blueagavenectar.com.
Stevia	Is a noncaloric natural herb. The taste isn't ideal, and stevia seems to lower sperm counts in some studies.	For the taste and the potential side effects, not our choice.

Chapter 5

Taking a Fat Chance

How Fat Ruins Your Health

Diet Myths

* Thin people are automatically healthier than fat people.
* A fat is a fat is a fat. All fat is equally damaging.
* Your ideal blood pressure is anything less than 140/90.

It doesn't matter whether you're just trying to shave a few inches from your waist or trying to morph your slushy belly into an ice-hard one, the fact remains: It's hard to forget about body fat. You see it when you get dressed, get washed, and get jiggy. You feel it when you sit down, when you walk up stairs, when you bend over to lick the last cake crumbs off the plate. And if you're a person who's struggled with weight for a lifetime, you likely stress about fat more than you stress about money, relationships, or anesthesia-free colonoscopies.

Fat is constantly right in our faces. And on our minds. And wrapped around our necks and arms. And hanging from our bellies, raining from our rears, and gyrating during twist contests. But you know what?

Oftentimes, we forget about fat. We eat a lot of food at one meal and go back to do it right again—because we don't see the health risks in the same way we see a slightly larger chin in the mirror. Now that our digestive journey is over, and you've learned how fat is stored, it's time to explore what that excess stored fat can do—to your heart, to your arteries, to your entire body.

Most of us assume that you have to be as skinny as a coaxial cable to be healthy, but the truth is that plenty of so-called thin **Myth Buster** people (especially over age seventy) are less fit and less healthy than so-called heavy people. **YOU-reka!** That's right: It's actually better to be fat and have few risk factors for bad health than it is to be thin and have a high number of health-related risk factors. Now, that's not to say we're ordering a round of fried pickles for everyone. When all else is equal, carrying extra fat will likely increase your risk of heart attacks, strokes, diabetes, and breast, prostate, and colon cancer. But our point is that we want you to stop thinking about pounds and pounds only; we'd rather you start thinking about the numbers that really matter—especially to your husbands, wives, children, parents, and friends. The real story of your body isn't measured by scales or wolf whistles. It's measured by your waist size—and what fat does inside your blood and arteries.

What Fat's Got to Do with It

Here's how many of us assess our health: If the pain's not severe enough to call the paramedics, then we tough it out, go on our way, and write off most of our general feel-bad symptoms to fatigue, stress, age, or the jug of vanilla fudge we downed during *CSI*. The problem with that approach? You're probably more in tune with the fall TV schedule than you are with your own body. Of course, if you're overweight, the extra fat is sure to manifest itself in some outward side effects like lack of energy or lack of self-esteem. But many of the risk factors associated with carrying too much fat don't have any outward symptoms at all—meaning that the only way to tell whether being overweight is threatening your life is by taking a microscope underneath the flub and chub and focusing on what's happening at your body's most core levels.

Sure, you know that fat lives on your hips, but it also lives in your blood. If you were to take a vial of blood and let it sit (we don't recommend doing this at home), you'd see a layer of clotty cream that would rise to the top of the vial, sort of like tiramisu. That's fat. How did it get there? (Half credit if your answer was tiramisu.) It's absorbed via your intestines. But the key player is the omentum. And why should we care about that organ that sounds like it's missing the letter *m*? Because the omentum can store fat that is quickly accessible to the liver (meaning it can cause lousy cholesterol and triglyceride levels to rise) and also sucks insulin out of circulation (making your blood sugar rise)—meaning that this cream-converted fat sets up shop in the omentum and puts your organs within very close striking distance of a hammer.

Myth Buster

See, fat is like real estate: it's all about location, location, location. We all have three kinds of fat: fat in our bloodstream (called triglycerides), subcutaneous fat (which lies just underneath the skin's surface), and that omentum fat. (The fourth fat, of course, is the fat in food). As you remember from the last chapter, the omentum is a fatty layer of tissue located inside the belly that hangs *underneath* the muscles in your stomach (it's why some men with beer guts have hard-as-keg bellies—their fat is underneath the muscle).

Because this omentum fat is so close to your solid organs, it's their best energy source. (Why go to the gas station on the other side of town when there's a station at the next corner?) Think of the omentum fat as the obnoxious eighteen-wheeler on a crowded highway—elbowing out the stomach, pushing away other organs, and claiming all the space for itself (see Figure 5.1).

What's most interesting—and encouraging—is that as soon as you make physiological changes to your omentum, your body starts seeing effects. That is, once your body senses it's losing that fat, then your body's blood-related numbers (cholesterol, blood pressure, blood sugar) start traveling in the healthy direction—within days, before you even notice any kind of physical sign of weight loss (especially when you consider that the size of your omentum is impossible to measure without a CT scan).

In addition, the fat released from the omentum travels to your liver rapidly and constantly as opposed to the more patient fat on your thighs. The processed material is then shipped to the arteries, where it is linked to health risks like high LDL (lousy) cholesterol. The other problem with omentum fat is that it secretes very little adiponectin, which is a stress- and inflammation-reducing chemical that's related to the hunger-controlling hormone leptin. When you have less fat, you secrete more adiponectin, which produces a product that reduces inflammation. But more important, higher levels of adiponectin are related to lower levels of fat. So the more omentum fat you have, the less fat-regulating adiponectin you'll produce. Those who have low levels of adiponectin have abdominal obesity, high blood pressure, high cholesterol, and other risk factors associated with coronary artery disease.

Those are the reasons why the fat in your thighs doesn't matter as much to your health as does omentum fat (even if it matters for your bikini pride), and

they help explain why omentum fat (or an "apple" body shape) is more harmful than subcutaneous fat (like thigh fat, which gives you a "pear" shape). Subcutaneous fat isn't supplying a feeding tube to the rest of your vital internal organs, and it's not messing up the levels of substances in your blood that are being supplied to your vital organs. And fat on your hips is actually a storage point for the good DHA omega-3 fat.

The closer your waist is to ideal, the healthier your arteries and your immune system will be. The healthier your arterial and immune systems, the longer—and better—you'll live. And the more energy you'll have every day.

Highways to Health

Before you know what's inside your arteries, you need to know how they're structured—so you can see what kind of damage they can sustain and what kind they can't. Made up of three layers, your arteries are the monorails of your body—they transport blood throughout your body and deliver nutrients to all of your organs (see Figure 5.2).

Inner layer: The innermost layer of your arteries (the intima) comes in contact with blood; it's slippery like Teflon so blood can easily flow through. This normally smooth layer helps protect the muscular middle layer (the media) and is the layer most susceptible to attacks from outside sources.

Middle layer: The middle layer of your arteries supports the entire arterial structure by working a little like a hand squeezing a hose or a boa constrictor squeezing a neck. When you're depressed or anxious, the layer can constrict, narrowing the amount of space where blood can flow through (the lumen). But it also has an

advantage; it can release tension by dilating (the hand releasing the hose) to pull the Teflon layer outward and open up *more* space in the part of the artery where blood flows—say, when you exercise. When that happens, it allows more red cells, oxygen, and other nutrients through. You feel more energy when that layer functions like it did when you were nine years old.

Outer layer: The outer layer (the adventitia) shields the artery from the rest of your body like sausage casing; it holds the artery together from the outside.

Under normal circumstances, the inner layer is lined with delicate cells, and blood runs freely. Think of the structure as a tile wall—it's a smooth wall made up of individual tiles connected together with little gaps throughout. In the tile wall, you have white gooey grout; in the artery, you have tight junctions holding the cells together.

Now, in your arteries, that wall will stay tight unless something comes along and starts chipping away at the junctions between those smooth cells. The most damaging tile buster—high blood pressure—is the arterial sledgehammer. But there is one other arterial sledgehammer, high levels of blood sugar, and plenty of other pickaxes can chip away at the arterial lining: cholesterol, nicotine, stress, anger, and about forty other smaller risk factors, primarily stemming from lifestyle choices you make. The effect? They chip away and cause little nicks in the intima of your arteries, and those injuries trigger the anatomical starter's pistol. As shown in Figure 5.3, the race to destroy—and repair—your arteries is on.

The Effects of Fat

For years, you've been used to looking down at a scale's needle to determine your health. Wrong needle, bucko. What you need: a needle in the hands of someone who can draw your blood. With results from a simple blood test, you'll find out what your current settings are and then be equipped with the data you need to take steps that will reset the settings to the factory originals.

Figure 5.3 **Clog Jam** continued.

Super HDL: The Future of Cholesterol Drugs

In a northern Italian village on Lake Garda, the villagers have low levels of HDL. Science would tell us that, without high levels of the protective cholesterol-carrying protein, they should all be dying of coronary artery disease. But they aren't. It turns out that these villagers have supercharged, Drano-like HDL (called apo-1a-Milano) that clears away the gunk from their arteries and allows blood to flow smoothly. This case study points to the next wave of cholesterol drugs: drugs that enhance HDL action to clear the bad LDL away, rather than those that work by lowering the LDL levels in the first place. This particular drug has proven difficult to make, but the principle remains: HDL is as good as sleep for your arteries.

Blood Pressure: These days, blood pressure machines are everywhere—at the pharmacy, in your gym, in mall kiosks. Even in Wal-Mart and McDonald's. That's good. Actually, it's great. (Get your BP, hold the fries.)

That's because you need to track your blood pressure—your most crucial vital sign—even more diligently than Anderson Cooper reacts to the news. High blood pressure still reigns as the leading cause of heart attack, stroke, heart failure, kidney failure, and impotence. While most of your other blood numbers reveal levels of substances inside your blood, your BP gauges how your blood travels through your body. Simply, blood pressure refers to the amount of force exerted by your blood on your arterial walls as it passes through. It's measured through the systolic pressure (the pressure being exerted when the heart contracts; the top number) and the diastolic pressure (the pressure on your arteries when your heart is at rest).

Now, if the force of that pumping required to push blood through is too great, it'll gouge holes between the tiles (cells) in the smooth inner lining of your arteries (see Figure 5.4), causing those nicks in the tile wall that trigger a chain reaction of grouting, then destructive inflammation and clotting (which we'll discuss in detail below). Think of it as the beating of a bongo. If you hit a bongo with your fingers, the drumhead will stay intact. But slug away with two baseball bats, and that bongo head will feel like a roach in an exterminator's crosshairs. Your goal: Treat your arterial walls with a nice steady rhythm—let your blood *tap tap tap* them; not *pound pound pound* them. (Blood pressure fluctuates throughout the day; the goal is to keep your total BP picture under control.)

Figure 5.4 **Pressure Situation** With hypertension, the arteries squeeze down so tightly that the heart struggles to keep the blood moving forward. To compensate, the heart gets too thick, like a muscle-bound weight lifter. It becomes so stiff that it loses flexibility and can't relax. The arteries have become so stiff that blood has trouble traveling through the arteries, and the resulting high blood pressure damages the arteries, gouging holes between the tiles (cells). The repair of these holes with LDL cholesterol further stiffens the walls, forcing blood pressure higher and continuing the lethal (but silent until the end) cycle.

Certainly, many factors can make your blood pressure soar higher than an Albert Pujols home run (stress, high levels of the mineral sodium, lack of the mineral calcium or potassium from not enough fruits and vegetables, lack of physical activity). But it's also clear that being overweight leads directly to high blood pressure. This happens in part when the kidneys, squashed by fat, feign death unless they are fed with a higher blood pressure. (Your kidneys are the organ primarily responsible for regulating blood pressure.)

Luckily, you can reduce your blood pressure quickly and dramatically by addressing your waist issues. Losing 10 percent of the weight you've gained since you were eighteen (that's only four pounds if you've gained forty) can result in a decrease of 7 mmHg (stands for millimeters of mercury to measure the partial pressure of a gas) from your systolic number and 4 mmHg from your diastolic one. The message is clear: Drop your waist and you'll drop your BP.

Cholesterol: Hear the word "cholesterol" and you're likely to think of eggs, heart attacks, and a mandate from your doctor. But cholesterol is part of your body's arterial repair kit; it's designed to help you, though it doesn't always happen that way.

Let's go back to those nicks in your arterial wall. Whether it's BP, nicotine, or too much sugar in your blood that damage the wall, your body gets angrier than a cinched-up bull—because it doesn't want the middle lining of the artery exposed to blood. So your body hires a handyman to patch up your nicks with grout, to cover the wounds in the inner lining.

What's that grout? Cholesterol, but not just any ol' cholesterol.

Your handyman—let's call him Lester—carries two things: a bucket of grout and a spatula. The grout can come in the form of lousy cholesterol, which is carried by low-density lipoprotein (LDL). It's big and puffy, and prone to breaking up and scattering bits of cholesterol when it hits the walls of the artery. When your LDL levels are too high to begin with (maybe from your diet or from your heredity), and then you nick the inner lining of one of your arteries, Lester goes crazy and slaps on more and more and more grout. He starts covering up the damage with the bad cholesterol—loads and loads of bad cholesterol.

But look inside Lester's tool belt. He's got a spatula that takes premium-grade grout in the form of cholesterol carried on high-density lipoprotein (it's the healthy HDL cholesterol). Compact and powerful, the spatula works with this slick stuff to take the extra gunk away.

Now, if you have too much of that LDL grout (this can be familial but is primarily a result of eating the wrong kinds of foods—simple sugars and trans and saturated fats—and especially *too much* food) and not enough premium-version HDL grout (from not eating enough of the right kinds of foods and omega-3 and omega-9 fats, not getting enough physical activity, or not having enough female hormones—yes, even men have them), it can lead to a chain of events that has potentially heart-stopping outcomes. We'll call it fat's domino effect.

Domino 1: Having too much bad cholesterol not only means you'll have too much junk (plaque) in your arteries. It also means that LDL cholesterol will get into the middle layer of your artery. That cholesterol in the middle layer acts like a drunk fan with courtside seats, making the environment much more hostile than it's used to being. The presence of LDL cholesterol in that middle layer stimulates the immune system to attract white-cell protectors to try to smooth out and calm down the rotten cholesterol.

Domino 2: Those white blood cells, in turn, spill some of their toxic contents that normally attack infections—and that causes generalized inflammation.

Domino 3: The toxic contents and cholesterol are soaked up by scavenger cells, building up blister-sized spaces in the walls of your arteries. They're called foam cells—and they increase the size of the plaque, or grout, even more to make the artery surface rougher.

Domino 4: Sensing something's wrong, your body responds with more inflammation, creating bulges and potholes in the wall, often in the area of weakness, where the initial nick was and a scar was trying to form over the dangerous plaque. If that plaque ruptures into the middle of your blood vessel, the next domino falls.

Domino 5: These rough patches in the wall then attract sticky blood platelets to form clots in your arteries. Normally, platelets are good (they help form scabs to heal wounds). But when they hit that rough patch in your arterial wall, they grab the lining and form a big clot on top of irritated, inflamed plaque. And this brings in more clotting proteins to the area that act to cement the platelets in place.

Domino 6: All of this gunk piles up faster and faster, and the inside of the arteries becomes so inflamed that the platelets and clots fill the entire artery. **YOU-reka!** This ruptured plaque process takes minutes rather than decades, so you can influence its likelihood today by making the right choices about food today.

Domino 7: The blood can't get through the artery, and nourishment to the heart is shut off.

Game Over: The chain reaction triggers a heart attack (or, depending where the process happens, causes a stroke, memory loss, impotence, wrinkled skin, or any number of health problems that happen when blood flow malfunctions).

As you can see, it's not the cholesterol by itself that's so bad; it's having high enough levels of healthy and low enough lousy cholesterol to thwart the process before it even begins. And, most important, it's doing things like normalizing your blood pressure and blood sugar to help decrease the chance of developing nicks in the first place.

While genetics dictates some of your cholesterol level, your physical activity levels and poor foods choices—trans and saturated fats, simple sugar, syrups, non-100 percent whole grains, and too many calories—really dictate whether Lester carries the right amount and kind of grout or moves the spatula fast enough to make for a nice, clean wall.

Blood Sugar: Yep, we know how it is. You don't have diabetes, so you're going to blow off thinking about blood sugar faster than a flight attendant blows off a flirty coach passenger. And that would be a mistake. Blood sugar is another substance that can nick your arteries if levels are too high. You may think your level is normal, but most blood sugar levels are recorded when you've fasted. Having "normal" levels for fasting (under 100 milligrams per deciliter, abbreviated 100 mg/dl) and for after meals (under 125 mg/dl) is important. Why? Because there's a good chance that even with normal blood sugar levels, your blood sugar may rise significantly throughout the day after you eat. Studies show that men with a waist of 40 inches or more have twelve times the risk of getting diabetes compared with men with a waist smaller than 35 inches. For women, having a 37-inch waist is that much riskier than having a 32½-incher. (The most sensitive way to diagnose diabetes is to measure the blood sugar fasting, and again two hours after taking 75 grams of sugar—to see how your body can deal with the sugar.)

Many people think that diabetes is a purely genetic disease, and of course it sure would be nice to blame Aunt Mabel for the medical condition, but it doesn't quite work that way. For type 2 diabetes (type 1 is the juvenile form), your environment (that is, your lifestyle, your behaviors, your macaroons) is a much more dominant trait than genetics. You turn those genes either up or down. Your genes are just protein factories, whether they are on a little (or not on) or producing a lot of proteins seems to be governed by what you feed them—that is, by the environment you provide them. And food is not "let's make a deal": *I'll have that sugared candy tonight and walk tomorrow.* It's not going to work, as what you feed your genes turns them up or down for several days to weeks. Just as in a factory, it takes some time to gear up to full production or wind down to little production.

Yes, type 2 diabetes is a genetic disease. But whether you turn those genes on or off is your choice. That is, if you are a twin and have an identical twin who gets type 2 diabetes, you have the genetics for it, but you don't have to express those genes. And it's a tough disease too: Diabetes ages you one and a half years for every year you live. For example, if you get it at age thirty and live to sixty, you're not really sixty; you have the energy and disability risks of a seventy-five-year-old.

Here's how it works (see Figure 5.5): Insulin in your blood normally takes sugar and puts it into the cells, but in people with type 2 diabetes, the transfer of sugar into your muscle and fat cells is inhibited. While nice in coffee, that sugar in your

blood chips away at your arterial wall by weakening the junctions between cells that form the surface lining of your arteries. Ultimately it allows holes to form in these junctions. By causing your insulin levels to go haywire and making proteins in your body less effective, sugar really behaves like nutritional cocaine.

Omentum fat (belly fat) contributes to type 2 diabetes by making it difficult to get glucose inside the cell and let insulin do what it does best: deliver glucose. Simply being overweight, especially having a waist greater than 37 inches (85 centimeters) for women and 40 inches (100 centimeters) for men, makes your body less sensitive to insulin; it acts directly and turns on genes that produce proteins that make the insulin receptors on the cells less likely to allow insulin to transmit the message enabling glucose transport into the cells, leaving the glucose to float around in your blood. That omentum fat is also selfish; it uses up the insulin so it can't do its job (one study shows omentum fat sucks up a quarter of the insulin that passes through the blood supply). By the way, waist size that affects health is absolute (37 inches or greater for women and over 40 inches for men) independent of height. If it makes you feel better, divide your height in inches by two. If your waist measurement is greater than that, you're getting into the aging, no-energy zone.

So your blood sugar level remains high because the sugar isn't being admitted to your cells readily and thus isn't broken down properly, meaning that sugar will hang out in your blood like a truant skipping school and causing mischief.

So what? Well, having too much sugar in your blood is like having too much rain in a small pond—the flooding can cause damage for everything around it. Too much blood sugar can:

❖ Weaken the junctions between those smooth endothelial cells lining your arteries, making the Teflon-like lining more vulnerable to nicks.

- Increase the power of the hammer, to cause greater high blood pressure effect. (Sugar turns the hammer into a sledgehammer.)
- Cause your white blood cells to stop fighting infections, thus weakening your immune system.
- Trigger a chemical process in your red blood cells, which transport oxygen in your bloodstream, that causes the cells to want to hold on to oxygen more tightly. That keeps oxygen from getting to your tissues. When that happens, the glucose, like a lost puppy, attaches to whatever it can find—most likely, proteins in your blood and tissues. These proteins deposit in tissues, leading to the development of cataracts, joint abnormalities, and lung problems.
- Get into your nerves and cause a reaction that makes your nerves swell, become compressed, and lose their ability to function—usually in the parts of your body farthest from your brain: your hands and feet.
- Flip off a switch in your small blood vessels. Normally your body automatically regulates the flow of nutrients into your small blood vessels. They sort of work on backup (like a generator for when the power goes out), so they can function even when your big vessels might be experiencing problems. But high levels of glucose turn off that automatic regulation—and let a little high blood pressure make more of those nicks and tears in the junctions between cells in your smaller blood vessels. This is like asking someone to use a sledgehammer to do the job of a jeweler's tool; it magnifies that effect and magnifies the size of the nick.

> **FACTOID**
>
> Monosodium glutamate (MSG), the additive found in many restaurant and supermarket Chinese foods (not real Chinese foods), may play a role in messing up the body's metabolic systems. A taste enhancer, MSG is used to overstimulate (some say poison) the glutamine receptors of the brain, so we sense salt and sweets more (but not bitter and sour tastes, interestingly). The downside? That may cause us to eat more and to have higher insulin levels.

But here's the thing. You can control your genes if you want to. To keep blood sugar levels down, you should avoid foods with simple sugar (including syrups) and lousy aging fats (trans and saturated fats). And about 1,000 calories' worth of activity a week—about thirty minutes of walking a day and twenty minutes of the YOU Workout three days a week—causes your muscles to be so much more sensitive to insulin, which allows sugar to do its duty inside your cells, rather than cause havoc in your bloodstream. A little physical activity goes a long way.

Arterial Inflammation: When we think of our arteries and what can damage them, we tend to think of that clog: the hunk of junk that stops the flow of blood like a lemon seed in a straw. If there's a roadblock in the way, then there's no way for traffic to move through. But that's only one mechanism for closing off blood flow. The other occurs through the process of inflammation. Typically, inflammation in our bodies makes us think of things that swell *out*—like a sprained ankle, or swollen gums, or the shiner from the 2 a.m. bar brawl. But when it comes to arterial inflammation, you have to think about swelling out and *in.* In response to all that clotting action we talked about with LDL cholesterol, inflammation occurs in the middle layer of your arteries. As the middle layer swells, it pushes into the inner layer because the outer sausage layer doesn't give easily or push out. Thus it pushes into the inner layer, reducing the size of the hole that blood can travel through (like drinking with a thinner straw).

One of the ways we determine potential cardiovascular risks is by measuring chemicals in the blood that signal inflammation. C-reactive protein (CRP) is one such chemical; elevated CRP indicates an inflammatory reaction somewhere in your body, from a sinus infection to gum inflammation. If it's high, your risk of heart disease is greater, because any significant inflammation in your body increases inflammation in your blood vessels. It's one of the reasons heart attacks and strokes are more common during flu season. The flu causes inflammation, which in turn causes plaques to rupture. Flu shots cause a little inflammation like exercise, with greater short- and long-term benefits than getting the flu.

Fat Chance: The Other Major Risks

We're not here to lecture you and pummel you with brochurelike statistics about health risks. But to put fat in perspective, remember that it's an all-body risk factor—with implications everywhere. Even if your numbers in some health categories are as perfect as a gold-medal triple toe loop, you're not risk-free. Being overweight or obese leads to the following:

Higher Risk of Cancer: The inflammation resulting from omentum fat also causes dysfunction in the system that protects you from cancer. In fact, there's a direct correlation between waist size and an increased risk of hormonally sensitive tumors, such as breast cancer in women and prostate cancer in men. Fat contains an enzyme, aromatase, which converts adrenal hormones into a long-acting kind of estrogen, which can cause increased breast cancer risk in women and infertility in men.

Higher Risk of Sleep Apnea: Fat around your waist correlates with a thick neck, and that can obstruct your breathing (you're at higher risk if your neck size is more than seventeen inches). In its benign form—snoring—you can still move air through your throat, but generate a kazoo sound that violates OSHA requirements and can cause permanent hearing loss and marital strife. In some cases, that obstruction worsens, until eventually no air can pass into the lungs for up to ten seconds at a time (see Figure 5.6). Fortunately, the body instinctively awakens prior to suffocation. As you get older, the tissue in your throat softens, and the area around your tonsils attracts fat. When you're asleep, and your muscles fully relax, the tissue collapses, so there's even less room in the back of your throat.

Sleep apnea makes you miss out on deep, restorative REM sleep. This leads to frequent awakenings at night (though your spouse may know it, you'll probably never feel yourself waking), lack of sleep, and daytime drowsiness. You're more likely to develop nick-causing high blood pressure (caused when your lungs hang on to carbon dioxide when you stop breathing) and, the bitter irony, you're more

Waist Not, Want Not

Everybody knows caloric cutback will significantly lower your risk of obesity-related problems such as heart disease. But new evidence suggests that the health benefits of seriously healthy eating may extend well beyond the usual suspect diseases. It looks as though lean living can lower your risk for all chronic diseases—from Alzheimer's to cancer—and as a result add years to your life, and life to your years.

How? Scientists speculate that calorie restriction causes certain genes to switch on and off. A gene manages the body much as you manage your household, but it's concerned with energy more than dollars. So a gene makes decisions based on how much energy it takes to reproduce (as when a mom is breast-feeding), to maintain the body (as when healing wounds or mending broken bones), and to grow (in height and weight). Using energy for one area limits the resources available for another. So if the gene is spending all its time repairing a broken body part or dealing with your continuing growth around the middle, it has fewer resources available to fight infection, keep the immune system strong, and keep all systems humming along nicely.

What do you think happens when the reverse is true? Bingo. If your body is in calorie restriction, it's better able to allocate its resources to many other systems in the body. The result of a leaner life is a longer one too.

likely to get fatter because of it. That's because sleep apnea is like a series of rear-end collisions—one accident after another. The lack of sleep makes you tired. You feel like you need more energy. You eat foods that give you quick energy but also have high sugar and fat. You get fatter. You continue to have sleep apnea. And the cycle continues. (As an incentive to embrace a good eating plan, most people will lose fat first in their faces and throats; so with a waist reduction of a few inches you'll probably be able to prevent or reduce these sleep problems by 30 percent early in your program.) Big waists also more than double the risk of asthma.

Higher Risk of Joint Problems: While strong, your joints are like parents trying to squash constant whining; they can take only so much before they break down. Your knees are some of the most powerful joints in your body because you use them to both push off and absorb force. But they're also prone to wear and tear if they have to carry a heavier load (that is, more fat in your body) than they're designed to. When you gain ten pounds of body weight, it feels more like a thirty-pound weight to your knees while you're walking. When you walk upstairs, the ten pounds of fat feel like seventy pounds to your knee joint. That extra weight makes you more vulnerable to developing joint-deteriorating conditions like osteoarthritis, which occurs when your joints get nicks in their smooth cartilage from bearing a load they're not designed to carry.

Fat Changes Your Genes: Most of us think we're condemned to obesity, or cancer, or heart disease because of our genes. Actually, it's the other way around: Your genes are the victim of your choices. Gather too much waist and you turn off good genes that prevent insulin resistance and diabetes, that work against heart and vascular disease (yes, wrinkling and impotence too), and that make cancer less likely. But lose a little waist and you gain a lot. We now have clues that a common pathway for these diseases is turning on the inflammatory-promoting gene DAF-2 and turning off DAF-16. DAF-16, nicknamed Sweet 16 because when you turn it on your outsides and insides look like you're sixteen, is turned on by the stuff in red wine or by calorie restriction. (Note: That's not an excuse to drink the wine; the ingredients are the key—and you'd need far too much wine to actually make a difference.) So you do get to control the genes of aging by having a thin waist or as we say, may you turn on Sweet 16.

When you reduce your omentum fat and your waist size, you'll automatically reduce your risk in so many areas of your health. Even better, you'll have the potential to see dramatic reductions in risk factors. **YOU-reka!** When overweight people (with an average weight of 225 pounds) lose about 7.5 percent of their body weight (about 17 pounds or 4 inches of waist size), they improve their HDL and LDL cholesterol levels, BP, and blood sugar numbers by—get this—20 percent. That's nearly three times the benefit compared with percentage weight loss. Take the following steps to help you get there in terms of both inches and risk factors.

YOU TIPS!

Know Your Fats. Fat in foods, like bosses, comes in two broad categories: those that are good for your well-being and those that want you to suffer. The strongest influence you can have on your levels of cholesterol (not to mention your waist size) is by watching what fats you're eating and what fats you're banishing from your life and your gut. Above all, you want to avoid saturated fats; a serving size should have no more than 4 grams of those villains combined (and no trans fats). They're the foods most associated with long-term weight gain and clogging your arteries. Essentially, bad fats are ones that are solid at room temperature: animal fat, butter, stick margarine, lard. Trans fat contains cross-linked hydrogen bonds, which make it stable for long periods of time at room temperature. Eating trans fat leads to abnormalities in cholesterol (decreasing your good and increasing your bad), increases inflammation, and damages your arterial cells, which makes you more prone to clotting. (By the way, trans fat was originally designed for candle wax, but the market died with the advent of electricity.) The value of trans fats is that they have a long shelf life (they are poison to insects—so insects smell them and avoid them, promoting long shelf life; our human smellers aren't that good). Food manufacturers would love to make foods with healthy fats if they could have the one-year shelf life of the unhealthy fats. The good fats, by contrast, are liquid at room temperature but get thick when cold, like olive oil. They help raise your HDL levels to clear away the guck. Far more important than the calories of fat are what fatty acids can do to your cell functions, and how they influence arterial function and inflammation.

Super (Youthful) Fats: Facilitate Spatula Action	Stupid (Aging) Fats: Cause the Clogs, Clump Up the Spatula
Monounsaturated Fats. They come in three forms: omega-3, omega-6, and omega-9 fatty acids, in the form of fish (3s) and nut (3s and 6s) and olive oils (omega-9). The omega-3s improve arterial and brain function. They're found in canola oil, fish oils, flaxseeds, avocados, and nuts (especially walnuts). They've also been shown to reduce blood pressure and lipid levels when used in place of carbohydrates. **Bottom line:** Make about 30 percent to 40 percent of your fats the monounsaturated variety.	**Trans Fat.** This is the fat that contains hydrogenated vegetable oil. It's the worst kind of fat and will stunt weight-loss efforts. Trans fatty acids are in all kinds of food—especially when long shelf life is important—from buttered popcorn and cookies to chips and margarine. **Bottom line:** Say no. Stay away from them the way you'd avoid highways on the day before Thanksgiving. Clog city. (continued)

Super (Youthful) Fats: Facilitate Spatula Action	Stupid (Aging) Fats: Cause the Clogs, Clump Up the Spatula
Polyunsaturated Fats. These are like monounsaturated except that they contain more than one unsaturated bond. They are usually present in vegetable oils and sesame oils. They may improve arterial and brain function, and will help keep up your satiety levels. **Bottom line:** Make 20 percent to 60 percent of your fats polyunsaturated.	**Saturated Fats.** Found in meats and dairy products, these fats will make you gain weight and clog your arteries. **Bottom line:** Limit saturated fat to lean sources like very lean cuts of beef and low-fat dairy products. Aim for less than 4 grams of saturated fat per meal. Less than 20 grams, or less than 30 percent of your daily allotment, should be from saturated and/or trans fats combined.

Note: The best oil to have in your home is extra-virgin olive oil or organic (or cold-press) canola oil. For cooking, you can also use sesame or peanut oil. That's because their smoking point—that is, the temperature at which the fat burns—is very high. Cook beyond it, and you'll end up with a burned, charcoal flavor. Once heated, oils can become rancid and also can generate toxic chemicals, so you lose the major benefit of eating these usually healthy foods. Also, it's best to cook the food, rather than the oil. So don't heat the oil directly in the pan; instead, roll your food in the oil first and then heat the food and the oil together so the oil doesn't become overheated.

Here are smoke points for some commonly used healthy oils:

Unrefined canola oil: 225°

Unrefined sunflower oil: 225°

Extra-virgin olive oil: 320°

Virgin olive oil: 420°

Sesame oil: 410°

Grape-seed oil: 420°

Refined peanut oil: 450°

Semirefined sesame oil: 450°

Clear It All Up. More and more evidence is showing that clog-free living is correlated with raising your amount of active HDL to thwart the clot-triggering process. By raising your active HDL, you increase the amount of healthy cholesterol that's available to clear away the lousy cholesterol. Things that have been shown to effectively raise HDL levels include:

❖ Consuming healthy fats found in olive oil, fish, avocados, and walnuts.

❖ Walking or doing any physical activity for at least thirty minutes a day—no excuses.

❖ Taking niacin. Take 100 milligrams four times a day. Regular (and OTC) niacin is much cheaper than prescription niacin, and there seems to be a beneficial effect of extended-release doses. Sometimes higher doses are needed, in which case your doctor needs to peek at your liver function to ensure that you avoid the uncommon toxicity. To reduce flushing (feeling hot and light-headed), take an aspirin a half hour ahead of time and take the niacin as you go to bed. Do not increase the dose above this level without talking to your doctor, and check with your doctor before using niacin at any dose if you have a history of liver problems. By the way, if you take large doses of niacin (without aspirin an hour beforehand) and do not flush, you are not receiving biologically active niacin.

❖ Taking vitamin B5 (pantothenic acid). We recommend a dose of 300 milligrams a day to decrease LDL and raise HDL with no side effects yet known.

❖ Having one drink of alcohol every night. You should not be drinking just to get your HDL up, but if you do drink alcohol, stick to one drink, and you may see some small beneficial effects.

❖ Substituting protein or monounsaturated fat in place of carbs. Recent research suggests that this can help reduce BP and modify lipid levels.

Just Say Yes to This Drug. If there were one magic pill for fighting fat and saving lives, the pharmaceutical industry would send everyone from scale makers to diet-book authors into bankruptcy. There's no pill that will do it all. (At least not yet. More on drug solutions in the appendix.) But that doesn't mean you can't use drugs to improve your health and reduce your cardiovascular risk factors. Our recommendation—and the closest thing to a pill with mystical powers—comes in the form of two baby aspirin (162 milligrams total) a day. You need two rather than one, since many folks, with or without excess fat, are resistant to the lower dose. (There is no measurable increased risk of stomach problems in studies with this small increase in doses from 81 milligrams to 162 milligrams, and the reduction in heart attacks or ischemic strokes goes from around 13 percent to around 36 percent.) Aspirin makes platelets less sticky and decreases inflammation that occurs to narrow the space where blood flows through your arteries. And it's been shown to reduce arterial aging and immune system aging, and that means decreasing your risk of everything from heart attacks, strokes, and impotence to colon, rectal, and esophageal cancers, and maybe even breast and prostate cancers. To reduce the gastric side effects, drink a half glass of warm water before and after taking the pill. (See your doc if you have any history of serious bleeding, are taking blood thinners, do extreme sports, or have your own or a family history of bruising, bleeding, or aneurysms.)

Have Regular Readings. Not just with your book club or by an astrologer. These regular readings are about tracking your health numbers. Instead of measuring your success through the scale, the real measurement—and test—of your success is seeing whether you are alive and vibrant, and if so, reduced your cardiovascular risk, as evidenced in the following test readings:

Myth Buster

Blood Pressure: Optimum level is 115/76. Blood pressure readings can be variable, so have your BP taken in the morning, during the day, and at night, as part of your normal activities (except for thirty minutes after exercise, when it will naturally be higher). Take the average of three readings to come up with your base number. After that, take readings every month to help you monitor your progress. (If your BP is high, then you can track it daily.)

Lipid Profile Blood Test: Have one now to establish your baseline measurement, then have your blood analyzed every other year so that you and your doctor can watch changes and make appropriate adjustments to your eating and/or drug plan.

HDL (healthy) cholesterol: You're at low risk if your HDL is greater than 50 mg/dl. But like basketball players, the higher the better. In fact, if your HDL is over 100 mg/dl (active, not fake HDL), the chances of having a heart attack or stroke related to lack of blood flow are smaller than the chance that a Hollywood celeb could walk through Boise unnoticed. (Except in some extremely rare cases where HDL malfunctions inside the body, there has never been a heart attack or stroke due to lack of blood flow reported in the entire medical literature in a person with a functional HDL over 100).

LDL (lousy) cholesterol: You're at a low risk if your LDL is less than 100 mg/dl. By the way, research shows that for all women, and for men over sixty-five years old, the LDL number isn't nearly as important as the HDL. So women and men over sixty-five don't need to obsess too much over LDL levels unless their HDL levels are too low.

Fasting blood sugar: Below 100 mg/dl.

C-reactive protein: Below 1 mg/dl.

Get a Lift. Muscle isn't just for football players, bouncers, and souped-up cars. Everyone benefits from adding some muscle to his or her body; in fact, adding some muscle will help lower your levels of blood sugar. The more muscle you have, the more you increase insulin receptivity—that is, the process by which insulin transports glucose into your cells. If you gain muscle and lose weight, you change the chemistry of your cell membranes so that you absorb more glucose throughout your body rather than having it stay in your blood. You add muscle by doing strength exercises (more coming up in the YOU Workout).

Stop Freebasing Sugar. One thing that causes blood sugar to spike is, uh, sugar. That is, straight, pure sugar—not eaten with any other substances like fat or protein around it. Though we recommend eating as few simple sugars as possible, if you do eat them, you should always be sure not to eat that candy bar or cookie dough by itself. Have a handful of nuts or some olive oil with 100 percent whole grain bread first; that slows your stomach from emptying and will keep sugar levels from creating a pyrotechnical effect in your blood.

Go Chrome. Chromium, a mineral found in a variety of foods (especially mushrooms), seems to help control blood sugar. Taking 200 micrograms a day of the supplement chromium picolinate can help aid the uptake of insulin, to help your cells use blood sugar for fuel. Though the studies aren't definitive at this point, many recommend the supplement for waist—and blood sugar—control. Chromium increases your cells' sensitivity to insulin and is depleted by refined sugars, white flour, and lack of exercise. One study showed users lost four pounds over ten weeks compared with no pounds in a control group. You should take it with magnesium, which reduces low-grade inflammation that can be associated with insulin resistance. A dose of 600 micrograms of chromium has been shown to be effective for those with type 2 diabetes, but for others, stick to the recommended dose of 200 micrograms. Just because a little is good doesn't mean that taking a lot more is better. Taking too much chromium can hurt your kidneys. Don't take it at all if you are even remotely going to be pregnant.

Become Sensitive. Here's a tantalizing observation: Cinnamon (with an *m,* not a *b*) seems to have an insulinlike effect, enhancing the satiety center in your brain while also reducing blood sugar and cholesterol levels. Just a half teaspoon a day can have some effect; feel free to enjoy more. Sprinkle it in cereal or on toast, or add it to a smoothie.

Get in the Zone. Studies show that meditation has a statistically significant reduction of risk factors for coronary heart disease, such as blood pressure and insulin resistance. Find a quiet room, take a few minutes, close your eyes, and focus on one healthy word or phrase, like "om" (or "omega-3 fatty acids").

Hey There, Good Looking, Can I Get Your Number?

In most cases, like a bike fall or a noodle-size hangnail, seeing your blood is not a good thing. But for our purposes, you need to look deep inside your blood to get an assessment of the effect of the extra weight you're carrying. That's where you'll find all the numbers that indicate the risks that may be associated with carrying extra weight. If you don't know these numbers, see your doctor for your latest blood results or request a blood test from your primary-care physician.

Blood Pressure: _____

(Measures the force of blood being pumped through your arteries. Ideal is 115/76)

HDL Cholesterol: _____

(Measures the amount of good clog-clearing cholesterol in your blood. Greater than 40 mg/dl is acceptable. And you've hit the lottery if you're above 60 mg/dl.)

Triglycerides: _____

(Measures the fat in your blood. Don't go over 100 mg/dl on this one.)

Hemoglobin A/C: _____%

(Measures the long-term glucose load on your body. Desirable is as much below 5.6 as you can go.)

LDL Cholesterol: _____

(Measures the amount of bad clog-forming cholesterol in your blood. Ideal is less than 70 mg/dl if you have any risk factors of heart disease, or 100 mg/dl if you are otherwise healthy as a horse and your ancestors never suffered heart disease.)

C-Reactive Protein: _____

(Measures levels of inflammation in blood vessels, a marker for many types of diseases. Ideal in most labs is less than 1 mg/dl.)

Chapter 6

Metabolic Motors

Your Body's Hormonal Fat Burners

Diet Myths

- ❖ It's your habits that are entirely to blame for fatness.
- ❖ Your body burns most of its calories through activity.
- ❖ You can't adjust your "slow metabolism."

Bad genes aren't something that you wore in high school. They're what can make you have a propensity for heart disease, baldness, mental problems, and putting on weight. Though diet and physical activity play the lead roles in losing fat and maintaining a healthy weight, your genes are part of the supporting cast. It is possible to eat like a guppy but grow bigger than a beluga. Simply, some people can have a bad genetic response to a good diet (that is, they put on weight), while other people (the scoundrels!) can have a good genetic response to a bad diet.

Myth Buster How do we know there's a genetic component to obesity? For one, studies of twins raised apart from each other show it. Two people with the same genes raised in different lifestyles and on different diets show about 30 percent of the same propensities for gaining weight. But genes don't just dictate how you metabolize fat—that is, whether you come from a "big-boned" family or one that could fit through slats in air vents. Genes help dictate many things regarding why you put on fat—like cravings for certain foods or the way you cope when you're stressed. And family ties also govern whether or not the homemade sauce has butter or olive oil.

Nevertheless, what we're trying to do is shrink the size of your jeans by shrinking the effect of some of your genes. While you have genetic influences that steer you toward a particular body type and behaviors, those dispositions and unhealthy decisions can be neutralized and minimized by eating the right foods, rebooting your body, and, in effect, changing which of your genes are turned on and which are turned off. That's right; your choices turn on or turn off specific genes you have. For example, the flavonoids (antioxidants, but they may work in other ways) in grape skins turn off the gene that makes an inflammatory protein that ages your arteries.

Now that we've discussed why you eat, how your food moves, and the effects of storing excess fat, you need to know how your body burns fat. In this chapter, we'll discuss the body's natural ways of doing so—ways determined by your genes—and in the next chapter we'll discuss ways you can add horsepower to your natural fat-burning engines.

Of course, the place to start is with your metabolism, your body's thermostat—the rate at which you burn off extra fat (metabolism literally means "change").

Most of the 1 million calories you consume every year are burned without your ever thinking anything of it. It takes energy for you to breathe, think, and sleep, and for all of your organs to function. The energy you consume and store is used primarily to power your anatomical systems and structures. **YOU-reka!** Only 15 percent to 30 percent of your calories are burned through intentional physical activity such as exercise, walking, or doing the wumba wumba on your anniversary. So while you may think that spinning class or Bikram yoga is the primary pathway to frying fat, physical activity is only a fraction of it. You burn most of your calories by keeping your heart pumping, your brain remembering your spouse's birthday, and your liver disposing of last night's vodka concoction.

Now, that doesn't mean there aren't many outside influences that slow down and speed up your burn rate. Any movement speeds metabolism, including fidgeting (called nonexercise activity thermogenesis in scientific lingo, or NEAT for short). Every increase in body temperature of one degree increases your metabolic rate by 14 percent (eating protein appears to do the same thing naturally, by the way). When you sleep, your metabolic rate decreases by 10 percent. **YOU-reka!** When you starve yourself for more than twelve hours, your metabolic rate actually goes down by 40 percent. When you skip meals, your body senses a dietary disaster and quickly goes into storage mode rather than burning mode. That's the primary reason why deprivation diets don't work. Your body panics about going into a famine, so it slows metabolism into emergency-storing mode rather than a steady state of burning. Breakfast eaters are on average thinner than those who skip breakfast. One reason is that breakfast eaters keep their metabolism genes turned on; this means that calories are more likely to be burned off before they can turn into fat.

In our battle to reduce our waistlines, we have several fearsome adversaries. And some of the greatest foes we will meet on the battlefield are our hormones. Sure, we all know that raging hormones can make a teenage boy become sex obsessed or give a menopausal woman hot flashes so bad she feels as though she's in Death Valley in August. But you may not know that your hormones have a lot to do with whether or not you're going to look good in a Speedo.

Is Something Secretly Making You Fat?

Before you hit yourself over the head with a stick of salami for lacking the willpower to resist aforementioned salami, or if you can't figure out why you eat less than all your friends but still gain weight, consider that your hormones may be influencing your body more than you think. Glands, which make up your *endocrine system* and produce your hormones, are responsible for the genetic conditions that could be influencing your metabolism and your weight. The primary metabolic glands are:

Thyroid gland: Thyroid hormone influences how quickly or slowly you burn energy. Too much hormone forces the body to waste energy too quickly (in extreme cases, it actually causes your heart muscle to become hypermetabolic and weaken). But if you don't produce enough, you develop a condition called hypothyroidism, in which your metabolic rate turtles way down. The best way to check levels of thyroid hormone? A simple blood test. You have elevated thyroid-stimulating hormone (TSH) if it's above 5 IU/liter. This means your body is desperately trying to build up your body's circulating free thyroid hormone levels but is failing. TSH is released from your pituitary gland and tells your thyroid to produce two hormones that help control metabolism. Though decreased thyroid levels are rarely the sole cause of being overweight, abnormal levels may indicate that you should see your doctor or an endocrinologist about whether you need to supplement your thyroid function in the form of a thyroid pill to boost your metabolism. (Symptoms of hyperthyroidism include anxiety, heart palpitations,

During the Muslim holiday of Ramadan, people eat only after sunset, so they consume all their calories at night. Should they lose weight? Anecdotal evidence, gathered by doctors watching residents working all-night shifts, indicates that people who eat all their 2,000 daily calories in one meal gain more weight than those who space those calories over three meals. Why? Because the one-timers are kicking in their starvation mode, making their bodies want to store fat rather than burn it.

sleeplessness, and fast-growing hair and nails. For hypothyroidism, you may be lethargic, gain weight, have a reduced appetite, or have brittle nails.)

Adrenal glands: Adrenal glands sit like a dunce's cap on the kidneys, but they are controlled by corticotrophin-releasing hormone (CRH), which is made by the hypothalamus. This valuable relationship enables the adrenal gland to be very responsive to sensory input from the world around us, like a charging woolly mammoth. When chronically stressed, your adrenal glands produce cortisol, and cortisol inhibits CRH—which is too bad, because CRH will decrease your desire to eat. High cortisol levels reduce insulin sensitivity, so diabetes becomes more common and adversely influences fat and protein metabolism. The kidney responds to high cortisol levels by retaining salt and water so that blood pressure increases. At the same time, other hormones created by the adrenal gland, including testosterone and its derivative estrogen, increase; this can lead to obesity-linked diseases like uterine fibroids and breast cancer. To measure cortisol levels, you need a blood test or a twenty-four-hour urine collection. Above 100 milligrams in twenty-four hours generally indicates a high level of cortisol. (Note: In some people, the cutoff number varies, depending on the lab.) By the way, this is also the reason why people on steroidal medications (for asthma, for instance) seem to gain weight; cortisol is a form of steroids. (These are not the same steroids that some athletes are abusing. Those *anabolic* steroids are related to testosterone.)

Pancreas: A normally functioning pancreas secretes insulin, the substance that helps glucose travel from the blood into muscle to produce energy and fat for storage. Insulin actually works a lot like leptin; it has a mechanism that tells you to eat less. But when insulin resistance occurs in cells, it negates the appetite-control effect. Especially in early diabetes, you can naturally avoid high blood sugar with your food choices. But when you eat high-sugar foods without adequate insulin secretion to overcome insulin resistance (type 2 diabetes), you have less feedback of being full and less appetite reduction than appropriate, so the vicious hunger cycle continues.

Hormones in Action

Now, your goal shouldn't be to burn all of your fat (though you may often consider it to be so). The average person has about 2,500 calories of carbohydrate reserves—stored mostly in liver and muscle—to use for all kinds of functions that need energy, especially immediate energy, like when you're trying to catch a bus or escape a charging rhino. An average person has about 112,000 calories stored in fat (that is, if you are at your ideal weight, you typically have about fourteen pounds of fat). The message: Your body fat isn't the enemy, unless you're carrying more than you need. We need fat to function; it's an energy bank account that we can withdraw from. (Remember how food is processed. See figures in Chapter 3.)

The trick, of course, is to make sure we don't let our banks open up branches in every single part of our bodies.

In all, you have nine known hormones that tell you to eat more and fourteen that tell you to stop eating. Hormones, like your own anatomical sports agent, are on your side. They're looking out for your health. But that doesn't mean you can't have genetic glitches. Maybe your body doesn't make leptin correctly, or your body has too much cortisol, or you can't get leptin to your brain, or none of your satiety-related hormones work at all. Those are problems no amount of willpower can overcome. Reprogramming your hormonal circuitry is the only solution. You can't beat biology, but you can make it work for you.

One perfect example of hormonal influence comes in the form of the hormone adiponectin, which we talked about in the last chapter. The more adiponectin you have, the lower your weight and body-fat percentages. (And it's directly related to omental fat, your gut fat. If you don't have omental fat, you'll have more adiponectin flying around.) It helps your muscles turn fat into energy and suppresses your appetite. Now get this: When you lose weight, *more* adiponectin is available to your body. **YOU-reka!** It's one of your body's greatest reward mechanisms. The more weight you lose, the better your body is able to deal with the inflammation we talked about in the last few chapters, because of the protective effect of adiponectin. It's one of the reasons why when you gain weight, you start increasing the irritation in your body—you produce less of this natural anti-inflammatory agent.

The Sex Factor

We all know what testosterone and estrogen do for things like body hair, breast size, and the desire to spend Saturday night rampaging between the sheets like a pair of Greco-Roman wrestlers. But your sex hormones can influence more than just the activity that goes on below your waist; they can also influence what happens *to* your waist.

Reproductive-hormone friendly fire: One of the most common causes of obesity in women comes from a condition called polycystic ovary syndrome. In fact, PCOS is responsible for 10 percent to 20 percent of weight problems among younger women and is often diagnosed by irregular periods and by physical appearance: abdominal obesity, acne, thinning hair, and malelike hair growth (for example on the face). In the end, sufferers lose their feminine appearance. What happens is this: Women with PCOS have stingy ovaries—they get an egg all primed and ready to go in its follicle, but they won't hit send and ship the egg out. The follicle, raring to go, keeps sending out its messenger, estrogen. Now, estrogen works great when it gets paired up with, or balanced

The Better Sex Diet?

There's an added benefit to healthful foods: Many of them can boost sex-related hormones that increase desire—including omega-3 fatty acids and foods containing the testosterone-boosting mineral zinc. Some additional foods (think asparagus and artichoke hearts) have been linked to sexuality because of their physical resemblance to certain anatomical parts. Since it's hard to complete a double-blind randomized trial on this theme, we'll just pass along the limited facts and let your imagination run. More information like this is in *YOU: Being Beautiful.*

by, another ovarian messenger called progestin, which gets released from the egg sac (called a corpus luteum) after the follicle ships out its egg. In PCOS, some of that excess estrogen running around gets converted to androgens, or male hormones; these cause that extra hair growth and increased appetite. That's when the pounds add on. To combat this drive for another slice of coconut cream meringue, many women go on the birth control pill, which stops the weight gain by giving finite doses of estrogen and progestin, telling the ovaries to quiet down. The pill alone won't cause you to lose or gain, but having less of a voracious appetite and reversing the hormonal burden of PCOS often will.

Testosterone: It may be what produces chin hair and male egos, but testosterone is also found in women and plays a role in weight gain in both genders. Testosterone levels tend to fall in postmenopausal women and older men; this reduces libido and can lead to weight gain because you have less muscle mass, and more calories get stored as fat. When the cause of weight gain isn't clear from other diagnoses (such as other hormonal deficiencies, including thyroid disease) and the cause of libido loss isn't clear (conflict in relationship, stress, vaginal atrophy), supplementation with testosterone patches or topical testosterone gels or creams could make sense not only to reverse a plummeting libido, but maybe—just maybe—to eliminate a paunch. And some argue that increased sexual satisfaction can help with satiety. Quick note: Testosterone is currently under investigation and not ready for prime-time use. So before you consider treatment, know that testosterone has risk factors and several side effects, including acne, facial hair growth, rage reactions, and prostate cancer in men.

YOU TIPS!

Myth Buster

If You Think It's Not You, Find the Cause. For some of you, it doesn't matter whether you eat like a worm or exercise like a thoroughbred; you just can't lose weight. "Hormones" are an appropriate scapegoat for some with knee-tickling guts. If you're convinced that your fat can't be attributed to your lifestyle, it's worth asking your doctor about blood tests that measure hormone and other chemical levels to see what medications may address hormonal issues. These are the levels we'd suggest learning about:

Test	Desired Level
Thyroid-Stimulating Hormone	Less than 5 mIU/l (milli-international units per liter)
Urinary Cortisol	Less than 100 mg/day
Potassium	Between 3.5 mg/dl and 5.6 mg/dl
Calcium	Between 8 mg and 10 mg
Luteinizing Hormone/ Follicle-Stimulating Hormone	The individual values aren't as important as the ratio, and you'd like a 3:1 ratio of LH to FSH, no matter what time of the month.
Free Testosterone	More than 200 mg/dl for men; 20–70 mg/dl for women.

Do a Once-over. PCOS can be diagnosed with a blood test that measures total free testosterone. If your ratio of luteinizing hormone to follicle-stimulating hormone is greater than 3:1 (see above), that can also indicate PCOS. Treatment comes in the form of birth control pills, to regulate the hormonal patterns, and the diabetes drug metformin—Glucophage—to help prevent a cross fire that happens between the ovary and the pancreas, and to calm the inflammatory responses in the liver, so that it helps the body become more sensitive to insulin.

Chapter 7

Make the Move

How You Can Burn Fat Faster

"Lats"

Rectus
Abdomenis
Six-Pack"

"Glutes

Diet Myths

❖ Lifting weights will make you bulky.

❖ The best exercise for losing fat is cardiovascular training.

❖ You need weights to build muscle.

We all know that muscles give us the power to lift boxes and babies. They give us the power to walk around the mall and sprint for the 5:32 train to Schenectady. And depending on your tastes in movie-star muscle, they have the power to make your tongue wag faster than a golden retriever's tail. But you don't have to be an appliance deliveryman, an Olympic shot-putter, or an oiled-up spring breaker to benefit from muscle. When it comes to waist management, the real power of muscles lies in their ability to work like an anatomical pack of wolves. While your hormones are responsible for a large portion of your metabolism, your muscles can expedite the process of burning extra calories.

YOU-reka! While muscles give us the metabolic ability to burn calories every time we move—during exercise, during gardening, during sex—their true advantage is that they constantly feed on calories, even when you're moving about as fast as a skateboard with a busted wheel. See, every pound of muscle burns between 40 and 120 calories a day just to sustain itself, while every pound of fat feeds on only 1 to 3 calories. Day after day, that's a huge difference in your metabolic rate and your daily calorie burn. When you add a water bottle full of muscle to your body, you're able to burn a refrigerator full of fat.

When we think about muscles, we tend to think about really big ones (Arnold's) or really nice ones (Brad Pitt's abs, Michelle Obama's shoulders). Working your muscles isn't necessarily about making you big, brawny, and eligible for the NFL draft.

Myth Buster

By focusing on the right muscles and following the right plan, you won't add bulk; you'll firm up, and you'll stimulate the amount of growth needed to help burn extra calories. Best of all? You don't need any expensive equipment or a gym membership to see the benefits of adding muscle. You need only one piece of equipment: your own body. Your body is your gym.

Your Muscles:
Strength Builders and Fat Burners

Your skeletal muscles—that is, the muscles attached to your bones by tendons and ligaments, not the involuntary muscles associated with working your organs, like your heart or esophagus—come in pairs. That allows one muscle to move a bone in one direction, while the other moves it in another (when you bend your arm at the elbow, your biceps muscle pulls your upper and lower arm together, while your triceps muscle pushes them away from each other).

Now, we could bore you to a pond's worth of tears by explaining the biology of muscle, so we'll summarize what you need to know: Skeletal muscle is designed to do two kinds of things—to make you fast and strong. It's made up of bundles of fibers, each of which is like a strand of spaghetti. These fibers have filaments that have to slide over each other like an expandable ladder.

When your brain sends the message for your muscles to move—to walk, to lift a couch, to kiss your lover's ear—your muscles contract the way an extendable ladder would contract, by ratcheting the poles up and down. And it uses a catch or hook to stop the muscle and keep it opened or closed (see Figure 7.1). Now, you can build up two parts of that ladder—the actual poles, which give you strength; and the force that it takes to move those poles up and down, which gives you stamina. The force-generating structures act like calorie-guzzling cyclers pedaling furiously to pull

FACTOID

Starting with the 1960s, the increase in time that the average American spends watching TV perfectly parallels the increase in the average person's waist size. Besides keeping us from running errands outside, TV frees our hands to engage in mindless eating as we plan for the next commercial-break run to the fridge. This is an especially big problem for kids, who on average watch seventeen hours per week.

FACTOID

Sure, protein is necessary for the building and repairing of muscle, but don't fall into the trap of thinking you're not getting enough. To meet your daily protein requirements, you need only two ounces; one small chicken breast includes that amount. Exercise does increase protein needs, but usually not much. More protein in your diet, as we mentioned earlier, does decrease appetite.

Scary Electron Microscope View

together muscle fibers (see Figure 7.1). Elastic recoil generated by the contraction and aided by stretching helps the muscle relax after exercise.

The two main forms of exercise—stamina training and strength training—influence the structure of the ladder differently. Stamina training increases your muscles' capacity to produce and use the energy they need to contract, since you are adding more powerful cyclers, but muscle strength requires strength training that builds up the ladder poles—making for a bigger, stronger, and sturdier muscle fiber structure. How? When you do any kind of resistance training (that is, pulling or pushing some kind of weight) you create tiny tears in your muscle fibers. Your body reacts to those tears by saying, "If you can tear down my ladder, I'm going to build a stronger, bigger one next time." And your body builds back bigger and stronger ladder poles. (Walking, by the way, increases both your energy capacity and your poles, which is one of the many reasons why it's a central part of this plan.) By regularly doing strength training, you create more muscle mass—muscle mass that you need to help you burn fat. In essence, you make the spaghetti strands a little thicker and stronger rather than making more spaghetti strands.

Muscle serves as a primary energy consumer for your body. Think of it as a raging fire. Toss a log into it, and it'll burn the log up pretty quickly. But your fat is more like one lit match—it would take years for that match to burn the log. In your body, muscle can fry up that cheese dog a lot faster than can fat—thus reducing the amount of fat you store.

Myth Buster

How Much Muscle Do You Have?

While some waist-related measurements are easily quantifiable (pounds, waist size, number of pants ripped since 1993), muscle mass is a little trickier to calculate. Sure, you can eyeball yourself in the mirror and see if your abdominals look like an alligator's back. One indirect way to estimate is through knowing your body-fat percentage: The lower your fat percentage, the higher your muscle mass (this percentage can be measured at a gym, or with at-home devices like calipers). The truth is that the amount of muscle mass doesn't matter in terms of health (most of us have between twenty and thirty pounds of muscle) and waist size does. What is important is that you do enough strength-building exercise to maintain your muscle mass, which otherwise decreases as you age.

YOU-reka! Add just a little more muscle, and you'll use more energy and store less fat. And that makes it an even more efficient exercise for burning fat than cardiovascular training.

That's pretty crucial when you consider that we lose an average of 5 percent of our muscle mass every ten years after the age of thirty-five—if we don't do anything about it. (Historically, hunters, gatherers, and carriers of children needed their muscular strength until they were about thirty-five, when kids were able to walk and younger tribesmen could hunt. But after they turned thirty-five, their bodies didn't give two tubers about whether they had any muscle, so their bodies adapted and allowed for that gradual loss.) Today we see drastic effects when we lose muscle—we gain weight. If you don't intentionally rebuild muscle through exercise, every ten years you'll need to eat 120 to 420 fewer calories each day to maintain your current weight.

So if you're at a stable weight at age thirty-five and don't do any kind of resistance training, while still eating the same amount of food, you'll gain weight.

Now, as your muscle ages, you also lose a little bit of the proteins that make up your muscle; they're what give your muscles the ability to have both strength and stamina. Exercise rebuilds and maintains proteins

FACTOID

Doing exercises for a particular body part will not burn fat at that very point. Your body decides where it wants to burn fat, so there's no such thing as spot-reduction through exercise. Otherwise, wouldn't we be seeing people doing double-chin crunches in the gym? Instead, by doing exercises for a specific body part, you're building muscle mass in that area—which, after burning fat, will have the appearance and attributes of lean, strong muscle.

and muscle mass to prevent you from gaining weight. Here's what you need to do:

❖ thirty minutes of walking *a day* to help rebuild the stamina- and strength-based proteins. That prepares your muscles for . . .

❖ thirty minutes of strength/resistance training *a week* to rebuild the strength-based proteins. (That's once a week for thirty minutes, or split up into two fifteen-minute sessions or three ten-minute ones.

In Chapter 13, we'll outline the specifics of the plan, but we also want to explain that muscle is a heavyweight prizefighter—not just in its ability to clobber fat but also because it's literally heavy. When people start to exercise and eat healthier, their initial reaction is typically frustration, because it seems like their weight doesn't change that much at first. **YOU-reka!** That's because fat floats and muscle sinks; muscle is simply a lot heavier than fat. So as you build a little bit of muscle mass and lose fat, you may not see a dramatic reduction in scale numbers right away, but you will see reductions in waist size and overall shape. After you make it through the initial transition into exercise, chances are that you'll continue to see more dramatic changes in your body composition, your metabolism, your weight, and your waist.

Now the question is: How do we add more muscle, rather than just maintaining what we've got? And how do we do it without ending up looking like a middle linebacker for the Bears?

The answer, of course, lies in exercise—but per-

> **FACTOID**
>
> Deciding between free weights and weight machines is like trying to decide between salmon and trout: They both have their strong points. Free weights (barbells and dumbbells) help you work on balance because your body has to work to balance the weights as well as lift them, while machines can help prevent injuries stemming from poor form because they're built in such a way that they force you to use proper form.

> **FACTOID**
>
> The supplement coenzyme Q10 is an essential part of your cells that is responsible for energy conversion (it converts glucose to ATP, the energy that powers your cellular functions). In a few, but not all, studies, CoQ10 improved muscular performance by 10 percent to 30 percent, and it can help protect muscles from oxidative stress.

haps not in the way you might think. Most of us break down exercise into two categories: stamina-based training (*aerobic*, like jogging or swimming) and strength-based training (lifting weights). Any kind of exercise burns calories while you're doing the activity, but the most potent and long-lasting fat burners are created not when you're swimming or running, as you might believe, but *after* strength training. That makes muscle one of your body's greatest anatomical allies. Here we're going to show you how to take advantage of your muscles' muscle—the right way, the easy way, the way that will not only get you more stares than a Monet masterpiece but also help you get the waist that you want.

While many diet plans don't discuss the role of exercise, we consider physical activity vital to inflate your health and deflate your waist size. Building muscle is one component, but cardiovascular training and increasing your flexibility are also part of your waist management plan. Together, the three components of exercise will have numerous effects on your body:

- ❖ Exercise increases your metabolism so that you burn energy at a higher rate than if you didn't exercise, and it reduces your appetite by turning on your sympathetic nervous system, which activates your fight-or-flight response. Do the experiment yourself. Take a quick walk or jog when you feel the first twinge of hunger. Presto, your hunger is gone when you return.

- ❖ Exercise will help you lose the extra weight that's stressing your joints. By dropping weight, you'll feel less pain in your knees, hips, ankles, and back. And that will put you into a positive cycle of behavior, so that you'll have the desire to exercise more.

Asian Invasion

Wake up any morning in Beijing, China, and you'll see hundreds of people of all ages greet the sun with awkward movements. They appear to be wrestling demons in the air, but they're practicing tai chi, a form of exercise used to balance, center, and relax the body. You can use tai chi as a meditative form of exercise or as a way to improve your balance. (See *YOU: Staying Young,* the workout.)

❖ Exercise stimulates the release of endorphins, which stimulate the pleasure centers in the brain. When they're stimulated, they give you a sense of control, which is associated with a decreased need to eat out of control.

❖ Exercise helps decrease depression and increases positive attitude, so you make other positive choices and don't have to use food as your medication. That will also help prevent your couch, chair, and bed from becoming anti–waist management devices.

❖ Exercise keeps your blood vessels open and clog-free, thus decreasing your risk of obesity-related morbidities like high blood pressure, elevated lousy cholesterol, memory problems, and heart attacks.

We could spend dozens of pages listing all the benefits of physical activity, but we think you get the point. You don't have to be an infomercial beefcake with a shaved chest to make physical activity a priority—and you don't have to spend three hours a day doing it to see the benefits.

Have You Gone Too Far?

Exercising is like nuts in at least one way: There is such a thing as too much of a good thing. While exercise has more pluses than a math workbook, you can take it too far. Burning more than 6,500 calories a week through exercise (that's roughly thirteen hours) or doing more than two hours in a row of cardiovascular training not only can stress your joints (depending on the exercise), but it also appears to be the level at which you induce too much oxidative stress in your body, and that decreases your longevity.

In fact, what's so wonderful about exercise is that unlike the things you have to take away from your life (junk foods, excuses), physical activity is something you can *add* (all while watching *Raymond* reruns). When you get your muscles moving in the right direction, your waist size will follow.

When you first start exercising, your body will respond with very outward signs: You'll sweat, you may feel sore, you may stink like month-old macaroni salad. Your body will also start responding on the inside, with changes in muscle size, blood flow, and blood chemistry. While exercise—even combined with a healthy diet—won't suck fat out of you instantaneously (more on liposuction in the appendix), you will see and feel changes in your body shape even within a week. And with the combined workout and eating YOU Plan, you may see a two-inch reduction in waist size within the first two weeks as your body composition changes. So get up and get moving.

FACTOID

As you increase the intensity of your exercise, the typical body utilizes a higher percentage of carbohydrate-fueled energy rather than fat-fueled energy. Some incorrectly interpret this to mean that as you increase exercise intensity, you are no longer burning fat, but burning only carbohydrates. Since the total number of calories burned during higher-intensity exercise is larger than the number of calories burned at lower intensities (even though a slightly higher percentage may come from carbohydrates than fats), you are almost always using (burning) more total fat than if you worked at a lower intensity.

YOU TIPS!

Know Your Fantastic Four. Physical activity and exercise are like vegetables; they come in all shapes, sizes, and tastes, and just about all of them are good for you. Depending on your health level and experience, you need to be thinking about including these components of activity in your life:

❖ **Walking:** We do it at the mall, around the house, and back and forth from the fridge to the water bed. And, yes, any walking is healthy (the optimum is to hit at least 10,000 steps a day). But you also need to dedicate a total of thirty minutes a day to walking (broken up into chunks of at least ten continuous minutes if you need to). It's the foundation for all other exercise because it not only increases your stamina but prepares your body for strength training. As a daily routine, walking is the psychological discipline that helps you stick with an activity plan. In fact, it has the highest compliance rate of any exercise. Commit to walking, and you'll start committing to more than just the TV lineup on Thursday nights.

❖ **Strength:** Even if the only barbell you've ever seen is the one that's piercing your buddy's tongue, that doesn't mean you should shy away from resistance training. Strength training—whether you use dumbbells, machines, bands, or your own body weight—helps rebuild muscle fibers and increase muscle mass, which will use up all those extra calories that you crave, so you can burn calories more efficiently

Myth Buster

and help prevent age-related weight gain. Now, here's the key to making it work: Many Americans tend to spend a lot of time working their peripheral muscles (like their biceps or their calves), but efficient strength training comes when you work the big muscles that make up the core axis of your body—your legs, the large muscles of your upper body (in your chest, shoulders, and back), your lower back muscles, and your abdominals. They're your *foundation muscles.* Best of all, you don't need a single piece of equipment to see the benefits.

One quick note about abdominal exercises: They won't burn fat per se, but they will strengthen your entire core to help flatten and tone your stomach when you do burn fat. And they'll give you a layer of muscular support that will also protect your lower back from injury. The tighter your abs, the less excess strain you'll cause your lower back. You can't build a house from the second floor down, and, in a way, your abdominal muscles and your entire core provide a base foundation that you can build upon.

❖ **Cardiovascular Stamina:** By doing cardiovascular exercise—that is, any activity that raises your heart rate for a sustained period of time (sorry, watching George Clooney movies doesn't count)—you'll increase your overall stamina, burn calories, and improve the function and efficiency of your heart, as well as lower your blood pressure. Getting your body to sweat also helps you to release toxins that would otherwise build up in your tissues.

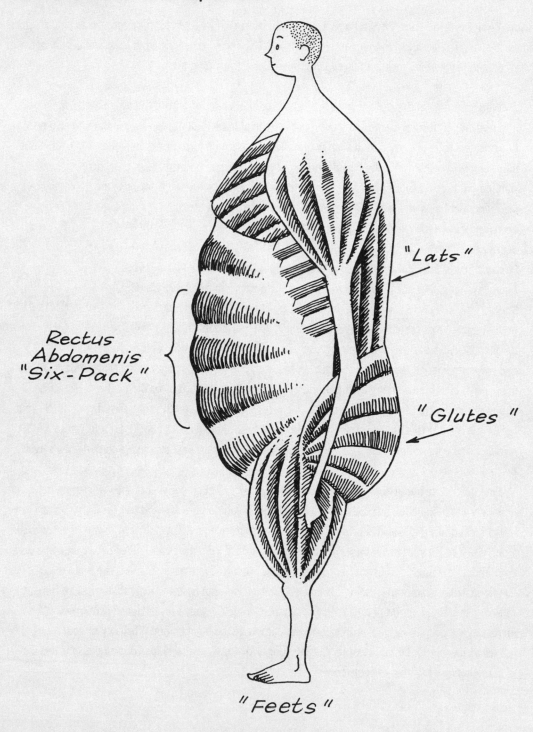

Figure 7.2 **The Tone Zones** Think of yourself as a homunculus with a studly torso, hips, back, and belly—your body's foundation muscles. When it comes to fighting fat, who cares about muscle-bound biceps and calves?

"Lats"

Rectus
Abdomenis
"Six-Pack"

"Glutes"

"Feets"

❖ **Flexibility:** Being flexible isn't just a good trait for yoga teachers and potential spouses; it's also what you want for your muscles. Good flexibility helps prevent injuries to your joints, because stretching works your muscles through a wide range of motion that you'll go through during exercise and everyday activity. Plus, being flexible just makes you feel better; it keeps your body from feeling stiffer than a week-old roach corpse, helps facilitate meditation, and allows you to center yourself as you focus on your body. Plus, the more pliable and loose you are, the less you're affected when you fall or get into accidents.

The YOU Diet Activity Audit

What You Need to Do	How Much You Need to Do
Walking	Ten thousand steps, total, accumulated throughout the day (with at least thirty minutes of continuous walking)
Muscular strength	Thirty minutes of resistance exercise a week
Cardiovascular stamina	Eighty percent of your maximum heart rate (calculated by 220 minus your age) for twenty minutes, three times a week. For a fifty-year-old, the target would be 0.8 times (220 minus 50), which equals 136 beats per minute. Also, you can measure it through exercise intensity. On a scale of one to ten, rate the intensity of your exercise. You should exercise at about a seven or eight on that scale—70 percent to 80 percent of your perceived maximum.
Flexibility	Five minutes a day

Excuse-Proof Your Life. When it comes to working out, most of us have two excuse cards we like to play: We have the ace of "no time" and the jack of "it's not convenient." Now, we know you're busy. We know you're juggling more balls than a twelve-armed clown. We know it's easier to sit on the couch than to do a push-up on the floor. But we also know this: Time and convenience aren't excuses. First of all, with this plan, you don't need a whole lot of time (thirty minutes a day to walk and thirty minutes a week to do some resistance training). If you don't have the time to do this, then you have to be willing to admit that the problem is not the fact that you're out of time but the fact that your life is so out of control that you can't budget enough time for your health and well-being. Plus, the newfound energy will enable you to do more than you could before.

And second, you don't need a gym or fancy equipment; heck, it takes more time to drive to the gym and change clothes than it does to actually work out. You can do all of this activity at home—with a few modest pieces of equipment or even by making use of items you already have. In fact, in the YOU Workout, you use your body as your weights. It sure beats spending your workout time waiting at the exercise machine for someone to finish her issue of *Quilting Quarterly*. Yes, it's easy to say you're too tired, too stressed, too busy, too this, or too that. We say, too bad. The only way you'll strip away the fat is to start by stripping away the excuses.

You Move, You Lose. One unsung form of exercise: fidgeting. Studies show that fidgety people are simply skinnier people. If you have two people working the same job and eating the same diet, the one who gets up to talk to someone down the hall rather than emailing her will be skinnier. Studies show that it isn't some mysterious food, organ, cell, or gremlin that makes these people burn up fat like an iron skillet, it's these fidgeting movements. Now, that's not to say that if you go on an all-fidgeting, leg-shaking, finger-tapping program (think Robin Williams), you'll be thinner than a Hilton sister. But numerous studies have shown that the more you move—in very subtle ways—the more calories your body will burn throughout the day. Find an excuse to move your muscles wherever you are. Clear the dishes. Stand up and walk in circles while you're on the phone. Walk down the hall to ask a coworker a question, rather then IM-ing her. Sit on an exercise ball for the first hour you work on your computer (a great core strengthener). Tap your toes in a meeting. Take every opportunity to move around, and you'll give your body subtle metabolism boosters that may just have more-than-subtle effects.

How Fit Are You?

There are lots of ways to gauge progress on a weight-loss plan: inches lost, Wendy's coupons tossed. But you can also measure your fitness levels in different areas of activity. Use these tests to see how you stack up. (Before doing each test, make sure to properly warm up by walking or doing light exercise for at least five minutes.)

Cardiovascular: You can measure your heart's efficiency by measuring your heart rate *after* exercise. After exercising for a period of eighteen minutes at 80 percent to 85 percent of your max (that's 220 minus your age), do three minutes at your maximum heart rate, then stop and check your pulse. Your heart rate should decrease sixty-six beats or more after two minutes of stopping. Do not do this without approval of your doctor unless you do it regularly as part of your workout.

Muscular: To gauge upper-body muscular stamina, do the push-up test (men in standard form; women can do it with knees on the floor). A thirty-year-old man should be able to do at least thirty-five (five less every decade after that, until he reaches seventy). A thirty-year-old woman should be able to do forty-five with knees on the floor (five less every decade after until she reaches eighty).

Flexibility: Measure lower-back flexibility by sitting on the floor with your legs straight out in front of you and slightly spread apart. With one hand on top of the other and fingertips lined up, lean forward and reach for your feet. Women forty-five and under should be able to reach two to four inches past their feet. Older women should be able to reach to the soles. Men aged forty-five and under should be able to reach to the soles. Older men should be able to come within three to four inches of the soles.

Squeeze Yourself. Here's an abdominal exercise you can (and should) do anywhere: Suck your belly button in tight and squeeze your butt in as if you're trying to pull up a pair of too-tight jeans. Pretend the top of your head is being pulled by a string to the ceiling. Now hold that position. Besides putting you into proper posture, it's working your transverse abdominis muscle (your supportive girdle muscles). Do it on the elevator, waiting in line, at work, and anywhere you walk.

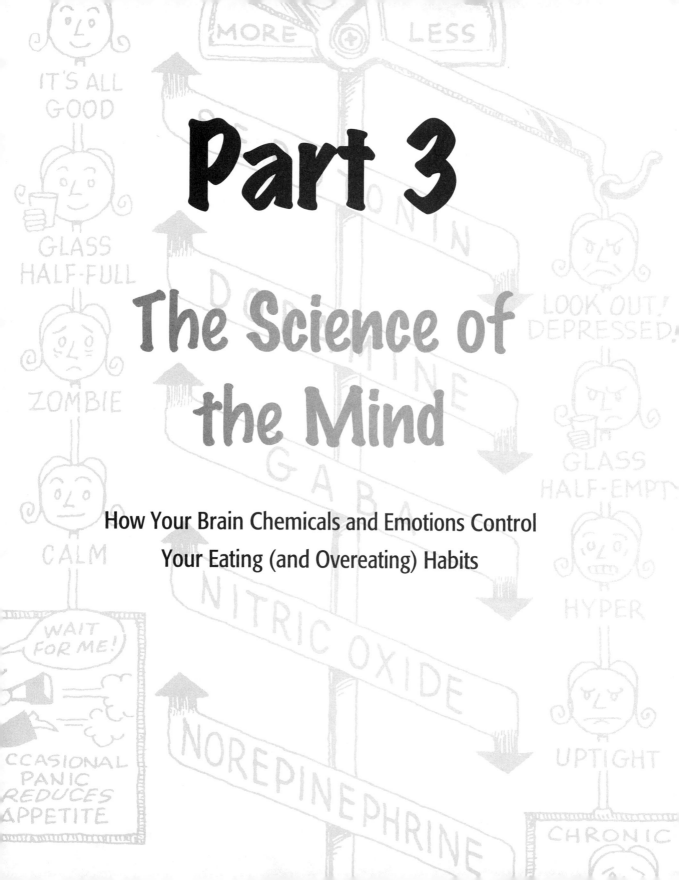

Part 3
The Science of the Mind

How Your Brain Chemicals and Emotions Control
Your Eating (and Overeating) Habits

Chapter 8

Shame on Who?

The Psychology of the Failed Diet

Diet Myths

- ❖ The diet would work if only you had the willpower of a lean person.
- ❖ It's better to have dieted and failed than not to have dieted at all.
- ❖ You can't make mistakes when you're dieting.

Most diets aren't about action; they're about thoughts. By their very nature, they force us to think, think, think, think. Diets make us think about food more than inmates think about escape. You have to think about calories or zones or the hour when you're next allowed to have half a cracker. You think about not having food so much that you develop only two sets of standards when it comes to eating: Either you follow your diet, or you don't. It's bean sprouts or it's prime rib. It's carrots or it's cookies. It's cucumbers or it's pepperoni. It's all or nothing.

Myth Buster

In a way, we've all been thinking too much about weight and what to eat, and not enough about how and why we eat. Just thinking about food causes us to eat more. The reality is that no matter how much we talk about calories and glycemic index, BMI and metabolism, we all know that the big battle over food is the emotional and psychological one.

And that's the next stop on our waist management journey: the brain and the mind. We've taken you through much of the biology of blubber, but now it's time to explore the aspect of overeating that many people believe is the real source of our troubles—that is, what happens between the ears is what drives what happens between the lips. In this chapter, we'll explore the psychology of why we eat; in the next we'll explore some of the neurological mechanisms that drive those thoughts and emotions. And in Chapter 10, we'll put it all together to help you learn how to manage the complexities of this perfect storm.

When most of us try to lose weight, we pull out the most powerful weapon we'd like to think we have—our minds—and launch a psychological attack in the form of discipline ("I can resist this food!") and ego ("I'm smart enough to avoid this food!"). But as you'll see in this chapter and the next, the truth is that there are very strong physiological (and thus chemical) triggers in our brains that make us eat—and make most diets fail. In many ways, our brains actually sabotage our minds' best dieting efforts.

The issue really comes down to our preconceived notions of what a diet really is. By trying the very thing that's designed to help us lose weight—a diet—we've created a no-win system of failure that spins us into a cycle of blame. And what's not to blame? We blame our societal fatness on free restaurant bread and meals with Mount McKinley–size portions. Or we blame our fatness on fast food (for the sugar, salt, and grease), magazine covers (for the unrealistic body images that taunt us to smear our self-esteem with daily fistfuls of cheesecake), sixty-hour workweeks (for making us sit down all day), cloud-soft recliners and reality TV (for making us sit down all night), sausage (blech!), or an intervention-worthy Velveeta addiction (double blech!).

But deep down in your gut (there, over by the sticky buns), there's really only one thing you honestly feel you can blame for the size of your gut:

You.

You blame you.

In your heart of hearts, you believe it's not the restaurants or food manufacturers or deep-fried cheese-stuffed peppers that are derailing your weight-loss efforts; it's your mind. The entire battle of the broken belt comes down to a flurry of mental "if onlys" and your perceived inability to control what food you shuttle down your esophagus year after year, day after day, meal after meal, bite after bite. If only you had the willpower to step away from the mayonnaise. If only you could stop after four Pringles. If only you had the power, the strength, the discipline, the chutzpah, the energy, the drive, and the motivation to control your mouth, you'd finally have the waist and energy you want.

System Failure

What you're really doing here is laying brain blame. We rely on our minds to resist temptation, to make smart decisions, to eat right, to know better, and to make healthy choices. So we naturally rely on our minds to combat the emotions we think we should be able to handle: stress, anxiety, and depression (studies show that those with higher levels of all these emotions are more likely to be overweight or obese). So when we give up on a diet and balloon to a size that makes doorways cringe, we automatically think that something's wrong with us, that our minds aren't strong enough to win over our waists.

The real reason we fail? Researchers theorize that indeed our minds may be mixed up, but not because of anything we're doing. At least scientifically, overeating may work a little bit like drug addiction: studies show that food lights up the brain reward centers of the obese in the same way narcotics affect the brains of drug addicts.

Let's say you're stressed. Stress activates neurotransmitters from a part of the brain called the locus coeruleus. Your body, in response, tries to calm those neurotransmitters and combat the stress. Some people do it with cigarettes, some do it with sex, some do it with drugs, some do it with food. When you combat stress with food, you're also activating the reward center of your brain. After that initial feel-good hit wears off, you'll reach again for the same thing that made you feel calm and relaxed: food. That's why stress and anxiety make it that more difficult, neurochemically, to stick to whatever plan you're trying to follow.

What's especially interesting is that right next to the hypothalamus, where the feeding and satiety chemicals NPY and CART are produced, is a part of the brain called the mammillary body (because it looks like a pair of breasts). That's where food memory is stored, so when you get the signal that you're hungry, you're also accessing your memory of and cravings for foods you've eaten in the past—which may have been bad foods (flip back to Figure 2.2). To make matters worse, the parietal region of the brain—the control center of the movement of the tongue, lips, and mouth—acts differently in heavy people than in skinny people. Brain scans show that in heavy people who are tempted with sugar, this region becomes activated and stimulates movements such as licking the lips, which reminds one to eat. In skinny people the region stays dormant, showing how sugar can play a role in emotional eating for people who are physiologically addicted to it by activating their brains.

The trick is to learn how you can make your brain (your genetic hardware) work with your mind (the software that can change as you change). Playing the blame game simply crashes your system, but adopting some of the behaviors we talk about in the next few chapters will help make the hardware and software work together to achieve what you want. Saturated fat, salt, and simple carbohydrates (non–100 percent whole grains—they turn to sugar fast) are addictive to most of us, not only psychologically but physiologically, as well. There are simply

Figure 8.1 **Food for Thoughts** When you eat sugar, you light up the motor cortex located in the parietal lobe of your brain, which controls your lips, tongue, and mouth. The hippocampus, which controls memories of food, lights up when people on rigid diets crave certain foods—overwhelming their willpower and ability to resist.

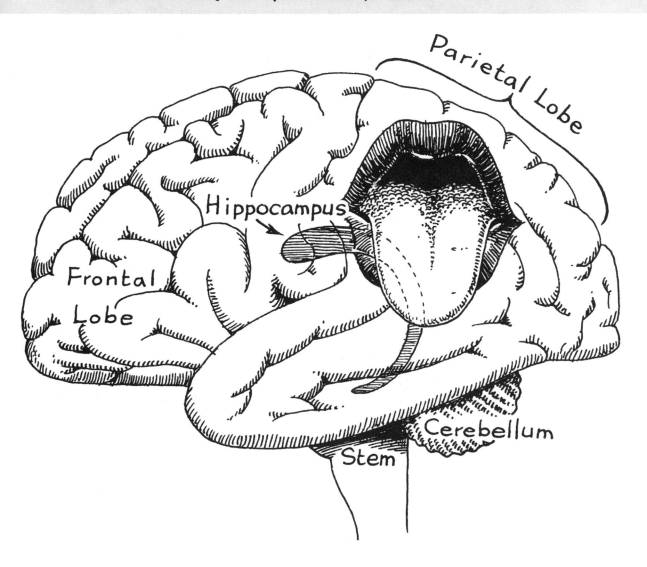

too many hormones and neurotransmitters whose jobs roughly translate to "Pass the pound cake." And to expect that your will or your fortitude can override these chemical messages is the equivalent of trying to stop a train with your pinkie. Remember the YOU Diet mantra: Diet Smart, Not Hard. Make your mind work in tandem with your brain, rather than letting it sabotage your efforts.

Dieting: Avoiding the Issue

For a second, think about one particular kind of person—the extreme example of fat gone wild. These people are often the stereotypical ideal—funny, kind, generous, charming, articulate, creative, and more brilliant than a perfect diamond—except for the fact that they're overweight. (We all say it: "He'd be so great if only he were thin.") That bothers us. It bothers us that we can't figure out the yin and yang of the situation. How can a person smart enough to know the difference between scrapple and apples or driven enough to have a successful high-tech career be the very same person who, night after night, gets clobbered silly by a helpless sleeve of Oreos hiding in the back of the pantry shelf?

Something has to be wrong.

And it is. But it's about as likely to be what you think it is as you are to find your true love in Las Vegas. The issues aren't at waistband level; they're at the level of the mind. You may know you have health problems and a waist circumference the size of Neptune. And you may even know that you struggle with the emotional issues of low self-confidence and lack of self-esteem that come as sides with the entrée of obesity. **YOU-reka!** But you may not know that you could be what's called an avoider, in that you suffer internally from the psychological turmoil that comes with the public and private disdain for obesity, and you avoid confronting your situation at all because of the internal fear of not being able to beat it.

Here's how avoiders think (nod if this sounds familiar): Once they deviate—even slightly—from a diet or healthy eating plan, they figure they might as well drop the whole thing. (Nodding?) And this starts a cycle that avoiders can't find a way out of: They're fat, they try to lose weight, they deviate just a little, they fear rejection for the perceived failure, they isolate themselves from people, they stop talking about it, they stop the diet, they mow through a pound of cheesecake, they get fat. And then they try to lose weight, and the cycle continues.

Avoiders at all levels (from the extreme cases to the milder ones) will see their weight bop up and down like a bull rider. Physiologically, it's a never-ending cycle of weight gain and loss (that's called weight cycling). But the real avoidance issues stem from the psychological effects of weight cycling. Instead of avoiding bad foods, avoiders tend to want to avoid other things—such as people who want to help them and the discipline of trying to eat healthfully. Above all, avoiders try to avoid these two strong emotions associated with dieting:

Guilt: "I Hope They Don't Find Out"

No matter what kind of diet you may have tried in the past, you've undoubtedly worked with a list of off-limits foods. High-protein diets might ban potatoes. Low-fat diets might ban cheese. Sugar-busting diets may ban you from ever setting foot in Aunt Thelma's kitchen again. Inevitably, like a child instructed not to touch the champagne flutes, you will want potatoes, you will want cheese, and you will find it incredibly rude to turn down Aunt Thelma's snickerdoodles three times in a row. So you cave. But because you've set yourself up with a list of banned foods, you perceive half a cookie, a hunk of Gouda, or three measly fries as first-degree diet homicide: The diet's dead. And that's where guilt sets in— from the fact that you know you deviated from a predetermined set of standards. That holds true for all levels of avoiders. We all identify with nutrition-induced guilt, and then we make a subconscious decision that it's easier to deal with the effects of being overweight than it is to feel the boulder-heavy guilt every time we want to smother a carrot in blue cheese.

Shame: "Oh Gosh, They Did Find Out"

For the person who feels he cheated on his diet—whether it was a simple kiss with a Kit Kat or an adulterous romp with a vat of cake batter—there's an even worse feeling than guilt. And that's the shame associated with dietary infidelity. You've cheated, so you now feel you lack the strength to succeed. So what are you going to tell your spouse and all your coworkers who've been watching you feast on iceberg lettuce at lunch for the past eight days? That, yes, you're a failure? That you could last on your diet for only a week? That you have one little thing you're doing, and by gosh, you can't even keep a stinking croissant out of your mouth? The public humiliation, or just the perceived threat of possible embarrassment, stems primarily from that societal disdain for obesity. This shame—a much more profound emotion than guilt—spins you back into the cycle of avoidance: It's better to not be on a diet and be fat, the avoider calculates, than to be on a diet and eventually prove to the world that you can't succeed.

So where does this leave us? Research actually shows that it's better for your health not to diet at all than to say you're dieting and steal spoonfuls of crème brûlée during every commercial break. That's because diets typically promote weight cycling and yo-yo dieting (gaining and losing, gaining and losing), which are actually more hazardous to your health than keeping a steady overweight weight. (That's probably because most weight cyclers eventually gain back more than they lost and suffer the slings of shame.)

So how does this all work for you, the person who knows she has to lose some weight but isn't necessarily breaking floorboards with every step? If you've spent years struggling with weight, it's likely you've experienced similar thoughts of guilt and shame and may even follow the same behavioral patterns. One of the strategies for bypassing the spiral of shame is to live and eat in the present, not being upset about what you ate in the past and not obsessing about what you'll eat in the future.

Why Our Brains Aren't Equipped for "Dieting"

Unfortunately, the very thing that's designed to help people lose weight is the very thing that promotes this behavioral and psychological pattern: diets that promote the all-or-nothing mentality.

It turns out that much of the diet dogma we've all accepted as fact is more hype than horse sense. Like a tantalizing trailer that creates expectations well beyond what a movie can deliver, the problem with most diets is not with the preview; it's with the plot. The typical diet drama opens to reveal the hero dieter preparing for battle—attacking the enemy head-on. Armed with grit, determination, and little else, the hero prepares for battle against flying chocolate sundaes in a quest for total domination over food. What our hero doesn't realize is that the secret weapon she was counting on will never arrive; the cavalry is nowhere in sight. So the battle becomes grueling, mentally and physically exhausting, and never-ending. All this hard work tends to create quite an appetite, and the energy halo from yesterday's feast of three stalks of celery and a cherry tomato is quickly fading. Our hero needs a pizza, and fast.

The camera zooms in tight as our hero quietly prays for the inner strength necessary to fend off yet another attack by the Food Insurgency. But just as she is reaching a state of inner peace, she is jolted back into reality by the unmistakable roar of a rapidly approaching truck. What she had hoped was a Humvee packed with volunteers from the local chapter of Foodaholics Anonymous turns out to be a minivan full of Girl Scouts offering free samples of their new and improved megamint cookies.

Unfortunately, much of the dieting mind-set comes from the initial expectation we set early on. When you're ready to go on a diet, you set the rules, you know the parameters, you know that veggies are nutritional G-men and cookies are nutritional mass murderers. That process and the anticipation of going on a diet can work in your favor, as long as you remember that the way your brain works isn't just psychological but chemical as well. But because of often-strict parameters, many diets leave you less wiggle room than one of Beyoncé's dresses,

Can You Spare Some Change?

We all know that making a change in your life is as mental as it is behavioral. Research shows that this is the best four-step process for making change:

Be Positive. It works for coaches, bosses, and parents, as well as waist managers. If you blame yourself for your weight, if you are depressed about your weight, if your mood is fouler than a subway station in August, then your first job is to refocus. You need to think about what you can do, how you can do it, why it's good for you, and how you'll succeed. In the weight-loss game, poker-faced confidence trumps negativity every time. By stripping yourself of the negative emotions of guilt and shame, you'll make the right rational (and long-term) decisions about your eating obstacles.

Add Some Support. You may not know it, but your world is full of saboteurs—people out to make you fatter than Microsoft's coffers. There's the boss who brings in sweets for every Thursday meeting. The friend who brings you a pie when you're upset. The spouse who suggests pitchers of margaritas and a plate of cheese nachos to celebrate the end of the week. Maybe there's nothing wrong with their intentions, but there is something wrong with the fact that their attempts to appeal to your heart are actually damaging it. What we want you to do—no, *need* you to do—is develop a support system of people who know your goals, know your obstacles, know your weaknesses, and know your strengths. (Don't have anyone? You can hook up on the Internet, at www.realage.com.) This person will be your sounding board, your comfort system, and your measure of accountability. With public accountability—that is, you reporting in on those daily struggles and successes—you're more likely to make a permanent change.

Make a Gesture. Small gestures (ones not involving individual fingers flung at passing motorists) can be viewed as anything from signs of love to signs of bribery. Token gestures can also help kick-start the psychology of change. Just making a seemingly small change will help determine your long-term success, whether it's buying a pedometer, a health-club membership, or new walking shoes; throwing away the unhealthy foods in your pantry; and even setting up a computer file to record your progress. **YOU-reka!** If you make one small move like this, research shows that you'll be three times more likely to follow through with the specific plan you intend to follow. This small change is your way of putting the key in your waist management ignition (www.mychoicescount.com can help).

Then Do It. Once you start with the small gesture, you're ready. Eat a full day's worth of perfect-for-you food. Walk thirty minutes today, tomorrow, and every day after that. That's right, thirty minutes of walking a day is the minimum commitment. (You can break it up into smaller segments if you can't do it all at once.) Then make a second action commitment: Commit to doubling (or tripling) your daily vegetable intake. With one foot, take one specific first step. The other foot has no choice but to follow.

so that there are only two options: rewards for compliance and no tolerance for failure.

In just about every other area of our lives, we allow ourselves margins of error. Baseball players who make outs 70 percent of the time are Hall of Famers. Basketball players need to make only half their shots to become all-stars. Lawyers don't win every case. Parents don't always make the right decisions. In fact, almost all of us make mistakes in our daily jobs. We learn from them and try to correct them so we don't repeat them again and again, or at least figure out how to minimize the damage. But when it comes to diets, we hold ourselves to the precision of a Blue Angels flight team. No errors. No mistakes. Once we've blown it and deviated even an inch from our plan, that's it. We head back to the locker room, take off the uniform, shower, game's over. Diet's dead. Pass the fondue pot.

Through the tips below and the strategies we outline in the next few chapters, you can learn to reprogram your mind to strip away the guilt that comes with eating, the guilt that comes with diets, and the guilt that comes with occasionally enjoying foods that aren't on the platinum level of healthy-eating charts. You also have to realize that it's not the first fry or first slice of cake that will doom your diet. It's the second, the third, and the whole dang shebang that lead to dangerous fat and waist gain.

At the beginning of our plan (which starts on page 255), you do have to listen to your body and respond intelligently to your cravings and your emotions. But over time, you'll learn how to eat right and manage your cravings automatically. At that point, you'll no longer obsess about eating right—and punish yourself for every obstacle you face. **YOU-reka!** The unrecognized truth is that when you stop overthinking—and, instead, program yourself to be on autopilot 95 percent of the time—you'll stop overeating.

YOU TIPS!

Make the Split. Clearly, some of us eat for physical reasons (we're hungry), and some of us gnaw on leftover Halloween candy for emotional reasons (we're steamed at the boss about having to start and finish a new report by 10 a.m., and it's 9:47). But sometimes it's not always easy to figure out the difference. To help, you need to start using the YOU Diet Hunger Test. Throughout the day, record your level of hunger as judged by this scale. Stay tuned to what your stomach is telling you, not what's happening outside with stresses (the car battery died), emotions (spouse is working late again), or habits (Conan equals bowl of Apple Jacks). This process will help you really feel your hunger, so that you can let your stomach, not your emotions, dictate your habits.

0 Tank = Hungry. It feels as if you haven't eaten since junior year of high school.

½ Tank = Edge is off. You're OK, not desperate, like maybe when you're driving home from work.

¾ Tank = Satisfied and not hungry. You can go much longer without food. You just ate nuts and had a drink before dinner.

1 Full Tank = Full and comfortable. It's the way you feel after finishing an average-portion, healthful meal.

Overflow Level S = Stuffed. You could've stopped two scoops of pudding ago.

Overflow Level OS = Overstuffed. Audible groaning detected.

Overflow Level BP = Button Pop/Exploding. It's the typical Thanksgiving gorge. You feel sick and even take the name of your momma's stuffing in vain.

The way the test works is, every time you find yourself reaching for the cheese sauce or cookie box, rate your hunger.
Then think about whether you're reaching for the leftover lasagna because you're truly hungry or for a reason that has absolutely nothing to do with hunger. Ideally, you'll want to stay in the ¾ to Full Tank range—satisfied at all times. And you'll get there by eating regularly throughout the day. (See Part 4 for

details.) After applying these gauges for two weeks, you'll start to instinctively know why you're eating, and, better, you'll train yourself to eat simply to keep your stomach satisfied—and not your emotions.

Pick, Stick, and Automate. Yeah, sure, variety may be the spice of life, but it can also be the death of dieting. When you have a lot of choices for a meal, it's a lot easier to slip out of good eating habits and into ham-induced bad ones. When you sit down at a diner and are presented with a menu that's the size of a phone book, it's easy to give in. One way to get away from fat bombs is to eliminate choices for at least one meal a day. Pick the one meal you rush through most and automate it. For most people, it's lunch. So find a healthy lunch you like—salad with grilled chicken and olive oil or turkey on whole grain bread—and have it for lunch every day. Every day. Yes, every day.

YOU-reka! More and more research is showing that putting a cap on the variety of foods and tastes you experience will help you control your weight. (Think of your dog: Penelope stays the same weight when she has her regular food every day. But as soon as she starts gorging on a variety of nightly table scraps, the puny poodle looks more like a massive mastiff.) How does it work? It seems that when you have meals rich in flavor variety, it takes more and more calories to make you feel full (think of Thanksgiving, when you eat a lot of different things, stuff yourself, and still have room for pumpkin pie). So when we experience meals with lots of diverse flavors—think Mexican or Indian cuisine—we tend to eat more to satisfy our taste buds. Now, we don't want you to become bored with food, but if you make this a habit for at least one meal a day, it'll decrease your temptations and help you stop thinking about food so often. In fact, we usually prescribe two meals and two snacks that are the same each day for our patients. It's one of the ways to automate your brain so that your habits follow. Of course, we don't want you to stop enjoying the wonderful diversity of flavors, but it will help control your appetite.

Another trick: Use extralight virgin olive oil, which has less flavor and may help control taste cravings.

Keep Your Hands Full. You'd think that being plopped in front of a TV playing Xbox would mean that you're destined for a life of fatness. But that's not the case; studies show that playing video games is actually not correlated with obesity. Why? Turns out that when you've got your two hands on the controllers and your fingers moving faster than Liberace's, that means one thing: Your paws won't be knuckle-deep in a bowl of chocolate-covered raisins. (Some games even have foot mats for you to make commands with your feet too, so you can get a complete workout; ask your kids about the Dance Dance Revolution craze. Wii Fit works too if you don't take too many breaks.) Now, that's not to say that an intimate relationship with Super

Mario should be your number one strategy, but it does prove an underlying point. **YOU-reka!** When you keep your hands and brain occupied—whether with video games, gardening, or removing a spleen—it means you're putting your brain into the state you want: not thinking about eating and not automatically reaching for something to put in your mouth.

Find a Substitute. For avoiders, we know that eating is about as rational as an inebriated sports fan. If we all had the ability to make rational choices, such as grilled zucchini over fettuccine—there would be no need for the multibillion-dollar diet industry. Eating is both an emotional action and an addictive one. The average person knows doughnuts are hand grenades to health. But we pass by a neighboring cubicle with a dozen cream-filled jobbies, and we've finished three before we've even turned the corner. Add to this the fact that research shows that people under the most work stress gain the most weight, and you've got yourself an obesity double whammy. So the question is really, how can you take irrational, emotional, and addictive actions and turn them into smart, rational, good decisions? For one thing, you can develop a list of healthful contingency foods and clear your fridge and pantry of waist-killing foods, which we'll show you how to do in Part 4. For another, you can look for other things to fill the needs that food is currently filling. Traditionally, so much of our self-satisfaction comes from how we see ourselves externally. But that satisfaction is fleeting, and we need to find and focus on the things in life we're truly grateful for—be it our family, our career, or a hobby that we're passionate about.

Chapter 9

The Chemistry of Emotions

The Connections between Feelings and Food

Diet Myths

- ❖ Hedonistic eating is triggered mainly by extreme hunger.
- ❖ Cravings are directed by taste buds.
- ❖ The best way to resist temptation is with willpower.

Our ancestors ate to survive; they ate because they were hungry or maybe to celebrate a victory over a warring tribe. Us? We eat because we're angry, bored, stressed, depressed, frustrated, watching a movie, busy, not busy enough, getting together with friends, or PO'd that the Lions lost. What we think of as an emotional reaction—where we substitute chocolate for a conversation, ice cream for a bath, or chips for a punching bag—isn't always as much about character as it is about chemistry.

We're guessing that you identified very strongly with some of the emotions and excuses we outlined in the previous chapter. They're all very real and very powerful, and they can be very destructive. But part of the equation is that those emotions also have a very strong chemical component. And when you learn about their relationship and look at the problem as a whole (as we do in Chapter 10), it's much easier to change your life and automate the good behaviors that will help you become healthier.

Early in the book, you learned about the chemical reactions that take place in your body that stimulate hunger. Leptin and ghrelin are the joysticks that control our eating actions. But the physical action of eating, as you know, can be triggered by emotions that coax us to wolf down a mustard-smothered dog. Your hypothalamus (remember, the site of your satiety center) is also the part of your brain where your mind and body literally connect. As the bosom buddy of the hypothalamus, the pituitary gland sends chemicals to talk to the rest of the body. It's really where the whole weight-loss game is won and lost—this connection between physiological and psychological needs for eating.

Myth Buster As you well know, emotional eating isn't about reaching for celery. Rather, it's out-of-control, hedonistic eating (which often comes from your food memory, banked in the mammillary body we mentioned in the last chapter), where you eat every cookie in the bag because they look good and taste even better. It's a craving, and usually for something that's starchy, sugary, salty, or loaded with fat. The following five brain chemicals are the ones that primarily influence our emotions, and not only do they provide the foundation for why we eat at certain times, but they're also the key chemicals in many of our current and future weight-loss drugs—because they tend to regulate some of the reasons *why* we eat certain foods (and certain amounts of foods).

❖ **Norepinephrine:** the caveman fight-or-flight hormone. It's what tells you to tangle with a saber-toothed tiger or hightail it to the safety of your hut.

❖ **Serotonin:** the James Brown of neurotransmitters. It makes you feel good (Hyah!) and is a major target of antidepression drugs.

❖ **Dopamine:** the brain's fun house. It's a pleasure-and-reward system and is particularly sensitive to addictions. It's also the one that helps you feel no pain.

❖ **GABA (gamma-animobutyric acid):** the English Patient of amino acids. It makes you feel like a zombie and is one of the ways that anesthesia may work to reduce your responsiveness to the outside world.

❖ **Nitric oxide:** the meditation-like chemical. It helps calm you. This powerful neuropeptide is usually a very-short-lived gas that also relaxes the blood vessels of the body.

Now, the real question is: What do all these chemicals have to do with whether or not you snack on a Hershey bar or a plum? Probably the best way to think about it is to use serotonin as an example. Picture your brain as a small pinball machine (see Figure 9.1). You have millions of neurotransmitters that are sending messages to and from one another. When your serotonin transmitters fire the signals (from the flippers), they send the message throughout your brain that

you feel good; this message is strongest when that feel-good pinball is frenetically bouncing around in your brain, racking up tons of yeah-baby points along the way. But when you lose the ball down the chute (that is, when cells in the brain take the serotonin and break it down), that love-the-world feeling you've

Mood Foods

Recent research shows what many of us knew all along: Our moods dictate what we eat. Researchers studied the diets of people to show how personality and foods collide—how our moods may steer us to certain foods on the basis of their physical characteristics. The study theorized that many moods send specific signals; for example, stressed adrenal glands could be sending salt-craving signals. So what does your favorite turn-to food say about you?

If You Reach For . . .	You May Be Feeling . . .
Tough foods, like meat, or hard and crunchy foods	Angry
Sugars	Depressed
Soft and sweet foods, like ice cream	Anxious
Salty foods	Stressed
Bulky, fill-you-up foods, like crackers and pasta	Lonely, sexually frustrated
Anything and everything	Jealous

just been experiencing is lost. So what does your brain want to do? Put another quarter in the machine and get another ball. For many of us, the next ball comes in the form of foods that naturally (and quickly) make us feel good, to counteract the drop in serotonin that we're feeling.

Unfortunately, the way we typically satisfy our urge to play another ball is to consume foods that provide an immediate rush of serotonin. That rush can come with a jolt of sugar: sugar stimulates the release of serotonin. Insulin facilitates serotonin production in the brain, which in turn boosts our mood, makes us feel better, or masks the stress, pain, boredom, anger, or frustration that we may be feeling. But serotonin is only one ball in play. You have all sorts of other chemicals fighting to send your appetite and cravings from bumper to bumper.

To see how the total picture works, think of those chemicals as parts of a scale. When the chemicals associated with positive feelings (such as serotonin and dopamine) are in the up (or activated) position, you're chemically high. But when they're down, you experience a big emotional and chemical downfall (see Figure 9.2). **YOU-reka!** And this puts you in a state of anxiety that sends you searching for the foods, especially simple carbohydrates, that get you back to the chemical high. That's how illegal drugs work too; users keep seeking the high not always for its own sake but to avoid the lows. You're constantly fighting to get back to that place of neurochemical comfort. When these chemicals are high, your weight gets lower, and when they're lower, you reach for the foods that eventually make your weight higher.

That's the reason why what happens inside your skull plays such a vital role in what happens under your belt. Knowing how your emotions affect your brain chemistry and direct your desire to eat will help you to resist your cravings and, ideally, avoid them altogether. Your goal: to keep your feel-good hormones level so that you're in a steady state of satisfaction and never experience huge hormonal highs and lows that make you search for good-for-your-brain-but-bad-for-your-waist foods.

Myth Buster

The Role of Soul

It's no secret that we use food as a medication for our acute emotional problems. Stress at work directs us to the box of doughnuts. Crazy kids send us to the snack shelf. A downer of a day puts us incisor deep into a half-pint of Edy's. But to end our discussion of how emotions and obesity collide right there would be like saying that Band-Aids and ice packs can cure all diseases. The reality is that a good number of us with weight problems have emotional issues that run deeper than the middle of the Pacific, and we try to satisfy our need for fulfillment by self-medicating with food.

Being overweight for some people is about lack of self-esteem—about the petrifying fear that you don't deserve to be thin. How do we know this? Not through studies or research but through real-life living, through our patients, through eavesdropping on a cavalcade of doughnut addicts. Here, we have to momentarily step out of the safety zone of hard science into an area that's typically not studied by the white-coat-and-goggles set, because the mental, emotional, and deep psychological issues involved with obesity are simply very difficult to "prove" in a Western sense.

So let's start here: Many people—women especially—lack the self-esteem for waist control. (In fact, the most common reason a woman doesn't take care of her own health is because she puts others' needs before her own.) But let's dive deeper: What is self-esteem? Let's assume that our general sense of self-worth comes from two forces: overcoming obstacles and accomplishing some kind of goal. In the case of waist management, what happens if you don't overcome an obstacle (a box of Ding Dongs) and don't accomplish something (your goal weight by your high school reunion)? Yep, your self-esteem plummets faster than the ratings of summer reruns. To resurrect it, you need to find ways to overcome and accomplish—without making the very standards by which you measure your life unrealistic weights, measurements, and stricter-than-boot-camp eating habits.

Now let's step back to see how the relationship developed between the emotional need for self-esteem and the physical need for baggy clothes. In our youth, many of us long for something in our lives that's deeper and greater than our everyday reality of work, home, sleep, repeat for 29,930 days. Maybe it's religion, maybe a calling to help others, or maybe a belief that the world revolves around the Cubs. Whatever the "it" is matters less than the act of finding something that gives you a sense of purpose and builds your self-esteem.

There are some chemical and biological foundations for the feeling of soul-level satisfaction that comes with finding your own special "it." One theory is that oxytocin, a hormone that is elevated in women after childbirth, also makes you feel a sense of community and pleasure within your family, during a religious experience, or when you have an epiphany about your existence. When levels of oxytocin increase, you feel calm. Another hypothesis argues that your sense of self-esteem and well-being is influenced by the chemical nitric oxide (not to be confused with the laughing gas nitrous oxide). Traits such as hopefulness and optimism are associated with the release of nitric oxide through the body. In the same way, the release of nitric oxide may serve to help reduce feelings of anxiety and stress. But this chemical effect lasts for only seconds, so you need to continually stimulate your body with the right cerebral karma.

Whether it's the result of oxytocin, nitric oxide, or both, soul-level satisfaction exists at a biochemical level as well as in your perceptible life. It's your deeper drive—not the drive to fill the needs of your stomach or your muscles or even your mind, but the drive to fill the needs of your soul.

OK, OK, OK, we know what you're saying: What does your soul have to do with the fact that you just mainlined an entire can of whipped cream?

A lot.

Many of us, instead of addressing—or even acknowledging—this deeper longing and the restlessness we feel for never quite fulfilling it, try to fill the emptiness with food and drink. We use a temporary fix (General Tso's chicken) to satisfy not only the chemical cravings but also the permanent void caused by not satisfying our spiritual needs (the "it").

Sound familiar? We bet it does. Of all the actions you pursue, one of the few things you totally control is eating. You have the freedom to chow down on what you want, where you want, how you want, and whether or not you want to do it

with or without clothes on. Because of that freedom, eating makes you feel good. Funny thing, though; food is like the paint you use to cover cracks formed in the foundation of your house. Two coats of robin's-egg blue may hide the flaws temporarily, but they're never going to fix the real root of the problem. **YOU-reka!** If this is you, your cover-up (emotional eating) is what starts that tornadolike cycle that keeps you from ever feeling satisfied physically or emotionally. Ask yourself: Could this be part of a cycle?

* You long for something deeper . . .
* And when you can't find it, you eat to feel better . . .
* But you feel lousy because you gain weight . . .
* Then you tell yourself you don't deserve to be thin because you can't keep the weight off . . .
* Then your self-esteem drops further because you haven't overcome obstacles or accomplished what you want . . .
* So you self-medicate with food . . .
* And then you medicate yourself with food when you can't find "it" . . .

What's especially interesting is that many people who use food as a cover-up *want* to live life in the tornado. They're terrified by the thought of being thin. Being fat gives them an excuse to fail, an excuse to be depressed, an excuse to tango with a Twix bar.

As to that total control, that's wrong. The processed food companies have discovered that some of us are genetically predisposed to become addicted to sugar or saturated fat, in the same way we can get addicted to alcohol or smoking. We're also not in total control because we're at the mercy of relentless advertising, ubiquitous fast-food joints, and a host of other circumstantial pressures that conspire to make us lose control when it comes to food (more on this in Chapter 10).

Still, there's a reason why many of us end up in that tornado. We may do so because this thought process is a safe one and because our fat serves as a literal and metaphorical protective layer that keeps us from interacting with reality. We don't have to play the game of life if we're constantly making excuses for living on the bench. *If only I could lose weight, if only I could fit into that bikini, if only I could take a hike with the family without breathing heavier than a prison escapee.* Though some people may say that fat is a failure, the truth is that fat—for many of us—is a way of avoiding failure, because it's an excuse for never competing and engaging in life to begin with. (Remember, "if only" are the world's two most dangerous words since "jalapeño popper.")

If this description fits you, where do you go from here, short of self-injecting oxytocin or inhaling high doses of nitric oxide? It's not as if you can turn this page and all of your self-esteem issues will vanish faster than Coney Island hot dogs on the Fourth of July. It will take some time, but it also will take some awareness. We're not asking—or expecting—you to fix your self-esteem all at once; we're asking you to be aware that this deep, in-your-gut feeling might be the reason why our society's belts are now being used to measure out 5K road races. Simply realizing that you may use food as a psychological painkiller is part of the solution for helping you break the cycle. So let's just consider that the warranty on this emotional baggage has run out. Now that you know this baggage doesn't serve you, it's time you dropped it off at a psychological landfill and got rid of it for good.

YOU TIPS!

Work Foods in Your Favor. Foods have different effects on your stomach, your blood, and your brain. These are some of the nutrients that may influence your hunger and the brain chemicals that affect it:

❖ Turkey contains tryptophan, which increases serotonin to improve your mood, combat depression, and help you resist cravings for simple carbs. But turkey isn't the greatest source of tryptophan. Try chicken soup and dark chocolate (preferably not in the same bowl).

❖ Omega-3 fatty acids, which are found in salmon and trout, have long been known as brain boosters and cholesterol clearers, but they've also been shown convincingly to help fight depression in pregnant women. Depression, as we'll explain in the next chapter, contributes to hedonistic and emotional eating. Since many of us have low omega-3 intake, it might explain some other cases of depression as well.

Savor the Flavor. If you're going to eat something that's bad for you, enjoy it, savor it, roll it around your mouth. We suggest taking a piece of dark 70 percent cocoa chocolate and meditating—as a healthy stress reliever and as a way to reward yourself with something sweet. Try to find small ways to make yourself feel good and increase your serotonin, so you don't plummet and scavenge for anything you can get your hands on. It's OK to eat bad foods—every once in a while. It's not the first piece that's going to Shamu you; it's scarfing down the whole bag that will.

Go to Sleep. Getting enough sleep keeps you thin. **YOU-reka!** That's because when your body doesn't get the seven to eight hours of sleep it needs every night to get rejuvenated, the neurons in your brain don't secrete the normal amounts of serotonin or dopamine. To compensate, your body craves sugary foods that will give you an immediate release of serotonin and dopamine. Lack of sleep throws off your entire system, even increasing your levels of NPY, which increases your appetite. Lack of sleep can become an even bigger factor as you age. When you get older, the pineal gland in your brain produces less of the sleep hormone melatonin, resulting in a craving for carbohydrates.

Get Touched. Both on a physical level and on a psychological level, seek out positive interactions with other people. (Remember to make a phone call to your buddy at the end of your walk.) Evidence shows that increased amounts of oxytocin may decrease blood pressure and lower the effects of stress. It happens by influencing CCK, which helps control your appetite. If nothing else, it's a darn good reason to schedule a weekly massage. And it may help explain why things such as meditation and hypnosis—which are suspected to increase oxytocin levels—can be helpful with weight loss. Also, while there's as much information on this as on obesity in elite marathoners, the fear of touch and lack of oxytocin release may be one reason why abused individuals often have problems with waist management.

Have Sex. It's not so that you have somewhere else to put your hands other than a jar of peanut butter. The reason is that having sex does a couple things: One, it activates the satiety part of your brain, so you don't hunger for food as much. Two, it also stimulates the release of oxytocin, which can help fulfill emotional needs. So if you have sex as part of a healthy, monogamous relationship, it can help your dieting goals in the end (not to mention that sex obviously burns some calories too). Just no whipped cream, please.

Breathe Deep. If you can take long, deep breaths through your nose, you'll stimulate a short-lived gas called nitric oxide, which opens up your arteries and relaxes you. That can help keep you calm when you're facing tough emotional situations. Inhale a deep, long breath. Then, to exhale, suck your belly button toward your spine to push the diaphragm up and empty all the air from your lungs.

YOU Test

Why Ask Why?

The fact is, you *know.* You know if you need to lose weight. You can tell by the way you look, by the way you feel, and by whether your clothes feel tighter than an unopened pickle jar. But to be able to make changes—sustainable changes—you not only have to know *what* you've done to your figure. You also have to know *why* you're abusing your body, in the form of the emotional and physical triggers that led you to gain waist. To start, perform a self-administered "why" test—that is, keep asking yourself "why" questions about your weight until you come to the real answer about why you want to lose weight and why you can't. It may go something like this:

Why do I want to lose weight? Because I want to fit into my old pair of jeans.

Why do I want to fit into my old pair of jeans? Because I'd have more confidence.

Why do I want more confidence? Because I'll feel better trying to meet new people.

Why do I want to meet new people? Because I'm recently divorced and hoping to start a new relationship.

Why do I want to start a new relationship? Because I'm feeling lonely . . .

And that's likely to be where the thread of questions stops—where you can link the first question to the last answer. You want to lose weight because you're lonely, but the likely cause of your weight gain is the very same thing: that you're lonely.

Chapter 10

Surviving the Storm

Make Biology and Psychology Work in Your Favor

Diet Myths

- You can fight temptation with brute mental force.
- You need to change your behaviors to be successful.
- Habits were meant to be broken.

Thanks in large part to the hit book and movie, the phrase "perfect storm" is tossed around more than fresh pizza dough. Bloggers, experts, and cocktail-party goers use the phrase to describe anything and everything in which a couple of factors cause one heck of a mess.

Get called into a meeting minutes before a crucial deadline? "Sorry I was late tonight, honey, perfect storm at work."

An accident at the very place where three lanes of traffic turn into a one-lane construction zone? "A perfect %#%@%#^-ing storm on the I-99."

Baby's tummy doesn't agree with the buffet of milk, prunes, and yams? "Uh, darling, perfect storm in the Pampers. Wipes! Now!"

Same holds true in the world of obesity research. Plenty of people offhandedly refer to our growing waistlines as a perfect storm of many factors—the increase of processed foods and the fact that our butts spend more time glued to the couch than they do performing walking lunges. Combine the dozens of factors, and the storm suddenly becomes fierce and relentless and is not going away anytime soon.

But before you batten down the hatches, hang on a second. We believe that the beauty of this ubiquitous metaphor lies in its subtleties. And it's in those details that you will learn more about the storm—and, more important, how to get out of it. In this final chapter before we move onto the nuts and bolts of the *YOU: On a Diet* plan, we want to pull together some of our big ideas about how you can ride out the storm and set your life back on course. Once you understand how emotional, psychological, and biological factors all swirl around your cola-craving brain, you'll be equipped with a true life preserver for when you find yourself in trouble—as well as the shelter you need to avoid it in the first place.

The Storm of the Century: Obesity

By now you'd have to have your head buried in the sandwich not to know that obesity is our society's top health problem. It kills people both directly and

indirectly and puts a huge burden on the health care system. This storm's a category 5XL.

If you take the definition of a perfect storm, you'll realize that it's not just a bunch of bad stuff that happens all at once. Rather, a perfect storm is a concurrence of events that, taken individually, are relatively insignificant but when combined can have powerful consequences. And that's absolutely the case when it comes to fat. Just look at all the factors that contribute to our growing size—biological, environmental, political, emotional, and so on. No matter their origin, there are a lot of them. Consider these individual reasons:

- We're hardwired to want sugar, salt, and fat. And they're readily available in every fast food joint and packaged food, even if you don't realize it.
- Our bodies store fat to protect against famine.
- We have mirror neurons that cause us to mimic the behavior of others (good when learning from Mom in the wild; not so good when the gang orders a large pepperoni pie).
- Our moods and social situations can dictate cravings. We feast on cream-filled goodies when we're stressed. When the family gets together on Sunday, it's a calzone feast.
- Junk food ads are all over the place (those mirror neurons kick in, making us crave what we see).
- The mass production of high-fructose corn syrup has made it easier to gobble down pounds and pounds of sugar every year in the plethora of processed foods that we eat.
- We have more desk jobs these days, keeping us inactive for a better part of the day.
- There are fast-food joints and convenience stores at every corner (one study even found that high schoolers whose school is within a quarter mile of fast-food places have a BMI higher than those who aren't as close).

- Schools and offices are littered with vending machines that are filled with foods that have empty carbohydrates.
- Our kids don't walk to school as they used to a few decades ago, and 40,000 elementary schools have eliminated recess from the schoolday, decreasing children's total time of activity.
- We've become a car culture—housing developments are often far from shops, and many neighborhoods don't even have sidewalks.

We—and we're sure you—could go on and on with other reasons as well.

Each factor by itself is no big deal. Put them all together, and this button-popping storm can destroy every organ in its path.

Why do we tell you this? Sorry to say, it's not to get you off the hook. You can't just chalk up your muffin top to muffin tops and call it a day. Our point is that we know darn well how hard it is to lose weight, maintain a healthy weight and waist size, and confront all of the challenges you face every day. We also know that it's impossible to outbrute, outpunch, and outwill those forces. Anybody who remembers the movie and the powerful wave that doomed the ship knows that you can't fight a perfect storm; you can't outslug it, and you can't stand stoically in the face of it. Instead, you have to get out of that evil sucker. A rowboat will get clobbered in a perfect storm no matter what measures it takes. But if you know the factors contributing to the storm and can track the storm to avoid it in the first place, you can beat it.

And that's the whole point. In order to ride out a perfect storm, you have to change your environment from stormy seas to calm ones. The rest of this chapter will give you the ability to do just that.

A Change of Attitude

If we've learned anything from the perfect storm, it's that the one thing we need to change is our approach to dieting. The way to outsmart the storm—the way to handle all of these factors that we've discussed over the previous nine and a half chapters—is to change your attitude about your attitudes.

Change . . . The Environment, Not the Behavior. In previous diet attempts, you may have sworn to make all kinds of behavioral changes: Not gonna snack, not gonna have dessert, not gonna eat bread, not gonna eat after 9 p.m., not gonna eat out. That's all well and good, especially if you snack on chips, have chocolate death for dessert, and eat 8,000 calories at the Big Butt Buffet. The savvier approach, though, is to realize that some of our behavioral urges are indeed hardwired and trying to suppress them is a recipe for failure. Face it, we need to eat every few hours, and we do have dopamine receptors that cause us to crave certain foods, such as sweets. So what should you do? Don't fight your biology; rather change the environment to make your biology work for you, not against you. In practical terms, that means you need to change your environment so you're less likely to be caught in a storm. Keep fruit in your pantry instead of chips. Meet your friends at a juice bar rather than a breakfast place known for its mile-high pancakes. You can't eat them if they're not on the menu.

And when you eat out? Choose a fish place rather than a burger joint. What's so wrong with a wonderful piece of grilled mustard-crusted salmon and a side of steamed veggies with garlic? While there's nothing earth-shattering about snacking on fruit or ordering a lean piece of fish, the aha moment comes when you learn not to fight the wave, by denying yourself the pleasure of dining out, for example, but to ride the wave, by adjusting the environment to your behaviors.

Fundamentally, you want to make it easier to do the right thing. Make the tough decisions when you are in a cold, calculating state rather than when you are in the heat of ravaging your pan-try. Choose what you're going to eat in the supermarket— actually, before you go to the supermarket (make a list in advance, stick to it, and *never* shop on an empty stomach)— rather than when the fridge door is off its hinges as you scavenge for food. By planning ahead, instead of finding leftover cheesecake in there, you'll find a bunch of fresh grapes. And make a workout (such as ours below) so seamless to the flow of your life that all the usual ex-cuses become even more embarrassing.

Change . . . Your Buddy System. As we discussed in the last chapter, we tend to put a lot of blame on ourselves for being overweight. We blame our inability to resist foods, and we carry that burden all by ourselves. Of course, every individual has the power to steer herself to make the right choices, but here's a concept we're betting you've never heard quite this way: Obesity is an in-fectious disease. No, no, no, it's not as if anyone's going to sneeze cheeseburger bits into your arteries. Nevertheless, there is a major infectious component of obesity: It spreads through social networks. Just consider one study that shows that if one of two friends is obese, the other's chance of becoming obese increases by 171 percent.

That's why it's crucial to consider what you surround yourself with—in terms of both food and people. If you socialize with the every-day-is-a-reason-to-eat-lasagna crowd, chances are you're going to be knee deep in ricotta without much chance of digging yourself out (except via fork). But if you're surrounding yourself with the let's-run-a-5K set, bingo, you're going to be spending more time running around the neighborhood and less time running to the convenience store. Does that mean we suggest you ditch any overweight friends? Of course not. But maybe it means you shouldn't schedule as many lunch dates with that person, or maybe you should become the ringleader to start a weekly hike along the local na-ture trail. Healthy living is as infectious as unhealthy living. And you can decide which bug you want to catch.

Change . . . Your Definition of Habits. Unfortunately, we've slipped into a cycle where we automatically think that habits are bad—and need to be broken. Smoking? Need to stop. Eating ice cream at eleven every night? Cut it out. In addition to breaking bad habits, we feel pressure to establish new ones: visiting the gym every day, chewing each bite twenty times. But the formation of good habits and the elimination of bad habits work best when you focus not on formation or elimination but on substitution. Habits are the mind's way of establishing a behavior without having to think about it. So take our discussion about changing your environment and apply it here. If you need to have a sweet late at night, forget the full-fat ice cream and really savor a small piece of dark chocolate. Or if you have to have something salty with your meals, sub out the fries for edamame. It's extremely difficult to substitute inaction for action; it's much easier to make a trade—one action for another. Before you know it, your new habits will be formed, ingrained, and automatic.

Change . . . Your Power Structure. You know who holds all the cards in your food-versus-you relationship? Yep. Tootsie rolls. And whipped cream. And fried eggplant. And anything else that constantly tempts you and teases you. Without sounding too much like a wrestling ring announcer, it's time to take on these temptations and change the power structure in this relationship. C'mon, a bag of chips is stronger than you? The truth is that feeling powerless over food is a superficial emotion that actually covers up many other deeper ones that are really frustrating you—whether you're feeling unsure, unsafe, angry, or empty. The minute you cross the line between seeing food as a source of energy and seeing it as a security blanket, you're in deep trouble. Remember how hard it was to give up your blankie?

By making yourself dependent on food for emotional support, rather than your relationships or your soul, you abdicate your power to control your eating. So we urge you to ask yourself some questions about your hunger: Do you demand immediate gratification from food because you are powerless in other parts of your life? Are you even aware of what you're eating, or is eating more like popping pain medication? The medical community can't concoct a magic bullet that dives into this deeper, emotional level of eating. And frankly, we're not even sure the words we (or anyone) say can inspire this change. This change is an internal one—but one that has some pretty major external benefits as well.

When you feel powerless in all other aspects of your life, the only remaining area that remains in your control is how you put food into your mouth, so this is how you express your desire for power. That's why telling people not to eat removes their one remaining pillar of independence, so they rebel by eating even more. So what you need to start doing is seeking power in your life—whether it's through spirituality, work, or even relationships. That way, you take the power away from the knife and fork and put it back into your heart and soul.

YOU TIPS!

Bust Your Desire. Whether in relationships, techie toys, or food, we all know how desire works: Want it, gotta have it, hurts so bad if you don't, so you want it even more. It's one thing if the other person isn't interested in you or the big-screen TV is too expensive; it makes it a lot easier to handle a letdown. But when the marshmallow spread is in the pantry, there's no need for a letdown. Just gobble away. So part of the trick for managing a perfect storm is learning the ways to adjust your desire, so you don't have those strong-pulling temptations. Of course, the main way to do that is to get harmful foods out of sight (and record your favorite TV shows so you can fast-forward through the food commercials!).

Delay the Game. Most hedonistic decisions are made on impulse. Tell yourself that you're going to wait until later in the day for your treat, and wouldn't you know it, most likely that desire will pass.

Pay It Forward. One of the big issues pertaining to so-called willpower is how you balance two competing forces—immediate gratification from the chips versus the delayed gratification of a better bikini body (not to mention a longer life!). That's a tough one, because the immediate gratification almost always wins. Instead, try flipping the immediate gratification into a long-term consequence and turning the delayed gratification into an immediate, visual picture. Think hard about the negative consequences of consuming that bowl of chips (picture a clogged artery; recall poor Uncle Joe, who died of a heart attack at fifty). At the same time, try to visualize yourself with the bikini body you desire. To make the impact even more immediate, stick a photo of yourself from the days when you had a bikini body to the door of your fridge.

Play Dominoes. Just one chip. Just one brownie. Just one more slice of pumpkin pie. Can't hurt a thing. And you're probably right—in many cases, just one won't hurt. But few people stop at one, and therein lies the problem. Instead of considering each temptation as being "just one," reframe it as one of many. So the cost of a simple dessert may be not 250 calories but 250 calories on top of the 250 you had on Tuesday on top of the 400 you had on Sunday. It's just one more entry on the dessert ledger that may ultimately total several thousand calories. Not so easy to rationalize when you think of it that way, huh?

Recognize the Addiction, and Enlist Your Mob. If your genes predispose you to be more likely to be one of the 50 percent or so of us who will become addicted to sugar or to saturated fat, the only way to avoid the addiction is not to have them near. That means whoever stocks your cupboards, fridge, hiding places, and so on, has to have your back—you need your mob to help you. Together, you have to make a family or group commitment to avoid the temptations that food companies are trying to entice you with. It isn't possible for you to diet smart with those foods beckoning you. You need your partners to help you change your habits, not help you feed your addictions.

Get Lost in Your Mind. Whenever you feel the urge to eat—no, don't sit down. Instead, walk around the block and think about your life and what's driving you to pick up a fork or open the fridge. Would you shove that stuff into a friend's or family member's body? It's OK to cry, it's OK to think, it's OK to meditate. In fact, maybe you can learn from your pain, not make it worse by thinking you can suffocate it with three extra inches of abdominal fat. For some, meditation or prayer enhances their power to satisfy the subconscious drive they have to eat.

Walk This Way. The root of the YOU physical activity plan is a minimum of thirty minutes of walking a day (broken up into three segments of ten minutes each if you need to)—and telling somebody about it after you're done (yes, every day, no excuses). You will do it not only for the physical effects but also (even more, actually) for the psychological effects. Remember what self-control (and esteem) comes from: the ability to overcome obstacles and achieve goals. Walking accomplishes both. **YOU-reka!** Walk for thirty; it's easy, doable, and maintainable—and it's a first step out of the tornado and back into the flow of life. A lot of people feel they haven't earned the right to lose weight. Walking every day earns you that right, and telling someone about it helps you feel proud of your accomplishment.

Plan. The big decisions about eating need to be made in the supermarket rather than your kitchen. Leave the storm brewing in the store. Don't create a home environment that's filled with junk, and it'll be easier to eat right and well. Shopping tip: shop the edges of the supermarket (rather than the middle aisles, where more of the packaged/processed food is sold). You can also make it a goal to find new places to shop so you are tempted by fresh locally grown veggies rather than salted pork rinds behind the soda drinks at the checkout counter where you buy gas.

Change the Temptation. Eating out at a colorful fast-food joint is like rowing out to a hurricane. The savory foods will flip you like a tidal wave. So the first trick to eating out is choosing a place that offers many healthy options (or will make them for you). You should be especially aware of danger zones—such as the first ten minutes of the meal (order veggies and olive oil, instead of bread) and the last ten minutes (have your glass of wine at the end of the meal, rather than a slab of chocolate mousse cake).

Make It Easy to Exercise. One of the reasons we find it so hard to be active is that we don't have easy access to activity. But how about taking your stationary bike out of the humid garage and putting it in front of the TV, so you can get thirty to sixty minutes in during your favorite show? (Plus, it'll keep you from eating mindlessly while watching TV.) Or changing your habits so that you do one exercise (such as an abs move or squats) during commercial breaks? Or keeping a set of dumbbells at work and doing an upper-body exercise for thirty seconds on the hour every hour? There are lots of ways to seamlessly incorporate activity into your life; all you have to do is be a little creative, and you'll find yourself easily substituting a good habit for a bad one.

The Personality Test

Yes, you could make the argument that those marshmallow-covered corn dogs at the carnival have a little something to do with your about-to-burst waistband. The more likely saboteur? Your excuses. Here, take this personality test to see what attitudes and behaviors may be preventing you from losing weight and getting healthy (Dr. Robert Kushner's full test is available at www.diet.com). Add up your check marks and see how your attitude toward eating and exercise influences the size of your waist.

Sound Like You?	Then Check Here	Because It Means You're a . . .
EATING PATTERNS		
"Day to day, I change my meal patterns more often than Martha Stewart changes fabric patterns."		**Meal Skipper:** You skip meals and have no pattern or routine to when you eat.
"I eat like a sardine during the day and like a humpback at night."		**Nighttime Nibbler:** You consume 50 percent or more of your calories between dinner and bedtime.
"The place I'm most likely to eat: one that has a waiter, a drive-through lane, or a delivery dude."		**Convenient Diner:** You're a brand-name eater. All of your meals are packaged, bagged, microwavable, or frozen.
"Fruits and vegetables have the same taste appeal as, oh, sewage."		**Fruitless Feaster:** With few exceptions, you're all about meat and potatoes (or pasta, bread, and desserts).

Sound Like You?	Then Check Here	Because It Means You're a . . .
EATING PATTERNS		
"I need a dietary restraining order. If there's any food within fifty feet of me, I'll eat it."		**Steady Snacker:** Besides your regular three meals, you snack anytime you come near food.
"My plate's so high, it breaks at least three city codes."		**Hearty Portioner:** You eat a lot, and you eat it quickly, whether it's healthy or not.
"I eat salads when I'm out with friends, then raid the pantry when I'm home."		**Swing Eater:** You eat a strict diet of good foods, but fall off the wagon and then overeat bad foods.
EXERCISE PATTERNS		
"I enjoy being physically active as much as I do making paper-clip chains."		**Couch Champion:** You don't like to sweat, and you don't really like any physical activity.
"I don't exercise because everyone else at the gym looks like a supermodel or Schwarzenegger compared to me."		**Uneasy Participant:** You hate exercising in public because of your body image.

(continued)

Sound Like You?	Then Check Here	Because It Means You're a . . .
EXERCISE PATTERNS		
"I like exercise, but if I have to miss it, I'm like a crashed NASCAR— it's hard for me to get back on track."		**All-or-Nothing Doer:** You work out hard for a few days or weeks, then stop and do nothing for even longer.
"For the past three years, I've been doing the exact same workout without changing it a bit."		**Set-Routine Repeater:** You're on a fixed exercise routine but aren't able to lose weight because your body has adjusted to the routine.
"I'm afraid I'll get hurt on the wrong end of the exercise machine, worsen my condition, or have a heart attack if I exercise hard."		**Tender Bender:** You either have an injury that prevents you from exercising or worry that you may suffer one because you're out of shape.
"I'd like to exercise, but I barely have enough time to shave, let alone step on a treadmill for twenty minutes."		**Rain-Check Athlete:** You're so busy and frustrated that you can't make time to exercise.

Sound Like You?	Then Check Here	Because It Means You're a . . .
COPING PATTERNS		
"Ahhh! I find food as comforting as a down pillow."		**Emotional Eater:** You eat when you're stressed, anxious, tired, or depressed.
"As for my clothes, I've got a bigger cover-up plan than a criminal—I'm ashamed of my body and how I look."		**Self-Scrutinizer:** You feel ashamed of your body and have trouble separating body image from self-esteem, and that affects your day-to-day decision making.
"I'm the Socrates of diets—I spend more time thinking about what I need to do to lose weight than actually doing it."		**Persistent Procrastinator:** You know the importance of losing weight and say you want to lose, but you never seem to make it happen because something always gets in the way.
"I'm juggling more than a circus performer. Last on my list? Time for myself."		**People Pleaser:** You are a good-natured person with responsibility and commitment to family, friends, and coworkers, but you always put them ahead of you.
"My life is moving fast, my to-do list is the length of a novel, and I can't find the brakes."		**Fast Pacer:** You multitask and don't take the time to think or plan how to improve your lifestyle.

(continued)

Sound Like You?	Then Check Here	Because It Means You're a . . .
COPING PATTERNS		
"I've tried everything to lose weight, but nothing ever works. Nothing! Nada! Zippo!"		**Doubtful Dieter:** You say you've tried everything and nothing works, so you develop a self-defeating attitude.
"My work? Great. Family life? A blast. I expect the same amazing results from my weight-loss plan—but my progress is never enough."		**Overreaching Achiever:** You're successful at home and work—and expect the same in your weight loss. But you never feel satisfied, and your high expectations make you feel frustrated and discouraged.

Adapted from *Dr. Kushner's Personality Type Diet* (St. Martin's Press) with permission.

Check Yourself: Add up your scores and get a score for food (eating), mood (coping), and movement (exercise). The dimension with the highest score is the category where you need to focus. A score of 4 or more in any one category means you need to focus on that area no matter what. So, if your food score is 6, mood score is 4, and movement score is 2, then you need to focus on food and mood, but don't forget your thirty-minute daily walk—no excuses.

YOU Test

Don't Avoid This Test

It shouldn't come as much of a surprise that avoiders typically have feelings of inadequacy and are hypersensitive to being negatively evaluated. Identifying with four or more of the following statements means you have strong avoidance tendencies.

❖ I avoid work activities that involve close interpersonal contact—not because of my deodorant level but because I fear criticism or rejection.

❖ Unless I know I'm going to be liked, I'm hesitant to get involved in relationships.

❖ When I'm in social situations, I feel more inept than an umpire with a detached retina.

❖ My shirt's not coming off unless the lights are going off.

❖ All of my social situations feel like high school; I'm preoccupied with being criticized or rejected.

❖ I don't engage in risky activities because my biggest fear is the risk of embarrassment.

❖ In new interpersonal situations, I feel the same way I feel at the beach: shy and inhibited, and I would do anything to be somewhere else.

Part 4

The YOU Diet
and Activity Plan

The Eating and Activity Plan
That Will Become Lifelong and Automatic

Chapter 11

Make a YOU-Turn

How to Change What You Thought You Knew about Dieting—and Change Your Life for Good

By now, you don't have to be Marie Curie to know the power of chemicals and realize that you're the clear-cut underdog if you try to take them on with brute force. You know that chemical changes in your brain and body play a big role in dictating everything from your actions to your emotions. But you can alter your chemistry in more subtle ways. For instance, take the act of positive thinking and interacting in social groups. There's evidence that those kinds of actions change serotonin levels to make you feel better and reduce appetite. That's really how you should be using your mind and all the intangible concepts like willpower, discipline, and motivation—to complement the chemical changes you're making in other, more concrete ways. They're the things that will help you overcome the occasional butter-laced obstacles that you'll face.

To show how you can use emotions to work for you as you're about to embark on the YOU Diet, let's step back into the mind of a typical dieter—let's say a woman. One of the psychological realities of being overweight is that many dieters—that is, people who know they need to lose weight and want to—are somewhat comfortable with their bodies. Yes, that body may be twenty, thirty, forty, or more pounds heavier than it was the day she turned eighteen. But maybe she's used to post-pregnancy weight, she enjoys Friday lunches with her friends, or she can't face a total wardrobe overhaul. **YOU-reka!** It's who she is—and she's more comfortable living her life at that level than going through the struggles and hard work (not to mention the guilt and shame) of trying to shed weight.

So the dieter has two choices: She can remain on top of the hill where she's currently standing and (relatively) comfortable. Or she can try to get to the top of that beautiful mountain in the distance—the ultimate destination for all of her weight-loss goals. There, on the mountain, she'll find smaller sizes, leaf-size bikinis, fewer doctor visits, and probably fewer health risks and an improved quality of life. Maybe that's where she'd *ideally* like to be. But the problem is that there's no easy bridge from the comfort zone of the hill to the peak of the mountain. To get there, she must travel all the way down from her current comfort level, hit some rough terrain along the way, and then climb, climb, climb her way up this

Figure 11.1 **The Right Route** Descending into the valley can make the trip up to the promised land daunting. Dieting smartly will build you the bridge you need to transition to your playing weight.

seemingly insurmountable incline. So she asks: Is it worth it to go through all the hard work to reach the top of the ideal mountain, or am I comfortable enough with where I'm standing right now?

That's how the dieter thinks after trying it once or twice. It's easier to stay at the current comfort level at a less than ideal size than it is go through a short period of somewhat uncomfortable change—doing things like developing a physical activity program, or avoiding drive-throughs, or changing menus, or going through periods of irritability and hunger. For many dieters, that path is hard to navigate, so they return—very quickly—to the original hill, the original place of comfort (often it is an even wider hill, psychologically and waist-size-wise). The fact is, most people aren't willing to face the challenges of finding the mountain peak, even if the peak reveals such vistas as better health and higher self-esteem.

So what we have to do is build that bridge—that bridge of smart food choices, of exercise discipline, or working smart, not hard. And we have to support the bridge with strategies and tactics that allow you to make wrong steps without falling completely into the abyss of chocolate nougat. How do we do it? By getting started. Right now. With small actions that lead to big changes.

Sometimes, we think the motivation to start a program has to come first, but oftentimes, the motivation comes after the action: Make a small change (be it walking thirty minutes a day, or eating nuts before dinner to keep you full), and suddenly you feel motivated to make more changes—and to succeed.

The point is that we want you to make it across the bridge as painlessly as possible, by giving you the tools to avoid the uncomfortable feelings associated with dieting, with hunger, with evil scales. The journey to the top of the mountain may feel like a little bit of a climb, but it shouldn't feel like you're starting way down there at the bottom. We'll build that bridge with these strategies and our YOU Diet and YOU Activity Plan.

YOU TIPS!

Adopt the YOU-Turn Mantra. If you've ever ridden in a car with a GPS satellite navigation system, you know how it works. Plug in your destination, and the system—using satellites to plot your current and final points—tells you exactly what to do when. Turn left after 400 feet. Stay straight. Get in right lane. But let's say you make a mistake and miss a turn or turn onto the wrong street. The GPS doesn't berate you, doesn't scold you, doesn't tell you that you might as well drive off a cliff, since you made a mistake and missed First Avenue. Instead, all it says, very politely, is this: "At the next available moment, make an authorized U-turn." **YOU-reka!** The GPS recognizes the mistake matter-of-factly and simply guides you back onto the right road. The GPS allows for mistakes and tries to help you correct them. That's the kind of mentality we want you to have. You're going to make wrong turns. You're going to turn left at the hot dogs, make a right at the blueberry pie, and occasionally merge onto the interstate of banana-nut pancakes with a side order of sausage patties. Does that mean you should steer off the dietary cliff and fall into the fatty crevasse of destructive eating? Of course not. What it means is that you need to pay closer attention to the road signs and the instructions about how to make it to your final destination. It also means that you can't beat yourself up with a basket of croissants every time you lick a little whipped cream off your finger. So what you're going to do—right now—is acknowledge that you will face obstacles. And instead of falling into the avoidant and defeatist mentality by drop-kicking healthy eating the moment you make one bad choice, you will confront it. How? By repeating the YOU Diet Mantra:

"At the next available moment, make an authorized YOU-Turn."

"At the next available moment, make an authorized YOU-Turn."

"At the next available moment, make an authorized YOU-Turn."

Get back on the right road.

What kills any regimen of healthy eating isn't the occasional dessert or slice of pizza; it's the cascade of behavior that happens after the initial indulgence. Use this mantra to steer yourself back—to understand that you can make mistakes but that you can correct and overcome them with some nonjudgmental coaxing. Why does it work?

❖ It gives you a mental crutch to carry when you're faced with difficult eating situations.

❖ It reminds you to be confident, to be positive, to know that the harm isn't in the first mistake, it's in not figuring out how to deal with it.

❖ It reinforces the grand scheme of this whole plan—the reason why you're trying to manage your waist. The long-term benefits to your health far outweigh what you're giving up in your Pyrex dish.

Know Your Fighting Weight. In all likelihood, the most common way you've measured your so-called dietary success or failure is by pounds lost. If you've lost down to your target weight, then you've won. If not, you've lost. But the reality is that over the long term, all of us will intermittently gain and lose small amounts of weight, even when we're trying to lose it. For one, our water weight often fluctuates depending on what we're eating. The reason why so many low-carb dieters lose weight fast is because the lack of carbohydrates causes them to lose glycogen stores from their muscles, and with this loss of glycogen comes a loss of a lot of water; as soon as they reinstate the carbs, the glycogen comes back to the muscles and attracts the water. That adds the pounds right back. So the first five to eleven pounds of weight loss on a low-carb diet is the fake loss due to a temporary loss of water.

Instead of tracking your weight by a single goal weight of, say, 145 pounds, what you're going to do is pick your weight class. You're going to pick a range of weight that's comfortable for you—say, 142 to 148 pounds (or 31 inches to 33 inches of waist size). When you divulge your weight to someone (not that anyone will be asking), it should never be in one number; you need to think of your weight as an ideal range. For one thing, this allows for the natural fluctuations that occur. For another, it also does something even more crucial to your psychological success: It stops you from focusing on some arbitrary number that promotes the idea of all-or-nothing success or failure. And it puts your mind in the right programming mode—to remind yourself that your body is supposed to change.

Stay Accountable. You can use your weight range to tell when you're pushing the upper boundaries of your ideal weight/waist with periodic checks using a measurement too—be it a tape measure around your waist, a scale, or, hey, how about a plastic waistband that you keep around your waist to alert you when you're getting too big, like a large version of one of those Lance bracelets? Whatever your accountability tool, we suggest checking it every Saturday around midday to keep yourself honest with your weight and waist class. Think of your body as a rubber band. Stretch it a little, and it can certainly snap back into shape. But once you stretch it too much, it's going to lose its shape and make it more difficult—if not impossible—to return to the original size.

Plan to Fail—and Develop Contingency Plans for When You Do. We keep tires in our trunks in case one goes flat. We keep candles in our drawers in case the power goes out. We keep backups of files in case our computers crash. (And some of us wish we backed them up more often.) And that's good; contingency plans give you the mental assurance that you'll be able to adapt to unexpected crises. But the one area where we don't make backup plans is in our diets. We eat broccoli, fish, and fruit for three days, then splurge on a double-fat burger with supersize fries on the fourth. For so many of us, that's grounds for euthanizing the diet right away—putting us right back in touch with our three favorite food groups of chocolate, chips, and chocolate chips.

Instead, start carrying a dietary contingency plan—a diet emergency pack for those times when you may experience a crash-causing blowout in one of your meals. Follow this three-step contingency plan to help you cope with occasional mishaps and potential catastrophes. Exercise it the moment you feel you're deviating from your waist management plan:

❖ **Mental:** Say the YOU-Turn mantra ten times. Let the mantra remind you that it's OK to stray occasionally, that you can take control of the situation and steer yourself back, and that the positive reinforcement and confidence that come with overcoming challenges will give you the mental strength of a tank. Plus, the relaxing aspect of it will help influence your serotonin levels in your favor. And it will help distract you, which is what you need when you're beelining toward the bonbons.

❖ **Physical:** Do a yoga pose or try the hippie stretch (see the YOU Workout). We suggest the downward dog pose (see below), balancing your weight on your hands and feet with your butt hiked toward the ceiling in an inverted *V*. Not only will it help you refocus, give you a few moments to take deep breaths, and remind you of your goals, but it will also work because it's sort of difficult to eat when you're upside down.

❖ **Nutritional:** Keep in your fridge a container of baby carrots, celery, or any crisp vegetable of your choice, or a favorite apple type (yes, types matter to our individual taste choices). Carrots and apples are perfect antistress foods because, one, they have just a tinge of sweetness to satisfy that craving, and, two, they give you something to crunch into at times when you really want to sink your teeth into your boss's neck. This will become your turn-to food—that is, the food you turn to when you feel angry, frustrated, mad, sad, or upset—as well as the one that will help you feel better about the nutritional mistakes you may have just made.

Many of us take the mental approach that the only way to "do a diet" is to do it perfectly. But that's a setup for failure and shame, because it never works. Success comes with persistence—persistence to overcome challenges, persistence to see the big picture, persistence to work hard enough in the beginning of the plan so that good habits become automatic.

Make It Automatic. Think of your waist management plan a little like the way you'd drive to work. Maybe the first day on a new job in a new city, you took the highway. But then you found out it was more clogged than Rapunzel's shower drain. So you experimented with a few back roads, shortcuts, and bypasses until you found the very best way to get to work. Now you don't need a map; you do it automatically, and you don't spend a single nanosecond worrying about what turn you take. It's automatic—just the way your approach to eating should be. When you're starting out on this plan, you'll experiment with different routes, get stuck in a few traffic jams, maybe even get a little lost along the way. But if you stick with it and find the right course, you'll automate your habits, regulate your chemicals, and make eating the easiest trip you've ever made.

How do we make it automatic? By using the tools that we've outlined in the book. (For those of you who've skipped ahead, the major ones are listed here.)

The 99-Second Edition

In the dietary gates and can't wait to start the race? Then skim through this cheat sheet of the YOU strategies—big and small—that you'll adopt and automate as your new eating, activity, emotional, and behavioral plan. It's the path to your new life. And your new body.

The Major YOU Principles YOU Need to . . .

Choose elegance over force.

Dietary battles are won not when you work hard, but when you work smart.

Make your eating plan automatic.

Train yourself over fourteen days to make appropriate choices, and you'll reprogram your body so that you never have to sweat over what you're eating again.

Remember that waist is more important than weight.

Belly fat is one of the strongest predictors of health risks associated with obesity. Ditch the scale in favor of the tape measure.

Know your body.

Understand the beauty of your internal organs to appreciate what you can do to influence them.

Stay satisfied.

To lose weight, you need to eat.

Add support.

Enlist a friend, family member, or new cyber buddy as your partner.

Know that it's OK to make mistakes.

As long as you quickly get back on the right road, you won't travel too far down the wrong one.

Eating Strategies for YOU

❖ To help make eating automatic, pick at least one meal a day to alter and have the same few food choices every day for all other meals.

❖ Eat throughout the day so that you're constantly satisfied. The less you eat, the more likely you are to sink into starvation mode and make your body want to store fat.

❖ Inspect food labels. Limit saturated fats to less than 4 grams per meal, and avoid all trans fats. Don't buy foods where high-fructose corn syrup (HFCS), or another simple sugar, is more than 4 grams per meal, or one of the first five ingredients. You're avoiding simple sugars in foods not just because of the calories but because they induce highs and lows in blood sugar that put you into a cycle of craving more high-calorie foods, and they cause atherosclerosis. They turn on genes that age you and turn off genes that keep you younger and decrease aging (see page 129).

❖ Eat foods with fiber, healthy fats (monounsaturated and polyunsaturated), whole grain carbohydrates, and protein, as well as fruits and vegetables. Eat a little healthy fat before your meal (such as one handful of nuts; that's six walnut halves) to allow the satiety signal to go from your brain to your stomach so you don't overeat during your meal. Eat fiber in the morning to help control afternoon cravings. Eat anti-inflammatory foods to help counteract the effects of obesity. Anti-inflammatory foods include green tea, omega-3 fatty acids (found in fish, chia seeds, canola oil, and walnuts), coffee, vegetables, and fruit.

❖ Drink a glass or two of water before you eat. Your perception of hunger signals may actually be thirst signals.

❖ Keep on hand emergency foods and items that can help you kill cravings, like V8, carrot sticks, an apple, or even Listerine breath strips.

❖ Keep a log of how hungry you are on a scale of one to seven (one being famished, seven being gorged). Try to stay in the three to four range at all times by eating moderate amounts of food throughout the day.

❖ Two spices have been shown to aid in waist management: red pepper and cinnamon.

❖ Realize that it's OK to make mistakes. The key is getting back on the right road, not beating yourself up over them. Use YOU-Turns to right yourself as soon as possible.

❖ Use nine-inch plates for meals. Smaller dinner plates equal smaller portions.

Activity Strategies for YOU

❖ Walk thirty minutes a day every day. No excuses. Then call your support partner after you do it.

❖ Start a strength-training program focusing on core muscles (legs, abdominals, and upper body) in the form of twenty minutes two or three days a week.

❖ Stretch every day after physical activity to keep your muscles loose and pliable, to help you prevent injury.

❖ Do this exercise any time you want: Suck in your belly button and squeeze your butt as if you're pulling up tight jeans. It helps with posture and strengthens your abdominals.

❖ Get up and go. Anytime you can move at work or at home, do it.

Who Woulda Thunk It Strategies for YOU

❖ Get seven to eight hours of sleep a night. Lack of sleep promotes hedonistic eating as you search for something to boost chemicals in your brain. Your brain needs sleep to regenerate these chemicals, and sugary foods help release the diminished supply of chemicals you have, to make up for the lack of sleep.

❖ Play video games. Keeping your hands full keeps them off the coconut muffins.

❖ Have healthy, safe, monogamous sex. Satisfying one appetite center of your brain can help satisfy another.

Measurement Strategies for YOU

❖ Measure your waist. Ideal is 32½ inches or less for women, and 35 inches or less for men.

❖ Ask your family what your parents and grandparents looked like when they were eighteen, to give you a sense of what your ideal body should look like.

❖ Get tested: blood pressure, cholesterol, blood sugar, thyroid hormone, and C-reactive protein (a marker of inflammation), and certain additional hormone levels, depending on your weight situation.

Medicine Cabinet Strategies for YOU

❖ Take two aspirin (162 milligrams), 600 milligrams of DHA, 1,200 IU of vitamin D3, and a probiotic every day to decrease arterial inflammation and health risks associated with obesity. Consult your doctor first.

❖ Take 600 milligrams of calcium citrate, 200 milligrams of magnesium, and half of an age-specific multivitamin (the last as an insurance policy against an inadequate diet) in the morning and again at night.

❖ See your doctor about prescription drugs associated with weight loss if you hit a waist plateau on the plan (see appendix).

❖ The following supplements have been shown to have effectiveness in some aspect of waist management: chromium picolinate, grapefruit oil, Garcinia, Hoodia, 5-HTP, L-carnitine, coenzyme Q10, turmeric, jojoba beans, simmondsin. Consult your doctor about which ones may be appropriate for you.

Chapter 12

The YOU Activity Plan

Physical Strategies for Waist Management

The world has all kinds of gyms: home gyms, hotel gyms, female-friendly gyms, muscle-head gyms, and gyms that look like spas. Though any of them may be perfectly decent places to pump your muscles, work your heart, or admire spandex, there's one gym that gives you absolutely everything you need:

Your own body. Your body can be your best gym.

Really, all you need are two things: your body and the knowledge of how to use it. No barbells, no dumbbells, no balls, no ankle weights, no machines, no infomercial equipment—just your body. By learning and using a plan that requires only your physiological barbells, you have all the tools you need to make exercise easy and automatic. That's because:

- ❖ Your body costs nothing to use.
- ❖ You eliminate the best excuses for avoiding exercise, like driving hassles or needing to buy equipment.
- ❖ Using only your body, you can work all of the muscles necessary for effective waist management—and that's for both beginning and advanced exercisers.

In fact, you can complete an entire workout that hits all three areas of activity—strength, flexibility, and cardiovascular—in one easy twenty-minute workout three times a week (or do it in smaller bits for almost as much benefit). And you can change that workout no matter what your skill level, simply by making small exercise adjustments to perfectly match your abilities.

Before we detail the plan, remember why you're exercising: Adding lean muscle through strength training, working your heart through cardiovascular training, and flexing your body with stretching help burn fat, reduce stress, improve health, and decrease your waist size. All without bulking you up to the size of a Miami condo. The other point of this program: You'll focus on your foundation muscles—the major muscles most responsible for fat burning, waist trimming, and injury prevention. Those key groups: your thighs, chest, back, and abdominals.

Whether you're a newbie to exercise or an old pro, the YOU plan starts with walking for thirty minutes a day—no matter what. Only when you've mastered that, no matter how long it takes—every day, no excuses—should you begin the rest of this program. Walking thirty minutes a day is as necessary and important as daily sleep, and it benefits you whether your exercise skills are those of a professional athlete or a potato chip. Most of us wouldn't entertain the nightmare of no sleep. From an aging perspective, it's as bad to skip a daily walk as it is to skip a night of sleep. As the nonwalking exercises get easier, and you get stronger and leaner, you'll be able to challenge yourself too, by adding exercises, or making slight but important variations of the positions.

The YOU Activity Plan

Every Day:

❖ **Walk:** Walk thirty minutes. No matter what. No excuses. It doesn't matter if you do this in one whole block or broken up into as many as three shorter sessions.

❖ **Stretch:** Once your body is warm (after walking, for instance), stretch for five minutes to help elongate your muscles. You'll find stretches detailed in the You Workout below and the yoga poses we've outlined later.

Three Times a Week:

Do the Twenty-Minute YOU Workout. Do the exercises in this order; in general, you'll strengthen a muscle and then stretch it. If you want to break the workout up into smaller sessions, pick and choose as you like, but always try to match the strength and stretch exercises for a particular body part—that is, work your legs with a strength exercise, then do the stretch exercise immediately after it. Also, on the other four days of the week, you can simply take all the stretches outlined below—denoted by the (*Stretch*) after the number—and turn them into the three-to five-minute postwalk total-body stretch.

FORM FIT: HOW TO EXERCISE THE RIGHT WAY

1. Look out at eye level or above to spare your neck and keep you from rolling your shoulders forward.
2. Assume the Botox pose: Keep your face relaxed and tension-free.
3. Relax your shoulders and lift up your chest.
4. Pretend the top of your head is being pulled up by a string to elongate your spine and keep you from rolling forward.
5. Count your reps of each exercise out loud; this counting will help you remember to breathe continuously and keep you from holding your breath.
6. Keep your abs tight and pulled in to support your lower back. (Practice sucking in every time you enter a car, bus, train, plane, elevator, escalator—that way it becomes automatic.)
7. Keep your knees slightly bent, so you don't lock them.
8. When doing shoulder exercises, make sure you can always see your hands (if you wanted to).
9. Breathe. Many people hold their breath while doing strength training.

How To Do It All Wrong.

10. Keep moving in between exercises to keep your heart rate fast, or move directly to the next exercise. If you're unable to hold a conversation, you're exercising too hard. If you can keep a conversation going and are able to fill the listener in on all the details, you may not be going hard enough.
11. As you get stronger, go longer rather than harder with cardio exercises, and stronger with weight exercises. That is, do more repetitions of any non-weight-bearing exercise. That will help prevent injuries from overexertion. If you really feel weak, just hold the exercise position without moving and slowly work up. It's more important to follow perfect form and do fewer repetitions than to do a lot of repetitions with form that's sloppier than spaghetti in a high chair.

The Twenty-Minute YOU Workout

Do the following movements in order. Make adjustments to time or repetitions as your ability level dictates. Each strength exercise is followed by a stretch to loosen the same muscle group and keep you limber. We recommend that women not do twisting during the menstrual period as the anterior cruciate ligaments (ACL) are vulnerable to injury at that time. See www.realage.com for video of each move.

1: Roll with It

Allows any kinks in your shoulders to be smoothed out.

Roll your shoulders forward for a count of ten and back for ten. "Swim" shoulders back for ten and forward for ten. Your goal is to get full range of movement with your shoulders. Notice any areas that you don't move fluidly and try to open them up by relaxing as you move your hands in full circles. Between sets, get into the habit of rolling your shoulders five times forward and five times back.

2: The Chest Cross

Strengthens chest and shoulders

(A) Reach your arms as forward as possible at shoulder height, and twirl your hands back and forth like you have a tennis ball in your hands. (B) Then, cross your straight arms in front of your chest in a series of quick horizontal motions with your palms facing each other (so they provide some wind resistance to your motion). (C) Next move your hands rapidly up and down with your palms facing the floor. Try to do each of these variations twenty-five times.

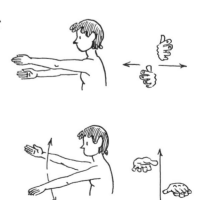

PREPARATION FOR PERSPIRATION

Before beginning an exercise program, you need more than a Lycra top. Exercise isn't dangerous, but your risk of injury will be less if you live with a few principles to protect your muscles and your entire body.

Warm Up. Before beginning any exercise, warm up your muscles for about five minutes to prevent injury. (The YOU Twenty-Minute Workout includes a warm-up, but if you're doing another activity, follow these guidelines.) Remember, your muscles are like spaghetti strands; they're pliable when they're warm, and more injury-prone if they're not. Jogging, brisk walking, cycling, or doing exercises with light weight or no weight will help prepare your muscles for activity. One good rule: Do the same exercise you will be doing but at a slower pace or with lighter weight. Your goal is to move your joints through the same range of motion as they will do with exercise—to raise your heart rate and to increase the temperature of your muscles, which will make them more viscous and less likely to be injured. Some advocate that at the end of exercise, you should cool down with a light jog, cycle, or walk, but there's no evidence that a cooldown will reduce injury or muscle soreness more than just stretching at the end. But if you are doing intense cardio exercise, you do need to do a cooldown, rather than stopping abruptly at the end of the workout. For a cooldown, do the same activity, like running, at a much slower pace than you were maintaining during your workout.

Focus on Your Muscles. Take special notice of where you tense up. You want to release tension in your body, not shift it somewhere else. Most commonly, people shift it to their shoulders and their foreheads. Notice this, breathe, and focus on the muscles you are working.

Listen to Your Body. Throughout stretching, make sure to keep breathing freely and slowly. If you ever feel pain during stretching, stop. (That's different from a little discomfort as you're loosening up; actual pain should be your warning to stop. We *want* burning in the muscles.)

Wear the Right Shoes. You'll need to invest in a good pair of lightweight running shoes for walking (the strength workout you should do barefoot, unless you use weights). Appropriate shoes are well cushioned and designed to handle the heel-to-toe movements for both walking and running. Best option: Go to a specialty running store, where the often underpaid salespeople are the experts; ask the pro there to analyze your stride and match up the best shoe for your feet.

3 (Stretch): The Clapper

Stretches chest

In a standing position and keeping your chest up, clap in front of you; then bring your hands behind your back and clap your hands together. Keep your hands as high as you can in front and back during the movement. Keep your chest lifted when clapping in back. Do ten times.

4 (Stretch): The Hippie

Stretches hips and hamstrings

With your feet flat on the ground, bend forward at your waist. Alternate bending one knee and keeping the other leg straight (but still keeping your feet flat), and let your head dangle down, releasing all your tension. Stretch each side for fifteen seconds.

5: Push-up Pride

Strengthens chest

Get in the appropriate "up" push-up position for you by either staying on your toes or keeping your knees on the ground. Lower yourself until your chest nearly touches the ground and push back up. As you straighten your elbows, push your spine toward the ceiling to exercise (to help engage your back muscles as well). Pull your heels away from your shoulders, keeping a long, solid body. Don't let your stomach hang down toward the ground; make your stomach active by pulling it in to support your lower back. This will help release any unnecessary tension on your lower back. Keeping your stomach tight in any exercise strengthens your belly muscles. If your lower back starts to hurt, raise your butt slightly and curl your tailbone by tightening your butt. Keep your chin slightly up and look six inches past your fingertips. This forces you to use your chest and not overextend your neck while doing push-ups. Do as many push-ups as you can (this is called exercising to fail-

Basic Training

Sometimes choosing a trainer can be like buying a car—it sure does look nice, but do you really know how well it runs? While a personal trainer isn't required, many people like working out one-on-one, specifically because of the trainer's knowledge and the accountability of having to regularly report to him or her. To make sure you get one who's qualified, take these steps:

❖ Make sure trainers are certified by a reputable organization like the American College of Sports Medicine (ACSM), the American Council on Exercise (ACE), the National Strength and Conditioning Association (NSCA), or the National Academy of Sports Medicine (NASM), as well as having Cooper Institute certifications.

❖ Check to see if they practice full-time, and aren't just doing training between acting jobs.

❖ Make sure their motivational style (including the voice) matches your workout style; some trainers are more vocal, while others are more soothing. If they're inspiring to *you,* you'll push yourself to get results and to show up, which is nine-tenths of the battle. If cost is a problem, try out our free program with New York City trainer Joel Harper or Tracy Hafen on www.oprah .com or www.realage.com. Get all of our YOU workouts at www.fitpackdvd.com.

ure, and it's what helps build strength proteins in your muscle). If these are too hard, just hold your chest off the ground without moving. Or you can do a pyramid push-up routine: Do five push-ups, then hold in the up position for five seconds. Then do four and hold for four in the up position, all the way down to one.

6 (Stretch): Pecs Flex

Stretches chest and arms

Sit up straight on your heels and interweave your fingers behind your butt, while keeping your arms straight. Lift your fingers up, knuckle side facing back, while opening your chest wide. Squeeze your shoulder blades together to open your chest more. Use your breath to your advantage here, by breathing into the muscles being stretched. Another option is to interweave your fingers behind your head and pull your hands away from your head. Face forward for all versions.

7: Steady on the Plank

Strengthens abs and shoulders

Get into a push-up position with your elbows and toes on the floor, while pushing the area between your shoulders toward the ceiling and keeping your stomach pulled in toward your lower back, to support it. Keep your buttocks tight and your eyes looking at the floor (ignore the fact that you suddenly realize you have to vacuum). Hold the position for as long as you can. If you can last more than one minute, make it more difficult by dropping your chin twenty times out in front of interweaved hands, or by trying to balance on one foot.

8: Whose Side Are You On, Anyway?

Strengthens obliques (the muscles at the side of your abdominals)

Turn to the side by putting an elbow on the floor and rotating the opposite hip toward the ceiling. Keep your body in a straight line and resist pushing your butt back. Keep your abs tight as you hold the position for as long as you can. Alternate sides. If you can hold for more than one minute, you can increase the difficulty by repeatedly dropping your hip, tapping it on the mat, and bringing it back into the lateral plank.

9 (Stretch): Up, Dog, Up

Stretches abdominals and obliques

From a down push-up position, with your hands below your shoulders, lift your chest and torso up into the air so that your upper body is nearly perpendicular to the floor as you come onto the tops of your bare feet. Lean backward to stretch your abdominals, but keep your butt relaxed. Hold for ten seconds. Then look over

FACTOID

It shouldn't be a surprise that the exercise and movements that require the most intensity are the ones that burn the most calories. Some samples of exercise and activities and how much energy they burn per minute for typical people (with a weight of 200 pounds for men and 150 pounds for women):

Exercise	Calories Burned per Minute (Male)	Calories Burned per Minute (Female)
Running, 9 min/mile	22	17
Swimming, moderate	14	11
Stationary cycling, moderate	14	10
Weight lifting, vigorous	12	7
Walking 4 mph	8	4.5
Activity		
Chopping wood	12	9
Shoveling snow	12	9
Gardening	9	6
Playing with kids	6	5
Watering plants	5	4
Job		
Firefighting	24	18
Construction	12	9
Masseur/Masseuse	8	6
Nursing	6	5
Computer work	3	2

your right shoulder for ten, then your left shoulder for ten, then back to center.

10: The Rickety Table

Strengthens upper back and butt

Put your hands and knees flat on the floor with your fingers spread apart and pointing directly forward. Keep your back flat and parallel to the floor and your supporting elbow slightly bent. Look down six inches above your fingertips. Reach your right hand forward and your left foot back and stretch them as far away from each other as possible, keeping your right hand higher than your head. The higher your arm goes up, the more work your back has to do, and the more effective the exercise. Now bring your right elbow to your left knee. Do twenty on this side, then alternate and do it with the other leg and arm. For more advanced exercises you can move your arm and leg out at a right angle from your body, keeping them above your spine, and hold them there for twenty seconds. Your stomach should be pulled in the entire time, supporting your lower back.

11: Superman

Strengthens lower back

Lie flat on your stomach, reaching your arms out in front of you with the palms down. Spread your extremities straight out in all four directions and lift your arms and legs simultaneously for enough repetitions to cause some mild fatigue. Continue to look down during the movement, and don't overextend your neck up. This exercise is about how long you can make your body stretch—not how high you can get it. Focus on squeezing your butt as you lift. Try to make it to one minute.

12 (Stretch): The Seated Pretzel

Stretches lower-middle upper back and hip

Sit down with your legs stretched in front of you. Bring your right foot up and set it down on the outside of your left knee. For back   support, put your right hand behind your right butt cheek. Bring your left toe straight up. Reach your left hand up as if indicating "stop" and drop your chin. Then twist to the right and bring your left triceps to the outside of the right thigh. To go deeper, twist more to apply pressure against your right thigh. Act like a string is pulling the top of your head up to elongate the spine. Breathe by expanding your rib cage like you are blowing up a balloon. Really concentrate on taking deep breaths every time.

Note for exercises 13 and 14: For all reclining abdominal exercises, keep your lower back flat on the ground. Pretend a quarter is trapped between the floor and your lower back, and keep your belly taut to train your stomach to be flat. As soon as you feel your lower back tenting up, stop and pull it back down as flat

Top of the Morning

Coffee, roosters, and shock jocks aren't the only things people wake up with. Many people enjoy starting their day with yoga's sun salutation: a series of movements that strengthen, stretch, and energize your body. Consider it your caffeine-free way to start the day. Do the sequence twice, switching legs on the second repetition.

Repeat and do the other leg

Sun Salutation

1. Stand with feet touching. Bring your hands together, palm to palm, fingertips pointing upward. Make sure your weight is evenly distributed. Exhale. Raise your arms upward. Slowly bend backward, pulling your abs in and up, stretching arms above the head. Relax your neck. Inhale.

2. Exhale while you slowly bend forward until your hands are in line with your feet, touching your head to your knees if possible. Press your hands down, fingertips in line with toes (bend your knees if

as possible before continuing. If this gets too hard, stop and hold it down as flat as possible for thirty seconds. Pretend there is a dumbbell tied to a string attached to your belly button, and it is pulling your stomach down toward the quarter.

13: Leg Drop

Strengthens entire abdominal area

Lie on your back with your hands on your chest and put your knees at a 45-degree angle and your feet in the air. Drop your heels down, tap the mat, and you have to), and touch the floor. Maintain a slight bend in the knees to take pressure off your back through your hamstrings, and extend and elongate your back, rather than arching it, to avoid lower-back issues. Relax your neck and shoulders; let them dangle down toward the ground. Use their weight to stretch your spine.

3. Move into an up push-up position with your hands and toes on the floor and your back straight.

4. Lower your body to a down push-up position with your elbows bent and your body remaining in a straight position from your legs to your head.

5. As you inhale, raise your head and bend backward as far as possible. while straightening your arms. To go deeper as you lift, arch backward and pull the top of your head up and out and come onto the top of your feet as you lift your pelvis off the ground. The four points would be your two palms and two tops of your feet.

6. Keeping your arms straight, raise your hips into down dog, pressing your armpits toward your knees, and align your head with your arms. Exhale throughout movement.

7. Keeping your leg straight, raise your right leg so it stays in line with your spine. Raise the left leg your second time through the sequence.

8. Return transiently to down dog position. Lunge your right leg forward.

9. As you inhale, keep your hands and feet on the ground, with your right foot between your hands. Reverse legs the second time through.

10. Raise your head and lift your hands straight up to the sky while maintaining the lunge position.

11. Open your hips by turning to the left and outstretching your arms right side forward and left side back so that they're parallel to the floor.

12. Bring feet together and stand up straight. Keeping your legs straight, bend at the waist and lower your upper body. Touch your head to your knees if possible. Exhale.

13. Return to position 1 by slowly rising, straightening your back into a standing pose. Stretch your arms above your head as you inhale. Exhale and then repeat the sequence so you can work the opposite muscles.

bring back up to 45 degrees. Do as many as you can (to failure). As soon as your lower back starts to arch up, return back to 45 degrees; keep pushing yourself a little bit further each time with your back glued to the quarter. Beginners, do one leg at a time. Advanced: Do it with straight legs.

14: X Crunch

Strengthens upper abdominals

Lie on your back with your feet on the ground and your knees at a 45-degree angle. Cross your arms behind your head, putting your opposite hand to the opposite shoulder to form an X behind your head. Rest your head in this X and keep your neck loose (in the beginning, you can put a tennis ball under your chin as a reminder). Using your abdominal muscles, crunch up about 30 degrees from the floor. Without holding your breath, you need to suck in your belly button to the floor to tighten the natural girdle you have (it's a muscle called the transverse abdominis) to keep the entire six-pack tight. Also pull up your pelvic muscles (like

when you are holding in your pee) to strengthen the bottom of the natural girdle. Do as many as you can, looking up toward the ceiling the entire time. Then repeat Up, Dog, Up (exercise 9) to stretch your abdominals.

15: Seated Drop Kick

Strengthens quadriceps

Sit with your legs straight out in front of you. Bend your right leg up with the knee pointing toward the ceiling. To keep your back straight, interweave your hands around this knee. Act like there is a string pulling from the top of your head, elongating your spine (and don't bob your head). Lift your straight left leg six inches off the ground, keeping your left toe pointed toward the ceiling. Lift twenty-five times, then switch legs. Do each leg twice. The only body part that moves is the leg; for variation, lift leg and move side to side.

Exercise Anywhere, Anytime!

Practice perfect posture—while sitting, standing, or walking—by tightening your abdominals (suck your belly button to your spine). Visualize a straight line from the top of your head down to your hamstring muscles in the back of your legs, making sure to keep your neck and shoulders back and relaxed down away from your ears. Visualize a string pulling you up from the top of your head, elongating your spine. Engaging in good posture not only will strengthen your core but will also add a small extra-calorie burn because you're working slightly harder to maintain the position. If you find your shoulders rolling forward, practice interweaving your hands behind your butt as you talk to people.

16: Invisible Chair

Strengthens entire leg

Sit in a chair position (with no chair!) with your back against a wall, and with your palms resting on your knees. Ideally, have a stool below you, so you can grab it or sit on it when you're done. Keep your heels directly below your knees and at a 90-degree angle; your relaxed shoulders should be rolled back and the back of your head should be against the wall. Hold for as long as you can, and try to work up to two minutes. Keep your face relaxed and breathe.

17 (Stretch): Nice Thighs

Stretches quadriceps

While standing on one leg, bend the knee of the opposite leg and grab the foot behind your back with interweaved fingers (or use one arm to hold something to keep balanced). Pull the foot toward your butt while lifting your chest forward and squeezing your shoulder blades together. Keep your knees together. Switch legs. Keep your abs pulled in the entire time, to support your lower back. Hold each for twenty seconds.

FACTOID

You can add a balancing element to almost any exercise by tweaking it slightly. Try doing two-legged exercises on one leg, or do an exercise lying on a stability ball instead of a bench.

Figure 12.1 **Picture this** To remove every possible excuse from your repertoire, the YOU Workout is summarized in three pages that you can post wherever you need to facilitate exercise. Remember, your body is your gym.

244 The YOU Diet and Activity Plan

12.

13.

14.

15.

16.

17.

246 The YOU Diet and Activity Plan

Are You Well Equipped?

Hooked on sweat? Then consider these add-ons to your physiological gym.

As You Get Stronger: Weights

Though you can use household objects for resistance exercises, it can be worth investing in a pair or two of dumbbells to use for lunges, squats, and other exercises as you get stronger. Weights usually cost about fifty cents per pound. See the *YOU: The Owner's Manual* workout at www.fitpackdvd.com.

Great Addition to a Home Gym: Exercise Ball

Once you establish a fitness foundation, these large, inflatable balls are wonderful to use for crunches and any other exercise in which you sit on the bench or floor. They help you develop balance and work your stabilizing muscles in your abdominal section. They are also great stretching devices. See www.realage.com for examples.

For the Traveler: Bands

Resistance bands allow you to increase resistance as you get stronger, and they're also small, so you can take them when you travel. See the *YOU: Being Beautiful* workout at www.fitpackdvd.com.

For Balance and Agility: Jump Rope

They're cheap and easy to use. While raising your heart rate, they'll also test and improve your agility.

For At-Home Cardio: Rebounder

Once you progress to doing cardio exercise, you can jog, swim, row, cycle, or do whatever you like to get your heart pumping. If you're one of our highly coordinated readers, one of the easiest ways to work your heart is with either a jump rope or a minitrampoline called a rebounder. You know about the jump rope, but for a rebounder, you can store it under your bed, pull it out, and do mini joint-safe cardio sessions by hopping and jumping on it for the allotted time. (Take a quick lesson before using it, so you can learn the safety rules.)

Versatile Bonus: Weighted Vest

This vest carries extra weight to give you resistance (many are adjustable so you can change the weights in one-pound increments), and you can use it for all of the central exercises, like lunges, squats, crunches, and push-ups.

Cardiovascular Workout

In a week, you need sixty minutes of an activity that raises your heart rate to 80 percent of maximum (220 minus your calendar age). You can choose from such activities as running, cycling, swimming, rowing, or using an elliptical trainer. (Vigorous sex also counts, but here it has to be continuous minutes, bucko, so it's unlikely this'll be a good alternative.) For the last one to four minutes, raise the intensity to the highest level you can for the maximum benefits. Then cool down for five to ten minutes on low intensity of the same exercise. If you do the YOU Workout above at a level that raises your heart rate, these twenty minutes of sweating can count toward your weekly cardiovascular exercise total of sixty minutes a week.

Note: When doing exercises with your own body weight feels too easy, you can add resistance by holding dumbbells or milk jugs filled with pebbles, sand, or water, or using other household products, like soup cans.

Amp It Up: Bonus Moves!

While the body-weight-only YOU Workout is a total-strength and total-stretch workout, we also believe that some of you may be looking for—or ready for— extra-credit moves. The following moves are ones you can do in addition to the basic twenty-minute workout, and are broken into the foundation areas of legs, chest, back, and abdominals. You can swap them in for similar exercises in the twenty-minute workout or add them in as extras. For you gym goers or home-gym owners, use dumbbells or other equipment. Aim for ten to twelve repetitions unless otherwise noted.

Legs Options

Lunges

Stand with your feet shoulder width apart, with your hands on your hips or holding weights. Take a long step forward with your left foot, like you're stepping over a puddle or stream. Now, for the best muscle burn, bend your left knee so that your thigh is parallel to the floor. (Make sure your

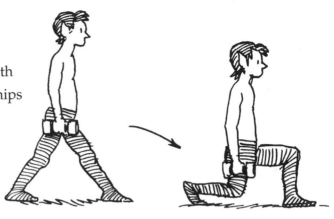

knee doesn't extend past your toes.) Pause, then step back into the original standing position. Repeat, by stepping forward with your right foot. This move will also build strength needed for better balance. If you have trouble balancing, turn the toes on your forward foot slightly inward, so you're not on such a tightrope. While doing lunges, pretend you have a broomstick attached to your spine so that you stay straight to the ground throughout the entire movement. You can also do these without alternating legs—do a certain number on one leg, then switch legs. That makes it a little easier on the knees.

Squats

Stand with your feet a little wider than shoulder width apart and with your hands holding weights or in *I Dream of Jeannie* style (elbows in line with shoulders, and hands crossed to opposite upper arm). Throughout, keep your elbows in line with your shoulders. Without curling your back, squat down to the point where your thighs are approximately parallel to the floor (or before that if you have knee or lower-back pain). It should feel like you're about to sit on the toilet seat, but just before your buns touch down. Pause, then rise up to the original starting position. Look forward throughout the movement. Keep your shoulders back and in line with your hips. Breathe in on the way down; breathe out on the way up. You can add resistance by holding dumbbells or other objects. You can do squats over a chair or sofa for safety in case you fall back. For variety, hold the lowermost position and pulse for a count of thirty and then continue your reps.

Step Taps

Stand in front of a set of stairs. Place one foot two steps up; leave it there as you raise the other foot, tapping that step twenty consecutive times and then switching legs. Use your arms to propel you up, as a sprinter would do. You barely want to hear your foot tap back down and back up. The softer it hits, the more burn you get, and the less impact on your knees.

Chest Options

Push-up Variations

As you get stronger, you can try these add-ons:

❖ Get in down-dog position: hands and toes on the floor and butt high in the air, like an inverted *V*. Look two inches above your shoulder-width hands and bend your elbows only, dropping your forehead to where your eyes are looking. Then straighten your arms. Keep your body in down dog the entire time.

- Wear a weighted vest (available at most sports-equipment stores, or try something like the ones at www .thexvest.com), which will increase the amount of resistance during the movement.
- Alternate lifting each foot a few inches off the floor and bending your knee on each repetition to incorporate balance into the exercise.
- One-arm push-ups. *Hooyah!* (If you can do this, uh, what are you doing reading this chapter, Rocky?)

Back Option

Bent-over Back Rows

Stand behind and to one side of a chair, bend over, and place one hand on the seat, and put a dumbbell (or water bottle) in your free hand. Keeping your back flat, pull the weighted hand up toward the outside of your chest, reaching your elbow toward the ceiling. Then lower your weighted hand as far as you can, keeping it extended to elongate the muscle, and repeat. As you're pulling up, keep your back parallel to the ground and your feet flat, not rocking, with your knees slightly bent. To get your heart rate up and an amazing burn, do 100 with a lighter weight. If it gets too hard, choose a lighter weight and keep going. But you have to maintain good form throughout. Better to use proper form than to do a lot of reps.

Abdominals Options

Crunch Variations

- ❖ At the same time you crunch your body up, curl your legs off the ground toward your head and squeeze your belly button to the floor. (Works the entire six-pack in three sets of two-packs: the upper, lower, and middle, respectively.)
- ❖ Place your arms loosely crossed on your chest. Lift your legs so that the soles of your feet are facing the ceiling. Keeping your legs straight, lift your tailbone one inch off the ground and then slowly lower it. (Works lower region of your abdominals.)

Exercise Ball Moves

- ❖ Lie back on an exercise ball. Reach your arms straight up toward the ceiling with your palms together. Keeping your arms straight, bring your biceps down to the sides or your ears praying hands way above head and back up. The only thing that is moving is your arms.
- ❖ Do a plank (facedown) with your elbows on an exercise ball and keeping your navel in the same spot. Alternate swiveling each hip down two inches toward the ground and then back to plank.

Bicycle

Lie on the floor with your hands resting lightly behind your head. Raise your feet off the ground and bend your right knee and pull it toward your chest. Simultaneously twist your opposite shoulder toward this knee, keeping your elbows out of your line of vision. Switch sides back and forth. Keep your lower foot suspended in the air as you switch sides. Then hold to one side, reaching your shoulder toward the opposite knee for thirty seconds. Switch and then hold to the opposite side for thirty more. The more you pull your stomach in, the more you can lift yourself up. For a harder version, stay in this last position, take the straight leg, and raise and lower it one inch for thirty times.

Remember, don't fall into the trap of thinking, misguidedly, that strength exercises are for *increasing* your size. You can do resistance exercises without making your muscles bulge more than a pug's eyes. The true payoff for strengthening your muscles is that you'll build a little more lean muscle mass, which will help you burn more calories throughout the day and speed your metabolism. The trick is to reduce your excuses (which we've done by eliminating equipment in the YOU Workout) so that you devote those sixty minutes a week to building, maintaining, and maximizing your body's natural fat burners.

Chapter 13

The YOU Diet

The Waist Management Eating Plan

IT'S CURLY LETTUCE!

Whether or not you're the kind of person who skips the plot to get to the ending, you've arrived. Welcome to the YOU Diet—our reprogramming plan provides you with the tools to make smart choices and with the strategies that allow you to make YOU-Turns after you've made bad choices. The specific program starts on page 264, but first, let's go over a few of our principles.

Whether it's at work, in school, or with sports, we praise the hard workers. If you bust your tail with hustle and sweat, then we'll want you to proceed immediately to the pedestal. You may not always score the promotion, the dean's list, or the championship, but, as a society, we place more value on effort than just about anything else (except maybe a 7 a.m. cup of Starbucks coffee). It's too bad that's the very reason why our societal waistband has exploded to the size of Saturn's rings. We expect that a little of X (hard work) and a lot of Y (suffering) should automatically lead to the promised land of Z (skinny waist). But our bodies don't work that way. In fact, you can't win the battle over waist size with do-or-diet effort: You have to get out of the two perfect storms (your environment, which makes addictive food choices irresistible, and the effect of your food choices on your liver's metabolism). The way to survive a perfect storm is to change your environment and enlist buddies to help keep you in less hazardous seas. The harder you try to diet (with deprivation, with willpower, with the sheer stubbornness to avoid pork rinds), the more likely it is that you'll drown in an industrial-size jar of marshmallow fluff. So you have to get out of the sea of addictive poison and into a sea of choices that provides you with energy.

There are many solid, smart diet plans available to you. *YOU: On a Diet* is meant not to compete with these worthy programs but rather to give you the tools to succeed no matter what you try. That's because the raw data from current research offer insights into the biology of your body that should enhance your decisions about food and exercise. Let the science-based explanations we offer serve as your operating system to which future diet and activity plans can be added like software programs. After reading *YOU: On a Diet*, you'll know enough to evaluate them all, and you shouldn't have to worry about yo-yo dieting ever again. You

A Portion of the Plan

Many experts will tell you that the key to successful dieting comes from two words: "portion control." That makes sense, but not in the way you might think. We emphasize that you eat healthy portions of food (about a fistful per serving) and use nine-inch plates not to restrict your calories per se but to slow you down. If you can slow your calorie intake, you'll give your brain a chance to keep up—and activate the right amounts of leptin and ghrelin to keep you satisfied. So, start with the right servings of food, take your time eating them, then gauge your levels of satiety (using our fullness gauge on page 177). If you're still hungry, then have another serving (the size of a fist, not the size of a head) of a good-for-you food.

will change your environment, and that will change how your genes function. No matter what your plan, you should know by now that waist management isn't about hustle. It's about the following two things:

Automation. The first thing you need to do is stop trying—and start living. Normally. Automatically. Intelligently. You can do that by reprogramming your body with the tools we provide you throughout this book (and the fourteen-day program that follows) so that your decisions, food choices, and lifestyle become an enjoyable, invigorating, energizing routine, not a burden.

Adjustment. To make the transition from a thick waist to a thin one, you also have to acknowledge that waist management isn't a success-or-failure proposition. It's a journey with some side streets, some dead ends, and a few metaphorical and literal forks in the road. That's why you must practice the psychological and behavioral actions that will help you develop routines to help you go from sidetracked to on track. That's our YOU-Turn—knowing that it's OK to face obstacles, and it's OK that sometimes they'll pound you square in the mouth. As long as you know the way back to the right road and can make YOU-Turns faster than a mouse darts from a cat, then you can plan for a lifetime of successful waist management.

Fill 'Er Up

About twenty-five minutes before dinner, eat ½ ounce of walnuts with 1 cup of your favorite YOU Soup. Or drink at least 8 ounces of water with 1 tablespoon of psyllium. Either will help fill you up so you won't want or need to eat as much to feel satisfied.

The YOU Diet Crib Sheet

Meal Strategy	Three main meals plus snacks, so you're never hungry. No eating within three hours of bedtime. Consider dessert an every-other-day treat.
Waist Foods (Eat 'em)	Whole grain carbohydrates; fiber; nuts, which include healthy monounsaturated and polyunsaturated fats; protein such as lean meats (two-legged preferred) and fish.
Waste Foods (Trash 'em)	Added sugars, simple carbohydrates, syrups (as in high-fructose corn syrup), trans fat, saturated fat, non-whole-grain flour, and enriched and/or bleached flour.
In a Hunger Emergency	Apples, almonds, walnuts, edamame (soybeans), sugarless gum, water, cut-up veggies, low-fat yogurt and cottage cheese, or premade YOU Soup.
Substitution Foods	In any recipe or meal plan, you can replace any fruit or vegetable with another to make recipes to your taste.
Meal Journal	You can keep track of what you eat at www.mychoicescount.com.

To go along with the foundation of a dietary operating system, we also want to offer you one "software" option—the YOU Diet, the food plan that can help reboot your body so that you learn to eat smart, not hard. With this plan, you can expect to lose up to two inches of your waist size within two weeks.

When you launch into this fourteen-day rebooting program, remember the YOU Detox Plan—you will detox yourself physically and emotionally—and your taste buds, body, and environment as well. (It's so easy that it's one seven-day plan done twice, so you can do it perfectly and learn to do it automatically). Your body is made up of hundreds of beautiful biochemical instruments, and they all play different notes, melodies, harmonies, and chords within your anatomical

Supplements	Twice a day, take half a multivitamin as an insurance policy against less-than-perfect food choices. Get 600 milligrams of calcium, 600 IU of vitamin D, 200 milligrams of magnesium, and 300 milligrams of pantothenic acid (vitamin B5) (all twice a day). Also, once a day take 2 grams of fish oil for omega-3 fatty acids (we actually take 600 milligrams of DHA omega-3 capsules) and ½ teaspoon of cinnamon. And make sure you get 10 tablespoons of cooked tomato sauce weekly.
The Team	Don't be afraid to enlist advice from qualified nutritionists and trainers. But one of your most important team members will be your support partner or buddy—someone who can encourage you and be a deterrent to failure too (you won't want to report to that person a four-doughnut binge). Remember, your buddy should be either someone who wants to be on the journey with you or is already on it.
The YOU-Turn	It's OK to make mistakes. The important thing is to catch them, recognize them, control them, and allow yourself the opportunity to get back on the right (waist management) road.

orchestra. As the conductor, you direct how those notes are played and what kind of sound they'll make. Like any new piece of music, the YOU Diet will take a week or two for you to learn, for you to feel it, for YOU to become ingrained. But once all this happens, your orchestra will play like never before.

The YOU Diet: Before YOU Start

Before you start anything—whether it's a new job, a 5K race, or putting together your daughter's 547-piece Barbie house—it always pays to prepare. You read the short form of the employee manual, you study the course route, you lay out the plastic pieces all over the floor while silently cursing the world's toy manufacturers. Before you start the YOU Diet, the same applies (minus the cursing). If you've skipped the intro, then we'll do a quick review here of the pieces you'll need to know before you begin. (If you've read the book, then this is just a quick refresher course.)

YOU Change the Inside to Change the Outside: This diet is about understanding and automating your biology to reboot your body back to its original factory settings that make you lean and healthy, not the settings that have caused an alarming increase in yearly Santa applications. This diet is about eating the foods that help all of your organs and systems function the way that they should. By focusing on the recommended ingredients and nutrients, you'll be helping your body's chemicals and hormones do what they want to do: get you to your ideal size. They're the ones that will make your body want to burn fat, not store it. And they're the ones that will turn on genes that fight cancer and keep inflammation out of your arterial system, brain, and joints. They make your body feel satisfied, not hungry. We call these YOU-th-FULL foods, because they keep you satiated and less likely to gorge on bad-for-you foods. Put together, that's the real recipe for a lean waist and a healthy body.

YOU Better Identify the Problem So You Can Better Solve It: We've tended to treat weight loss as more art than science: more trial and error than predictable cause and effect. Through recent advances in molecular genetics, neurology, and biochemistry, we're finally able to learn what really causes us to gain weight and lose it, and what causes us to stay full and become hungry. Because of that, weight loss is revealing itself as a complex yet predictable and controllable pro-

Best Blade Plans

When following any eating plan, what you do and don't do with your fork and spoon are your most crucial actions. But don't underestimate the power of a great knife—to make what you do in the kitchen as enjoyable as what you do at the table. Overpay to buy the best eight-inch chef's knife (without serrations) you can afford. And follow these rules, to avoid leaving a finger in the guacamole:

Always keep the pointed edge on the cutting board; just lever from the point and cut sliding away from you under the back end.

Always cut away from yourself.

As you're lining up foods with your noncutting hand, tuck the tops of your fingers under the bottoms, so you let your knuckles, not your whole fingers, be the guide.

See www.realage.com for more cutting instructions, or watch the technique on *YOU: On a Diet,* the PBS special.

cess. Simply put, working smart means clearly defining the problem—that is, by understanding how your body works—before you set about solving it. A problem well defined is half-solved.

YOU Automate the Process: One of the reasons why we're a society of shot-putters instead of a society of milers is that we have millions of choices about what to eat. And while that variety is a win for the food industry, it is a miserable defeat for our waists. One of the ways that you'll be able to reboot your body is by stripping away the thinking and debating about eating. For a few meals a day, you'll take away the millions of choices to automate your actions. You'll eat essentially the same meals for breakfast, lunch, and snacks, and change up options for dinner. By decreasing the variety of foods eaten throughout the day, you'll decrease the chance for the hedonistic rampages that can be so dangerous.

YOU Stop Beating Yourself Up for Every Mistake: Somewhere and sometime, you've been led to believe that the only way you can lose weight is to eat perfectly all the time. That's not realistic. That's not fair. And that's why almost all diets fail. Perfection is impossible. One of the ways you can avoid the all-out Alfredo-fest is to activate your contingency plans: ready-made meals and snacks that you can turn to when you're stressed, tired, or bored. These foods will help you through cravings, they'll help you make YOU-Turns, and they'll help you make good decisions to avoid bad foods.

YOU Make It Easy on Yourself: We all know that the only way you'll be able to automate eating is if it's easy and fast. Almost all breakfast, lunch, and snack recipes take less than ten minutes to make, and no dinner takes more than thirty minutes of prep time.

YOU Eat to Stay Full—Not to Hit a Specific Calorie Count. Before we outline the meals, recipes, and strategies for succeeding on the YOU Diet, we want you to remember this one principle of eating: Eating isn't all about calories, it's about staying satisfied. The key to this program is eating nutritionally rich foods, avoiding the toxic ones, and using your body's clues about satiety to help you stop eating when you should.

It's about eating the foods that will help keep you full—and what "feels right," so that you can achieve and maintain your ideal playing weight. That said, we know some of you are members of the math/stat/calorie squad, so we'll indulge your number-loving selves for a moment.

We've designed this diet and its serving sizes based on a person with a metabolic rate of 1,700 calories. That is, the person who burns 1,700 calories a day through normal processes and activities can eat this to maintain his or her weight. To lose weight, this person would have to have a slightly smaller portion for dinner, for instance. If you burn 2,000 calories a day, you'll lose weight using these portion sizes, but if you burn only 1,400 calories a day, you'll consume more calories than you burn. To find your approximate no-waist-loss point, find your resting metabolic rate and add your physical activities.

❖ An easy way to estimate your resting metabolic rate is to multiply your desired weight in pounds by 8 and add 200, but this is very variable, so if anyone ever offers to measure your real metabolic rate, accept the offer.

Be Prepared

Here's a waist management fact: Bad foods aren't bad just because of the ingredients they contain but also because many of them are fast and easy, which are the exact traits that can get you into a whole lot of trouble. The key to successful dietary contingency plans is to have premade foods ready for those times when you've been conditioned to reach for bags of sugar-containing waist killers. Instead, choose your favorites of these options to make once a week so you'll have something to grab when you need it.

Cut-up Vegetables: Your choice. Cut them, bag them, eat them. Nothing wrong with baby carrots, grape tomatoes, and broccoli florets, but if you prefer jicama, sugar snaps, and orange pepper strips, go for it.

Sautéed Vegetables: Your choice. Sauté them in olive oil with chopped garlic, red pepper flakes, or a good dash of tumeric. Refrigerate and use for side dishes or hot (microwaved) snacks.

Soups: Make one or more of our filling YOU Soups (see recipes) once a week and store them in serving-size cups in the refrigerator. Eat 1 cup as a predinner appetizer, to take the edge off, or have a cup of soup as a snack.

Steel-cut Oats: If you're worried about time, cook up one week's worth of oats per directions and store in the refrigerator for up to a week. For some people, that may seem as appetizing as a slice of baked wrapping paper, but reheated oats actually taste great.

Emergency Foods: Every house needs fire-extinguisher foods—good-for-you foods that will put out three-alarm starvation fires. Our list of foods that you can reach for when you're hungry include any of the above foods as well as a handful of almonds, peanuts, or walnuts; bags of store-bought, prechopped fruits and veggies; dried fruit (apricots, cranberries); and edamame (soybeans—look for microwave bags in the frozen food section). Avoid the foods with added sugars. In a real pinch? Pop one of those mint breath strips—they can help turn off appetite by making food less appetizing.

❖ To find the calories you burn from physical activity, multiply the number of minutes you walk by 4, and your cardiovascular and strength minutes (not the time watching others) by 8. So that's about 300 calories for 30 minutes of walking and 25 minutes of strength or cardiovascular exercise. You can also use the readouts from cardiovascular machines you use if the machines have them.

So let's see how it works.

Say you want to weigh 150 pounds and do an average of 300 physical activity calories per day—about what you do on our plan (more on some days and fewer on others). That means:

Your basic calories used are $8 \times 150 = 1,200$
$+ 200 = 1,400$
$+ 300$ in activity $= 1,700$

So to maintain your desired weight, you'd need about 1,700 calories a day. To lose a pound a week, you'd need to decrease that by about 500 calories a day, or increase your physical activity by 500 calories a day, or a combination of the two. But tracking calories is a lot of work if you do not automate your eating. (There are also programs for handheld devices that can do it for you, such as at www.my choicescount.com.) The point, though, isn't to track calories; it's to let your body, your stomach, and your brain give you the signals to stop when you're satisfied, and not stuffed.

The YOU Diet Meals: YOUR Choices

Think of this rebooting program as the training wheels in waist management. It will help you find your eating balance. The plan is all about using body chemistry, not willpower, to succeed. For example, lots of fiber and lots of protein are included in the morning. (In case you skipped from the first chapter to this one, fiber in the morning helps control afternoon cravings. Extra protein decreases appetite.) More body-chem help comes from all the good fats—nuts, olives, olive oil, omega-3-rich oils—which help keep your sense of fullness and healthy HDL cholesterol up and your lousy LDL cholesterol down. We've limited simple sugars because they set off sharp swings in blood sugar levels that put you into a cycle of craving high-calorie foods. Plus all of these food-moves fight the destructive inflammatory effects and gene activations that make you hungry, your arteries unhealthy, and your waist larger, not smaller.

At a glance, you'll see lots of raw veggies and 100 percent whole wheat toast. In fact, the same-old-same-old routine actually is the point. Studies show that people who eat the same meal for at least one meal a day lose more weight than those who have more variety. And if you're like our patients, you won't be hungry on this plan. Having a lot of food choices is what makes us live life like we're in a never-ending speed-eating contest. But decrease your food choices, and you'll automatically decrease your appetite and waist size. Pick the one meal you rush through most and automate it. For most people, it's lunch. So find a healthy lunch you like—salad with grilled chicken and olive oil, turkey on 100 percent whole grain bread—and have it for lunch every day. Every day. Yes, every day.

On the following pages, we've listed your options for every food moment of the day (except dinner, which you'll find outlined specifically in the daily schedule). You can choose any of the options listed, but ideally choose just one or two to eat on most days. We've found that the most successful people are those who pick just one—and stick with it.

YOUR Breakfast Choices

For Cereal Lovers	For Egg Lovers	For Bread Lovers	For Breakfast Haters
Cooked oat cereal with 4 ounces of skim milk, or soy milk fortified with vitamin D and calcium, and 1 fistful of your favorite fruit OR 1 cup Kashi high-fiber or cold-oat cereal (like plain Cheerios) with 1 fistful of your favorite fruit, with 4 ounces of skim milk, or soy milk fortified with vitamin D and calcium	Egg-white omelet (3 egg whites and 1 whole egg), plus cut-up mixed veggies OR 2 scrambled, poached, or hard-boiled eggs with 2 pieces of lean turkey sausage or tofu sausage (scramble with a little canola Pam spray, not butter)	1 slice toasted 100% whole wheat bread with 1 teaspoon peanut butter, or 1 teaspoon apple or walnut butter or avocado spread	Magical Breakfast Blaster (see recipe, page 290) OR Pineapple-Banana Protein Blaster (see recipe, page 289)

YOUR Lunch Choices

Meal-Size Salad	Soup and Salad	Healthy Burger	Fast Food
Chopped salad: 6 chopped walnuts, chopped veggies (your choice), and chopped mixed greens tossed with 4 ounces of salmon, turkey, or chicken breast; with balsamic vinegar (2 parts) and olive oil (1 part) dressing OR One of the YOU Salads (recipes follow)	1 cup of one of the many hearty YOU Soups plus any of the YOU Salads (recipes for both follow) or a non-Caesar salad using olive or canola oil, or balsamic vinegar and olive oil dressing	Veggie burger or Boca Spicy Chik'n Patty on a toasted whole wheat English muffin with 1 tablespoon of fructose-free olive oil–based marinara sauce, sliced tomato, romaine lettuce or spinach leaves, plus slices of red onion	See best options for fast-food meals on page 284.

YOUR Morning and Afternoon Snack Choices

Fruit and Nuts	Grains and Berries	Revved-up Veggies	Fruit and Yogurt
½ ounce raw nuts with an apple, banana, plum, pear, orange, wedge of melon, cup of berries, 2 kiwis, ½ grapefruit, or any other fruit	½ cup whole grain cereal mixed with ¼ cup almonds and ¼ cup dried berries, apricots, or raisins	1 cup of cut-up sautéed veggies, warmed in microwave and stuffed into small whole wheat pita OR Cut-up veggies dipped into 4 ounces plain, low-fat, no-sugar-added yogurt or low-fat cottage cheese mixed with lots of dill, chives, ginger, red pepper flakes, or other spices (your choice) OR Just plain cut-up veggies	Low-fat probiotic (live culture) yogurt covered with ½ cup of canned, unsweetened peaches or mandarin oranges and some raisins

YOUR Dessert Choices

Eat Every Other Day
1 Lifestyle 180 Bar (see recipe) OR Cinnamon Apple Sauté à la Mode (see recipe) OR Roasted Pear with Raspberry Coulis, Chocolate, and Pistachios (see recipe) OR Sliced Peaches with Raspberries, Blueberries, and Chocolate Chips (see recipe) OR 1 ounce of dark chocolate (made with real cocoa), approximately three or four bites

YOUR Evening Snack Choices

(But Don't Eat after 8:30 p.m.)

Simon's Popcorn (see recipe)

OR

Any snack option

OR

100 percent whole wheat pita toasts and Tomato-Avocado Salsamole (see recipe)

YOUR Drink Choices

Plain or sparkling water (with fruit slice if desired), skim milk, coffee, hot or iced tea (decaffeinated is best if you have problems sleeping), diet soda (but only 1 to 2 a day)

For breakfast, you may include an 8-ounce glass of fruit or vegetable juice, such as tomato juice or 100 percent grapefruit juice or orange juice with pulp, fortified with calcium and vitamin D

For dinner, you can include one glass of alcohol, which we prefer you to drink toward the end of the meal so it does not hinder your satiety center's ability to slow your voracious appetite. If you're a nondrinker, it's OK to swap for a teetotaler's cocktail made with low-sugar grape juice, sparkling water, and lime

Dish List

Nowadays, foods have more labels than a clothes rack, ingredient names look like the names of Greek goddesses, and cunning marketing lingo makes sugar-drenched cereal appear as if it's healthier than a bundle of prunes. And that's just not the case. Prince Nutrition sounds great until you read the label and find no nutrient other than sugar and saturated fat neatly disguised. The trick to navigating through store aisles is not only to shop for value and whisk the kids past the Admiral Nutrition candy bars and potato chips but also to shop for content—for the ingredients and nutrients that allow you to eat smart, not diet hard. Here is our guide for ingredient inspection:

Look for less. Generally, fewer labels and ingredients equal better foods. Natural foods that come directly from the ground generally don't require labels. (Ever seen a marshmallow bush?) That's why any produce is generally OK for you. (One caveat: Make sure it has a great feel, a healthy smell, and has not been waxed; waxed versions are like a Barbie doll—look great, but not much substance. These versions often have less taste and less nutrition.)

Turn the package. Ignore what's on the front of the package and go directly to the food label and ingredient list. "Fat-free!" or "zero trans fats" may sound like a dieter's dream, but fat-free foods (especially salad dressing) can be loaded with more sugar than a baker's bowl. Another caution: Just because something "contains whole grains" doesn't mean it's made entirely or even mostly with whole grains (more on deciphering "whole grains" on page 281). Bottom line: The front of the package isn't even as revealing as the outside of a new car. It might look seductive, but you really have to check what's under the hood to see what it's all about. The ingredient list is where all the answers are.

Beware of the imposters. Many foods contain cheat words in their ingredient list—the words don't clearly scream "imminent heart attack!" as some other words may, but they indicate danger all the same. Some notable clues to watch for:

For sugar: Dextrose, sucrose, or anything with "ose." And mannitol, or anything with "ol." Those are alcohols that are quickly converted to sugar. Stay away from foods that have more than 4 grams of sugar in them. Even natural sugars such as maple syrup and molasses are sugar, so you should also keep them to fewer than 4 grams per serving, unless it's pure fruit (we make that exception because fruit has so many nutrients).

For fats: Besides saturated fats (fewer than 4 grams per serving) and trans fats (avoid them all), you should avoid foods with other fat code words, like partially hydrogenated, palm, and coconut oil.

Relax. We don't want you to spend more time in the store than you did in freshman economics class. If you haven't inspected labels before, it'll just take some time before you know exactly how to ID the nutritional heroes and the imposters. We also don't want you to be a paranoid shopper or paranoid about eating—some dangerous-sounding foods such as walnuts or real peanut butter or even honey (fewer than 4 grams per serving here) are OK in moderation.

The Fourteen-Day YOU Diet

During these two weeks, we'll give you the meal guidelines, the tools, the strategies, the tricks, the plan, and the help you need to change your diet and live it. By the end of the fourteen days, you'll have developed eating patterns and behavioral habits that will help get you on your way to changing your body from the inside out. Here we outline the seven-day plan and strategies for making smart decisions about food and eating. In week two, you'll repeat the first week, making appropriate food substitutions where you wish.

Day One: Saturday

1. **Walk:** Thirty minutes. Walking—whether you do it by yourself, with a friend, with your dog (only actual walking time counts, not time spent waiting for the dog to sniff), or around the dining room table—gives you your first dose of physical success. Walk every day for thirty minutes, and you'll establish the behavioral and motivational foundation for the YOU Diet.

2. **Stretch:** Do three to five minutes of stretching after your walk. See Chapter 12. While stretching keeps your muscles limber and flexible to help prevent injury, it also has a meditative element to it, helping you refocus and cope with cravings. "No pain, no gain" does not apply here.

3. **Dump Your Fridge:** To make room for all the new, good food you're about to buy, it's time to rid your kitchen of the nutritional felons. The appeals are up; it's execution time. Read the label of everything in your kitchen cupboards, your refrigerator, your secret boxes, and everywhere else you stash food. If something has any of the following in one of the first five ingredients, throw it out. This is the *YOU: On a Diet* Rule of 5. Don't have any of these five ingredients in the first five ingredients on the label:

    1 and 2. Simple sugars and syrups. This includes brown sugar, dextrose, corn sweetener, fructose (as in high-fructose corn syrup), glucose, corn syrup, honey, invert sugar, maltose, lactose, malt syrup, molasses, raw sugar, and sucrose. Keep a little table sugar handy, and honey, and maple sugar, because you'll use some for recipes. (See the box on other sweeteners on page 107.)

    3. Saturated fat. This includes most four-legged animal fat, milk fat, butter or lard, and tropical oils, such as palm and coconut.

    4. Trans fat. This includes partially hydrogenated fats, vegetable oil blends that are hydrogenated, and many margarines and cooking blends. (If you must, use cholesterol-fighting sterol spreads such as Promise and Benecol.)

5. Enriched flours and all flours other than 100 percent whole grain or 100 percent whole wheat. This includes enriched white flour, semolina, durum wheat, and any of the acronyms for flour that is not whole wheat—they should not be in your kitchen.

4. **Go Food Shopping:** Your current kitchen is most likely like a prison—it's filled with a lot of bad dudes. We want to turn your kitchen into a nutritional honor society, so that it's filled with good-for-your-waist foods that make it easy (and automatic!) to eat right. The first week, you'll have a larger-than-normal shopping list because you'll stock up on essentials as well as ingredients you'll need for this week's recipes. For a specific shopping list that works with our suggested seven-day schedule, see page 277.

5. **Make Your Weekly Staples:** Your choice of vegetables or soup. See above.

Eat!

Follow guidelines for breakfast, lunch, and snacks. For dinner, have . . .
Asian Salmon with Brown Rice Pilaf

Day Two: Sunday

1. **Walk:** Thirty minutes.
2. **Stretch:** Do five minutes of stretching.
3. **Partner Up:** If you try to undertake this alone, there's a much higher risk that you'll end up lips-first in a bowl of creamed corn. Find your YOU partner—be it a spouse, a friend, a coworker—someone you can talk to about your goals, your meals, your new plan. Make a plan to talk (or email) five minutes every day—to tell him or her that you walked that day and to tell about your day's meals. If you prefer a cyber friend, log on to www.realage.com and match up with a partner there.

   Better yet, try to find a partner or partners who are in this *with* you, on the same journey to good health. Share this book; share the knowledge you've learned; embark on a "work smart, not hard" journey together. It's one thing to lose three, four, or five inches yourself, but quite another when you can help contribute to America's collective loss in waistband size. After all, what's better than experiencing the satisfaction of helping yourself achieve your goal? Helping others do the same.

Eat!

Follow guidelines for breakfast, lunch, and snacks. For dinner, have . . .
Spicy Chili or Stuffed Whole Wheat Pizza

Day Three: Monday

1. **Walk:** Thirty minutes.

2. **Do the YOU Workout:** Follow the twenty-minute no-weights YOU Workout, which includes both strength and stretching exercises, on page 233. Strength training helps you add muscle, which will help speed your metabolism and burn fat. Also start tightening your abs when you walk, which will help improve your posture and make your clothes fit better. Walk at a pace that raises your heart rate, or include twenty minutes of another cardiovascular exercise.

3. **Write It Down (or Type It In):** Generally, we're into guilt trips as much as we're into bourbon as a topical anesthetic, but we also think there's a fine line between guilt and motivation. One of the ways you can help reprogram yourself is by writing down (or recording, for you technophiles) everything that you eat. In a way, it holds you accountable; you won't want to eat bad foods, because you won't want the visual reminder that you ate them. For these two weeks only—just to establish your new routine—write down *everything* you eat. Yep, even the three M&M's you just swiped. (For the technically savvy, some handheld devices have programs that allow you to scan the bar codes of the foods you eat. You enter the quantity you eat, and the program will keep track of your calories—see www.realage.com or www.mychoicescount.com.)

4. **Go Shopping:** With three days of walking under your soon-to-be-loose belt, it's time you made another trip to the store. This time, make it the sports store—for a good pair of running shoes. Use them for walking only. Running shoes are lightweight, and they provide lots of heel cushioning (because they're made for people who pound the ground with more force). Your best bet: Go to a running specialty store, where the staff can not only measure your feet but analyze your stride and determine what kind of walker you are. (Note: Go shopping in the late afternoon when your feet are more likely to be swollen, to ensure the best fit.) If you like, you can also add these to your list:

   ❖ Socks with extra padding on the bottom. (Avoid cotton; you need socks that wick moisture away from your feet.)
   ❖ A yoga mat, so you don't slip and slide while enjoying the deep poses (and dumbbells or resistance bands if you're already advanced enough to use those; see page 247).

Eat!

Follow guidelines for breakfast, lunch, and snacks. For dinner, have . . .
Mediterranean Chicken with Tomato, Olives, and Herbed White Beans

Day Four: Tuesday

1. **Walk:** Thirty minutes.
2. **Stretch:** Do five minutes of stretching.
3. **Make Any Needed YOU-Turn:** It's not uncommon at this point for you to have already dabbled in the neighbor's cake, picked at the kids' chips, or snuck a few bites of a butter-covered pretzel from the mall. And that's OK. Just get yourself back together.

   At the next available moment, make an authorized YOU-Turn.

   The next time you find yourself dancing with the Devil Dog, try these coping strategies:

   ❖ ***The Lip Lick.*** Breathe in, lick your lips, swallow, and breathe out slowly, saying "ohm." Let the cool air flow across your lips. The soothing move—which takes all of about three seconds—helps you to reset, calm down, and refocus.
   ❖ ***The Waist Hang.*** Stand up straight, bend over at your waist, and let your lower back relax. Reach for the floor, grab your elbows, or hold the back of your knees. The important thing is to let all of the tension you have stored in your back and hips unwind. Relax your neck completely. If you feel tight, don't straighten your knees.

Eat!

Follow guidelines for breakfast, lunch, and snacks. For dinner, have . . .

Royal Pasta Primavera Provençale

Day Five: Wednesday

1. **Walk:** Thirty minutes.
2. **Do the YOU Workout:** Follow the twenty-minute no-weights YOU Workout, which includes both strength and stretching exercises, on page 233.
3. **Call Your Doctor:** Remember, waist management is a team game, and your doctor is one of your MVPs. So schedule an appointment for thirty days from now (or sooner if you have a great relationship). You can use him or her to help you in many different ways:

   ❖ Update your vitals such as blood pressure, waist size, and heart rate. If you need a baseline for such numbers as HDL and LDL cholesterol (HDL is more important for women and men over sixty), now's a good time to schedule a physical, get a few blood tests, and talk to your doctor about your new plan.
   ❖ Having a physical will also prove helpful when you reach a plateau—when your waist and weight loss will seem to have stalled. (Your doctor may then be able to prescribe medication that can help you get over a hump; see appendix A.)

Eat!

Follow guidelines for breakfast, lunch, and snacks. For dinner, have . . .
Apricot Chicken and Green Beans with Almond Slivers

Day Six: Thursday

1. **Walk:** Thirty minutes.
2. **Stretch:** Do five minutes of stretching.
3. **Do a Little Bragging:** If you go public with your success, it makes turning back more difficult. Tell a friend or a coworker about the progress you've made and the changes you've noticed.

Eat!

Follow guidelines for breakfast, lunch, and snacks. For dinner, have . . .
Turkey Tortilla Wraps with Red Baked Potato

Day Seven: Friday

1. **Walk:** Thirty minutes.
2. **Do the YOU Workout:** Follow the twenty-minute no-weights YOU Workout, which includes both strength and stretching exercises, on page 233.
3. **Restock Your Kitchen:** Check your pantry for ingredients you've run out of and make a shopping list for next week's recipes.
4. **Grade Yourself:** Whether it's with work or a first date, it's always nice to have some way to know how you're progressing. Now is the time to take your waist measurement and weigh yourself, just to see what changes you've made. In your first week, you may see up to a one-inch waist reduction and a two- to four-pound weight reduction. You might even be able to drop one clothing size.

Eat!

Follow guidelines for breakfast, lunch, and snacks. For dinner, have . . .
Broiled Trout, Orata, or Branzini with Rosemary and Lemon

Day Eight to Forever: Your Reprogrammed Body

There you have it. We've given you all the tools, actions, and adjustments you need to take your body back to its factory settings, with a healthy waist and a healthy weight. Now just repeat the steps for the second week, making meal substitutions as you like (see additional recipes starting on page 289). Work smart, not hard. Week one puts you in motion and allows your body to adjust. Week two gives you seven days to practice the plan, feel what it's like to eat well, and figure out what to do if you don't. Research shows that it takes two weeks of repetitive action to make the action become automated, so now you can take the plan and tweak it. Or repeat it. Or try new dinner recipes that you can find on our website, www.realage.com. Make adjustments based on our nutritional guidelines as well as your tastes. This isn't the end of your waist-management plan; it's just the beginning.

Somewhere between the second and third weeks of the program, data show that the behavior changes that are crucial for sustained waist loss will start to become ingrained in you. About the same time, your newly detoxified body will become more sensitive to poor-quality foods. Instead, as you adopt the *YOU: On a Diet* habits, you will crave the foods similar to the ones we list. Your liver will enjoy not having to manage toxic elements and will pass along the love to the rest of the body by reducing inflammation. All the data we have on folks who have lost a lot of weight and kept it off points to using a steady, resilient program. You can make mistakes but still bounce back if you keep moving and keep making calm YOU-Turns without a lot of emotional baggage. The types of foods we advocate will always come to your rescue even if you make a few wrong turns, anyway.

When you reach a plateau—which you will—you will have three choices: drop another few calories from your daily intake, increase your physical activity, or see a physician about extra help if appropriate. But remember that the purpose of losing weight is to gain health, so when you reach your playing weight and your body is loving the feeling, just stay the course.

Sample Eating Schedule

Above, we've given you all the tools you need to reprogram your kitchen, your body, and the biochemicals that will keep you from going hungry and that will keep you from storing fat. Below, we put it all into action by giving you a sample week showing how the YOU Diet works. Want a plan that requires absolutely no thought at all? Then follow this schedule and the shopping list on page 277.

Note: Because we all have higher or lower caloric needs (depending on genes, metabolic rates, activity levels, and other factors), we do not dictate serving sizes here. Your goal is to eat the amount that makes you satisfied—that's a level three or four on our satiety scale (see page 177), not feeling more bloated than a puffer fish. For some people, portions may be a little more than a traditional serving size. For others, they may be a little less.

Sunday
Breakfast: Egg-white omelet; juice and coffee or tea
Morning Snack: Revved-up Veggies with dip
Lunch: Healthy Burger with the works

Afternoon Snack: Yogurt with fruit

Dinner: Asian Salmon with Brown Rice Pilaf

Dessert: 1 ounce dark chocolate with a sliced orange

Drinks: Water, coffee, tea, etc., as you wish (see proposed broader list)

Monday

Breakfast: Magical Breakfast Blaster

Morning Snack: ½ ounce raw nuts

Lunch: Chopped salad of walnuts, veggies, greens, and salmon/turkey/chicken

Afternoon Snack: Yogurt with fruit

Dinner: Stuffed Whole Wheat Pizza

Evening Snack: Simon's Popcorn

Drinks: Water, coffee, tea, etc., as you wish

Tuesday

Breakfast: Cheerios with skim milk; juice and coffee or tea

Morning Snack: Apple

Lunch: Cup of Garden Harvest Soup; Cranberries, Walnuts, and Crumbled Cheese over Greens

Afternoon Snack: Yogurt with fruit

Dinner: Mediterranean Chicken with Tomato, Olives, and Herbed White Beans

Dessert: Cinnamon Apple Sauté à la Mode

Drinks: Water, coffee, tea, etc., as you wish

Wednesday

Breakfast: Magical Breakfast Blaster

Morning Snack: 1 ounce raw nuts

Lunch: Chopped salad of walnuts, veggies, greens, and salmon/turkey/chicken

Afternoon Snack: Yogurt and fruit

Dinner: Royal Pasta Primavera Provençale

Evening Snack: Tomato-Avocado Salsamole and pita toasts

Drinks: Water, coffee, tea, etc., as you wish

Thursday

Breakfast: Cheerios with skim milk; juice and coffee or tea

Morning Snack: Plum

Lunch: Cup of Garden Harvest Soup: Cranberries, Walnuts, and Crumbled Cheese over Greens

Afternoon Snack: Revved-up Veggies in ½ whole wheat pita

Dinner: Apricot Chicken and Green Beans with Almond Slivers

Dessert: 1 ounce dark chocolate with a sliced orange

Drinks: Water, coffee, tea, etc., as you wish

Friday

Breakfast: Magical Breakfast Blaster

Morning Snack: 1 ounce raw nuts

Lunch: Chopped salad of walnuts, veggies, greens, and salmon/turkey/chicken

Afternoon Snack: Yogurt with fruit

Dinner: Turkey Tortilla Wraps with Red Baked Potato

Evening Snack: Simon's Popcorn

Drinks: Water, coffee, tea, etc., as you wish

Saturday

Breakfast: Cheerios with skim milk; juice and coffee or tea

Morning Snack: Yogurt with fruit

Lunch: Cup of Garden Harvest Soup; Cranberries, Walnuts, and Crumbled Cheese over Greens

Afternoon Snack: Revved-up Veggies with dip

Dinner: Broiled Trout, Orata, or Branzini with Rosemary and Lemon; Rock Asparagus

Dessert: Cinnamon Apple Sauté à la Mode

Drinks: Water, coffee, tea, etc., as you wish

Your Shopping List

The first week, you'll be buying more stuff than all other weeks, as you're gathering the building blocks for your new fridge and pantry (including spices, oils, and other long-term ingredients). We believe in working from the inside of the store out so that heat and bacteria have less time to grow on your produce before you get it home. This list includes both your staples and your ingredients for the recipes on our seven-day sample schedule (see page 275) for two people. You can make weekly or biweekly shopping lists for any of the recipes and snack choices and for any number of people (one to twenty-four) at www.realage.com.

Shopping List Basics

Serves two for one week:

❖ The shopping list has been subdivided into categories to make shopping easier (grains, refrigerated items, protein, dried fruits and nuts, fresh veggies, and so forth).

❖ A general condiment list has been included below for seasonings, spices, oils, and so on, needed to complete the recipes. You may already have many of these items in your pantry.

❖ Tomato or cranberry juice can be substituted for any or all of the orange juice.

Inside Aisles: Grains

1 box cold oat cereal (Cheerios)

1 package 100 percent whole wheat or 100 percent whole grain English muffins (try to find a brand without sugar, honey, or high-fructose corn syrup added)

One 12-inch or 10-ounce prepared thin 100 percent whole grain pizza crust

1 box short-grain brown rice

1 box 100 percent whole wheat rigatoni or linguine pasta

1 box steel-cut oatmeal

1 bag small 100 percent whole wheat pitas

1 bag 100 percent whole wheat tortillas

1 jar (1–5 pounds) of chia seeds

Inside Aisles: Canned/Jarred Items

2 quarts (8 cups) low-salt vegetable or chicken stock or broth

1 can (15 or 16 ounces) white beans

2 cans (14½ ounces each) stewed tomatoes

1 can whole, crushed, or diced tomatoes

16 ounces tomato sauce (with olive or canola oil and less than 4 grams of sugar per ½ cup)

1 jar kalamata olives, halved

1 jar olive relish or tapenade

1 can sundried tomato bits or finely chopped sundried tomatoes (not in oil)

2 cans unsweetened peaches or tangerines

1 small can jalapeño peppers

1 jar popping corn (enough to make 8 cups)

1 jar unsweetened apple juice or cider (preferably organic)

1 jar apple butter (keep in fridge)

1 jar all-natural peanut butter (no trans fat, no added sugar or fructose)

Inside Aisles: Dried Fruits and Nuts

1 bag raw walnuts (at least 8 ounces)

1 bag raw hazelnuts (at least 4 ounces)

1 bag raw almonds (at least 4 ounces)

1 bag slivered almonds (at least ¼ cup)

1 bag dried cranberries (at least ¾ cup)

1 bag dried apricots

1 package chopped pistachios (enough for 1½ tablespoons)

Staple Condiments/Spices: Buy these or make sure you have them in your pantry. Refill as needed.

Olive oil

Canola oil or canola oil fortified with DHA

Salt

Pepper

Fresh garlic

Low-sodium soy sauce

Balsamic vinegar

Wine vinegar

Maple syrup (look for a brand that doesn't have high-fructose corn syrup listed in the first four ingredients)

Marinara sauce or other red tomato sauce

Dijon mustard

Hot red pepper sauce

Pam spray-on canola oil

Nutmeg

Cinnamon

Your favorite coffee or tea

Dark chocolate bar with at least 70 percent cocoa, or 1 small bag mini semisweet all-cocoa chocolate chips (not milk chocolate and without milk fat)

Refrigerated Items

1 half gallon skim milk or low-fat soy milk fortified with calcium and vitamin D

1 quart 100 percent orange or grapefruit juice with pulp, fortified with calcium, magnesium, and vitamin D

1½ cups (6 ounces) crumbled farmer cheese

6 eggs

1 bag finely shredded part-skim mozzarella cheese (enough for 2 ounces)

eight 4-ounce containers of probiotic low-fat yogurt

Chicken/Turkey/Fish

2 bone-in chicken thighs without skin

2 skinless, boneless chicken breast halves (about 4 ounces each)

12 ounces sliced cooked salmon (or white turkey or chicken from deli)

8 ounces skinless salmon fillets (or skinless chicken or turkey breasts)

1 whole fish (trout, orata, or branzini, about 4 ounces per serving; we prefer trout as its the only fish in the United States other than salmon to still contain "fish fats," or DHA).

Frozen Food

1 box Boca Spicy Chik'n Patties

1 bag frozen unsweetened blueberries

1 bag frozen unsweetened raspberries

1 small container nonfat or low-fat vanilla frozen yogurt

Health Food Aisle or Health Food Store

Soy protein (like Nature's Plus Spiru-Tein)

Psyllium

Flaxseed

Other

1 bottle white wine

Produce Area (shop last)

Wild Card: If you especially like particular fruits or vegetables, buy them in whatever quantities you want and eat them as substitutions or additions to your recipes (especially in season).

three 10-ounce bags of salad mix (classic romaine or other mixed-green salad)

10 cups mixed mesclun or spring greens

1 pound cut-up stir-fry veggies (asparagus, broccoli, cauliflower, mushrooms, multicolored bell peppers, red and white onions, zucchini)

Sliced carrots, apples, broccoli and/or celery in a package

2 pounds other veggies (your choice) to sauté, dip, mix into omelets, chop into salads

5 small apples (Jonagold or Ambrosia)

2 small plums

3 tomatoes

1 bunch of carrots

1 bunch bananas

2 red bell peppers

1 yellow or orange bell pepper

1 small head cabbage

1 cup thin green beans

1 pound asparagus spears

1 small eggplant

3 shallots

2 large cloves garlic

3 medium yellow onions

1 red onion

1 small bunch green onions

1 small dried ancho or pasilla chili pepper

1 large russet baking potato

1 bunch each fresh parsley, basil, rosemary, thyme (or lemon thyme), chives, oregano, and chervil

1 piece ginger

1 lime

1 avocado

1 small basket fresh raspberries (if available; if not, substitute frozen)

1 small basket fresh blueberries (if available; if not, substitute frozen)

The Whole Truth

It used to be that the only thing with a hole in it was a doughnut. Now, it seems, everything is touted as "whole" this or that. Whole grains, whole wheat, a whole lot of health: It's the latest in food marketing. Why? Because food manufacturers know that whole grains are, in fact, one of the healthiest ingredients you can eat. Surely, more and more foods are made with them, but that doesn't mean all are created equal. Why? Because those marketing words don't always present an accurate picture of what's inside the food.

To decipher the whole mess, you first need to understand what exactly whole grains are and how they work. "Whole grain" means the grain still has all three of its original elements: the outer shell or bran, which contains fiber and B vitamins; the germ, which contains

To make sure you receive the health and dietary benefits of whole grains and wheat, the labels should read "100 percent whole grain" or "100 percent whole wheat." Anything else means that the food is also made with the less beneficial enriched or refined flour. Remember to avoid those with added sugars like high-fructose corn syrup or honey.

phytochemicals and B vitamins; and the endosperm (what a name), which contains carbohydrates and protein. The key is that they're "whole" and not "refined," by stripping away the bran and germ, which leaves you eating only the aptly named endosperm. Instead, the whole grain should be left intact—meaning you get more fiber and more micronutrients that help protect against disease. These whole grains are also healthy for you because they're absorbed more slowly than enriched or bleached flour and thus raise glucose and insulin levels less—keeping you fuller longer and slowing your digestion. But not all foods that tout whole grains or whole wheat are the healthiest form. Some fake-out words you should watch out for:

Made with: It may have a drop of whole grains, but unless it's made entirely with them, you won't reap all the potential benefits.

100 Percent Wheat: This means it could have some or a lot or no "whole" wheat.

Multigrain: This tells you nothing about whether the grains are whole or refined. Even if you're getting 38 grains, that isn't much good if they are all refined.

Whole Grain: If the label doesn't say "100 percent whole grain," it may have many blends. Bad words to see: *enriched, bleached, unbleached, semolina, durum,* and *rice flour.*

Blends: "Whole grain blend" means it usually doesn't have much whole grain at all.

Good Source: This means it has 8 grams of whole grains per serving or as little as 13.5 percent. Don't confuse whole grain with fiber; 8 grams of whole grain may have less than 1 gram of fiber.

Excellent Source: This means it has 16 grams per serving or as little as 27 percent.

Supports Heart Health: Any food can say that it "supports" an organ. What you want to see on the label: "May reduce the risk of . . ." This means that the food has ingredients clinically shown to be effective in reducing the risk of, say, heart disease or high cholesterol, depending on the food.

*YES, YOU'LL GO STERILE IF YOU DON'T EAT YOUR BRAN FLAKES!

The Perfect Eating Environment

Research shows that your surroundings may play a role in determining how much you eat. Specifically, the more comfortable and relaxed you are, the more you lower your inhibitions. If you want to create the mood to keep you the fullest, make this your dining-room feng shui:

- ❖ Choose bright lights over soft lights.
- ❖ Choose a warm room temperature over cold.
- ❖ Choose conversation over music or TV, which can distract you into eating more.

When You Need the Fast-Food Fix

We understand how it is. Sometimes you need the absolute quickest path from food to belly. While most fast-food options are more destructive than a 4 a.m. vandal, you can still make smart choices in the drive-through lane. Some things to remember:

- ❖ There are some main dishes that can be good for you, but you have to be careful. Some slight name variations can make the difference between causing your fat and keeping you flat.
- ❖ Avoid side dishes and desserts unless indicated below. They're all loaded with bad fats and simple sugars, and they often have more calories than the main dishes.
- ❖ Choose low-calorie dressing, not low-fat. Low-fat dressings are steeped in HFCS, which has plenty of calories, and the fructose tricks your body into staying hungry.
- ❖ Don't eat breakfast at fast-food places. There are virtually no healthy options on any breakfast menu we could find.

When life steers you out of the kitchen, these are your best bets at these places, which offer some decent alternatives.

	Main Dishes*	Best Salad Dressing	Best Sides
Wendy's	Mandarin Chicken Salad with roasted almonds (but without the crispy noodles)	Reduced-fat creamy ranch	Plain baked potato (ask for marinara sauce to top it), mandarin orange cup, Caesar side salad without croutons, chili
McDonald's	Fruit and walnut salad Caesar salad with grilled chicken	Newman's Own Cobb dressing	Fruit and yogurt parfait
Burger King	BK Veggie Burger (without cheese) Tendergrill Chicken Sandwich (without sauce)	Ken's light Italian dressing	Side garden salad
Taco Bell	Spicy Chicken Soft Taco	Bring your own	None at this time
Arby's	Arby's Chicken Breast Fillet	Raspberry vinaigrette	None at this time
Domino's Pizza	Pizza with green pepper, onions, mushrooms with crunchy thin crust	Use your own	None at this time

* And always ask for 100 percent whole wheat buns. If not available, consider ditching the bun and eating the meat with a knife and fork.

Restaurant Tricks

Eating out can be a great experience—for everyone except your gut. With Rushmore-sized portions and dietary disasters in every plate, basket, and spoonful, restaurants are dangerous places. While you should always follow our guidelines for good foods (the waist foods, not the waste foods, in our crib sheet), you should also know that most dietary mistakes are made within the first and last ten minutes of any restaurant experience. Some tips for bookending your meal the right way:

❖ Return the free bread and ask if you can have cut-up raw vegetables instead. (Do this four times in a three-week period, and we've found that most good restaurants remember the trick and automatically make that change every time they see you—if they see you at least once a week.)

❖ Order oil and vinegar in separate containers and on the side for salad dressing, and put a little on. (You have to do this; relying on the waitstaff or chef to do so gets you about 400 extra calories per side salad.)

❖ Ask to replace the potato or rice with sautéed vegetables.

❖ If you're going to have dessert, order one for the table and have just a few bites.

❖ For a quick guide, use this chart to make smart eating-out choices:

Menu	Order It	Avoid It
American	Salad with oil and vinegar; veggie burger; grilled chicken without any sauce or spice on top (savings of 100 to 400 calories); any vegetables, boiled and seasoned or sautéed with onions and garlic; baked potato with marinara sauce	Hamburger, grilled cheese, fries, anything that has *fried* in the name
Italian	Sautéed vegetables, salad, seafood salad, fish with olive oil, whole wheat pasta in small amounts with marinara sauce	Fried calamari and zucchini, stuffed mushrooms, baked ziti, fettuccine Alfredo, anything with bread crumbs, pizza with meat toppings and lots of cheese (continued)

Menu	Order It	Avoid It
Eastern Mediterranean	Hummus (chickpeas), tahini (sesame paste), tabbouleh (parsley salad), bean soup, lentils	Phyllo dough, meatballs, fried and breaded meals
Asian	Seaweed salad; sea vegetables; miso soup; edamame; sashimi; any vegetables that are not fried, such as bok choy, bamboo shoots, sautéed green beans; green beans with snow peas and water chestnuts made without lard (you have to ask for it that way); broiled chicken; fresh spring rolls; moo shu chicken or vegetables; spicy eggplant; tofu (not fried); whole steamed fish; chicken soup; drunken chicken	Tempura; noodles (most are dried and drenched in saturated fat); white rice; smoked foods; anything described as "fried" or "crispy," including fried rice, General Tso's chicken, fried noodles, and fried egg rolls; pickled food; food with too much soy sauce; egg dishes, such as egg foo yong, salty soups and monosodium glutamate on dishes for anyone younger than fourteen or any pregnant woman
Mexican	Fajitas, black beans, refried beans cooked without lard, guacamole as a condiment, brown rice, jicama, grilled chicken or fish, ceviche, avocados, chicken enchiladas without cheese, arroz con pollo (request brown rice), camarones	Fried flour or corn items such as tortillas, taco shells, sour cream, cheese, quesadillas, chalupas, nachos, ground beef or pork

Ready-made Meals

Sometimes it's easier to reach into the freezer than it is to pull out the pots, even when you do have drag-race-worthy recipes. That's OK. Plenty of ready-made choices are available for you to sub for one of your lunches or dinners, if that's easiest for you. You should still follow guidelines we've outlined (look at labels to avoid high levels of waist-busting ingredients, like more than 4 grams per serving of sugar or saturated fat and any trans fat). These are some of the ones we favor.

Soups:

Check sodium to make sure it's less than 400 milligrams per serving, and avoid soups with noodles, since they may be cooked in saturated or trans fats.

Dried: Healthy Valley and Fantastic Always Natural

Canned: Eden Organic, Health Valley, Amy's Organic Soups, Muir Glen Organic, Wolfgang Puck, Campbell's "Select"

Snacks:

Low-calorie cheese: Horizon Organic part-skim mozzarella sticks and veggie singles

Meals:

Check to make sure a meal is low in trans and saturated fats.

Lean Cuisine, Healthy Choice, Amy's Kitchen

The YOU Diet Troubleshooting Guide

If YOU . . .	Then YOU . . .
Eat something you shouldn't	Don't worry, but don't keep eating. Use one of our YOU-Turn techniques (a stretch, a meditation technique, or the lip lick) to refocus so you don't turn one mistake into a buffet-clearing gorge. Call your buddy and get help.
Stall with weight/waist loss	Talk to your doctor about using medication to help you get past the plateau to lead to further weight/waist loss (see page 453, appendix A). (continued)

If YOU . . .	Then YOU . . .
Can't find a support partner	If you can't blackmail a partner with all the benefits she'll also receive (she too will learn about elegant solutions she can apply to her own life), then match yourself with one at www.realage.com.
Have a family that decides to go to the buffet tonight	Before you go, have a cup of soup, a handful of nuts, and one glass of water. That will fill you up before you eat, so you eat sensibly and automatically. And limit yourself to one trip with a seven- or nine-inch plate, and keep it to single-story servings.
Feel foot pain and find it hard to walk	Stop walking and find an alternative activity such as biking or swimming. See a podiatrist to diagnose your ailment. Stretch your plantar fascia. See *YOU: Being Beautiful.*
Travel all the time and have to eat on the road a lot	Rely on more snacks rather than gorging on big meals. Travel with easy-to-carry (in plastic baggies) snacks such as nuts, cut-up apples and carrots to take the edge off your hunger.
Are diagnosed with a serious illness	It's not always the time to lose weight when you're sick, but it is the ideal time to get food on your side. But if you're prescribed a drug that may slow weight loss (such as a beta-blocker), talk to your doctor about a more aggressive weight-loss approach that's ailment-appropriate, since subsequent weight loss is more difficult.
Might have a food allergy (for example, irritable bowel syndrome or unexplained lethargy)	Do the elimination diet found on page 104.

The YOU Diet Recipes

YOU Drinks

Pineapple-Banana Protein Blaster

2 servings ❖ 207 calories per serving

1 large ripe banana, broken into chunks

½ cup low-fat (1 percent) soy milk

1 can (4 ounces) crushed pineapple in juice, undrained

½ cup "pineapple-passion" sorbet, such as Select brand
　　(a Safeway brand)

1 tablespoon soy protein powder (8 grams protein)

Combine all ingredients in blender. Cover; blend until fairly smooth.

What's in it for you?	
Total fat	2 g
Saturated fat	0.8 g
Healthy fats	1.1 g
Fiber	2.1 g
Carbohydrates	38 g
Sugar	17 g
Protein	11 g
Sodium	31 mg
Calcium	39 mg
Magnesium	40 mg
Selenium	1 mcg
Potassium	428 mg

Magical Breakfast Blaster

2 servings ❖ *136 calories per serving*

½ large ripe banana, broken into chunks (or other fruit of your choice)

1 scoop (⅓ cup) Soy Protein (like Nature's Plus Spiru-Tein:
   naturesplus.com)

½ tablespoon flaxseed oil

¼ cup frozen blueberries

½ tablespoon apple juice concentrate or honey

1 teaspoon psyllium seed husks

8 ounces water

Combine all ingredients in a blender. Optional: Add a few cubes of ice, as well as powdered vitamins. Cover; blend until fairly smooth.

What's in it for you?

Total fat	2.6 g
Saturated fat	0.3 g
Healthy fats	2.4 g
Fiber	6.3 g
Carbohydrates	16.8 g
Sugar	11.1 g
Protein	29 g
Sodium	380 mg
Calcium	93.5 mg
Magnesium	33.1 mg
Selenium	1.8 mcg
Potassium	195 mg

Lifestyle 180 Choose Your Fruit Pancakes

Makes 12–14 pancakes, 110 calories per serving (2 pancakes)

1⅓ cups whole wheat pastry flour

1 tablespoon baking powder

¾ teaspoon salt

½ teaspoon cinnamon

1 tablespoon ground chia seeds

1⅓ cups water

1 tablespoon vanilla extract

½ cup toasted walnuts

1 apple, grated

1 pear, grated

1 banana, peeled, halved, and thinly sliced

In a large bowl, combine the flour, baking powder, salt, cinnamon, and ground chia seeds and mix well with a wire whisk. In a separate measuring cup, combine the water and vanilla extract. Add the mixture to the dry ingredients and mix well with a wire whisk. Add the walnuts, grated apple and pear to the pancake mixture; then add the banana. Mix well, and if the batter seems a little thick, add two tablespoons of water. Make the pancakes in a preheated, nonstick pan that has been wiped with a light film of vegetable oil. Cook over medium heat.

What's in it for you?	
Total fat	4 g
Saturated fat	0 g
Healthy fats	3.7 g
Fiber	3 g
Carbohydrates	18 g
Sugar	4 g
Protein	2 g
Sodium	280 mg
Calcium	49 mg
Magnesium	13 mg
Selenium	0 mcg
Potassium	88 mg

Lifestyle 180 Tofu Scramble

2 servings ❖ 170 calories per serving

2 tablespoons extra-virgin olive oil

½ cup diced extra-firm tofu

½ cup blanched broccoli florets (or any leftover cooked vegetables)

¼ cup chopped onion

¼ cup diced red bell pepper

¼ cup sliced shiitake mushrooms

8 egg whites

2 whole eggs

¼ teaspoon salt

¼ teaspoon freshly ground black pepper

Heat oil in a large nonstick skillet over medium heat. Add tofu; cook until light golden brown, about 2 minutes. Add vegetables; the broccoli, onion, pepper, and mushrooms; sauté 3 to 4 minutes or until softened. Beat together the egg whites, whole eggs, salt, and pepper and add the mixture to the skillet. Continue cooking, stirring occasionally, until eggs are set.

What's in it for you?	
Total fat	11 g
Saturated fat	1.5 g
Healthy fats	11 g
Fiber	1 g
Carbohydrates	6 g
Sugar	2 g
Protein	13 g
Sodium	280 mg
Calcium	76 mg
Magnesium	13 mg
Selenium	16 mcg
Potassium	180 mg

Lifestyle 180 Banana Steel Cut Oatmeal with Cinnamon

3 servings ❖ 200 calories per serving

2⅓ cups fat-free milk

⅔ cup steel-cut oats

⅛ teaspoon salt

1 large banana, thinly sliced

½ teaspoon ground cinnamon

Place 2 cups of the milk in a medium saucepan. Bring to a gentle simmer over high heat. Stir in the oats and salt. Reduce heat to low; simmer, stirring frequently, until most of the milk is absorbed and oats are tender, about 25 minutes. Remove from heat; stir in banana and cinnamon. Pour into two cereal bowls and serve with remaining ⅓ cup milk.

What's in it for you?

Total fat	2 g
Saturated fat	0 g
Healthy fats	0 g
Fiber	4 g
Carbohydrates	37 g
Sugar	12 g
Protein	11 g
Sodium	170 mg
Calcium	190 mg
Magnesium	8 mg
Selenium	0 mcg
Potassium	106 mg

Lifestyle 180 Berry-Banana Smoothie
2 servings ❖ 130 calories per serving

1 small banana, broken into chunks

1 cup fat-free plain yogurt

½ cup orange juice

½ cup fresh or frozen raspberries

¼ cup fresh or frozen blueberries

½ cup fresh or frozen blackberries

Combine all ingredients in a blender. Cover and blend until fairly smooth.

What's in it for you?	
Total fat	0.5 g
Saturated fat	0 g
Healthy fats	0 g
Fiber	4 g
Carbohydrates	28 g
Sugar	20 g
Protein	6 g
Sodium	65 mg
Calcium	176 mg
Magnesium	37 mg
Selenium	4 mcg
Potassium	435 mg

Lifestyle 180 Chia Muffins

Makes 12–14 muffins ❖ 150 calories per muffin

1 tablespoon ground chia seeds

1½ cups whole wheat flour

2 teaspoons ground cinnamon

½ teaspoon ground nutmeg

2 teaspoons baking soda

½ teaspoon salt

15 ounces canned pumpkin

¼ cup canola oil

2 tablespoons agave nectar

1 tablespoon vanilla extract

¾ cup chopped walnuts

¼ cup water or no-sugar-added apple juice

1 cup fresh apple, peeled and grated (5½ ounces by weight)
(grate apple on large-hole side of the grater)

Preheat oven to 350°F. Combine the chia seeds, flour, cinnamon, nutmeg, baking soda, and salt and mix with a wire whisk. In a separate bowl combine pumpkin, canola oil, agave nectar, vanilla, walnuts, and water or juice, mix, and then fold into dry ingredients. Fold in the grated apple. Scoop into paper cups in muffin tins and bake for 33 minutes, or until inserted toothpick comes out clean. Remove from muffin tin and cool on wire rack.

What's in it for you?	
Total fat	9 g
Saturated fat	1 g
Healthy fats	8 g
Fiber	3 g
Carbohydrates	16 g
Sugar	4 g
Protein	3 g
Sodium	270 mg
Calcium	29 mg
Magnesium	36 mg
Selenium	10 mcg
Potassium	152 mg

Lifestyle 180 Vita-Mix Green Smoothie

3 servings ❖ *120 calories per serving*

2 cups ice

½ cup cold water

½ cup packed spinach leaves

1 cup chopped cooked kale leaves

1 orange, peeled and seeded

1 cup green seedless grapes

1 small ripe pear, peeled and cut into chunks

1 large banana, peeled and broken into chunks

2 teaspoons chia seeds

Combine all ingredients in a blender. Cover and blend until fairly smooth.

What's in it for you?	
Total fat	1.5 g
Saturated fat	0 g
Healthy fats	1.5 g
Fiber	5 g
Carbohydrates	28 g
Sugar	17 g
Protein	3 g
Sodium	30 mg
Calcium	89 mg
Magnesium	47 mg
Selenium	1 mcg
Potassium	520 mg

Garden Harvest Soup

10 servings (about 1 cup each) ❖ 176 calories per serving

1 tablespoon extra-virgin olive oil

1 medium onion, chopped

1 carrot, chopped

4 garlic cloves, thinly sliced

1 red bell pepper, chopped

2 quarts (8 cups) low-salt vegetable or chicken stock or broth

1 can (28 ounces) whole, crushed, or diced tomatoes, undrained

2 cups water

1 small head cabbage, thinly sliced

½ teaspoon hot red pepper sauce (optional)

Salt and freshly ground black pepper (optional)

Optional garnishes: chopped fresh parsley, chopped fresh cilantro

Heat a large saucepan over medium-high heat. Add oil, then onion; cook 5 minutes, stirring occasionally. Stir in carrot, garlic, and bell pepper; cook until tender. Add stock, tomatoes, water, and cabbage; simmer uncovered 20 minutes. Season to taste with hot sauce and salt and pepper if desired. Garnish with parsley or cilantro if desired.

What's in it for you?

Total fat	4 g
Saturated fat	0.8 g
Healthy fats	2.85 g
Fiber	3.6 g
Carbohydrates	15.9 g
Sugar	4.6 g
Protein	7.1 g
Sodium	374 mg
Calcium	73 mg
Magnesium	35 mg
Selenium	5.6 mcg
Potassium	631 mg

Lisa's Great Gazpacho

4 servings (about 1 cup each) ❖ 120 calories per serving

1 can (28 ounces) crushed or diced tomatoes, undrained

1 cup tomato juice

1 cup *each:* diced (¼ inch) red or orange bell pepper, unpeeled cucumber

¼ cup finely chopped red onion

2 green onions, finely chopped

1 bunch cilantro leaves, chopped

3 tablespoons red wine vinegar or apple cider vinegar

3 tablespoons extra-virgin olive oil

2 dashes (or to taste) hot red pepper sauce

2 garlic cloves, minced

Salt and freshly ground black pepper (optional)

Optional garnishes: chopped fresh parsley, diced avocado

Place all ingredients except salt, pepper, and garnishes in large bowl and combine. Coarsely puree about half the mixture in a blender or food processor and return it to the bowl; stir well. Season to taste with salt and pepper if desired. Refrigerate for at least 2 hours and up to 8 hours before serving. Garnish as desired.

What's in it for you?	
Total fat	12.1 g
Saturated fat	1.8 g
Healthy fats	10.2 g
Fiber	4.6 g
Carbohydrates	19.2 g
Sugar	5.2 g
Protein	4.4 g
Sodium	207 mg
Calcium	74 mg
Magnesium	53 mg
Selenium	0.9 mcg
Potassium	780 mg

Spicy Vegetable Lentil Soup

10 servings (about 1 cup each) ❖ 94 calories per serving

1 tablespoon extra-virgin olive oil

1 medium onion, chopped

1 carrot, chopped

1 red bell pepper, chopped

5 garlic cloves, sliced

2 quarts (8 cups) water

1 cup dried lentils

1 can (28 ounces) crushed tomatoes, undrained

2 bay leaves

2 tablespoons balsamic vinegar

Salt and freshly ground black pepper (optional)

Heat oil in a large saucepan over medium-high heat. Add onion; cook 5 minutes, stirring occasionally. Stir in carrot, bell pepper, and garlic; cook 3 minutes. Stir in remaining ingredients except salt and pepper; bring to a boil over high heat. Reduce heat; simmer uncovered 18 to 20 minutes, or until lentils and vegetables are tender. Season to taste with salt and pepper if desired. Remove bay leaves before serving.

What's in it for you?

Total fat	1.6 g
Saturated fat	0.2 g
Healthy fats	1.4 g
Fiber	2.8 g
Carbohydrates	8 g
Sugar	1.6 g
Protein	1.9 g
Sodium	82 mg
Calcium	26 mg
Magnesium	16 mg
Selenium	0.6 mcg
Potassium	228 mg

Two-Onion Delight

8 servings (about 1 cup each) ❖ 129 calories per serving

1 tablespoon extra-virgin olive oil

2 onions, sliced

2 shallots, sliced

1 leek (white and light-green part only), sliced

2 quarts (8 cups) low-salt chicken stock or broth

Salt and freshly ground black pepper (optional)

½ cup (4 ounces) grated low-fat Swiss cheese

1 bunch chives, finely chopped

Heat oil in a large saucepan over medium-high heat. Add onions; cook 5 minutes, stirring occasionally. Stir in shallots and leek; continue cooking until golden brown, about 5 minutes. Add stock; simmer uncovered 15 minutes. Season to taste with salt and pepper if desired. Ladle into shallow bowls; garnish with cheese and chives.

What's in it for you?	
Total fat	5 g
Saturated fat	1.2 g
Healthy fats	3.4 g
Fiber	0.3 g
Carbohydrates	12.3 g
Sugar	5.7 g
Protein	8.5 g
Sodium	385 mg
Calcium	84 mg
Magnesium	16 mg
Selenium	6.4 mcg
Potassium	321 mg

Curried Split Pea Soup

8 servings (about 1 cup each) ❖ 155 calories per serving

1 tablespoon extra-virgin olive oil

1 onion, chopped

1 carrot, chopped

4 garlic cloves, sliced

1 quart (4 cups) low-salt vegetable stock or broth

1 quart (4 cups) water

1 cup dried yellow split peas

1 teaspoon curry powder

1 teaspoon ground cumin

½ bunch parsley, chopped

Heat oil in a large saucepan over medium-high heat. Add onion; cook 5 minutes, stirring occasionally. Add carrot and garlic; cook until softened, about 5 minutes. Add remaining ingredients except parsley; bring to a boil. Reduce heat; simmer uncovered 30 minutes, or until peas are tender. Ladle into shallow bowls; garnish with parsley.

What's in it for you?	
Total fat	3.6 g
Saturated fat	0.7 g
Healthy fats	2.7 g
Fiber	6.8 g
Carbohydrates	22 g
Sugar	5.1 g
Protein	9.5 g
Sodium	183 mg
Calcium	30.8 mg
Magnesium	38 mg
Selenium	3.4 mcg
Potassium	432 mg

Quick Black Bean Soup

8 servings (about 1¼ cups each) ❖ 445 calories per serving

1 tablespoon extra-virgin olive oil

1 onion, chopped

3 garlic cloves, sliced

1 carrot, chopped

2 stalks celery, chopped

2 quarts (8 cups) low-salt vegetable stock or broth

2 cans (15 or 16 ounces each) black beans, rinsed and drained

1 teaspoon ground coriander

¼ teaspoon cayenne pepper

1 tablespoon balsamic vinegar

1 bunch cilantro leaves, chopped

Heat oil in a large saucepan over medium-high heat. Add onion; cook 5 minutes, stirring occasionally. Add garlic, carrot, and celery; cook until soft, about 5 minutes. Add stock, beans, coriander, and cayenne pepper; simmer uncovered 10 minutes. Stir in vinegar. Transfer to blender or food processor; process to desired consistency. Reheat if necessary. Ladle into shallow bowls; garnish with cilantro.

What's in it for you?	
Total fat	6 g
Saturated fat	1.4 g
Healthy fats	2.8 g
Fiber	15.3 g
Carbohydrates	71.8 g
Sugar	7.4 g
Protein	27.4 g
Sodium	360 mg
Calcium	139 mg
Magnesium	180 mg
Selenium	1 mcg
Potassium	1,771 mg

Minted Fresh Pea Soup

8 servings (about 1 cup each) ❖ 157 calories per serving

1 tablespoon extra-virgin olive oil

1 onion, chopped

1 carrot, chopped

2 garlic cloves, minced

2 cups frozen or fresh peas

2 quarts (8 cups) low-salt vegetable stock or broth

1 cup low-fat plain yogurt

Salt and freshly ground black pepper (optional)

1 small bunch mint leaves, chopped

Heat oil in a large saucepan over medium-high heat. Add onion; cook 5 minutes, stirring occasionally. Add carrot and garlic; cook until soft, about 5 minutes. Add peas and stock; simmer uncovered 20 minutes. Transfer in batches to blender or food processor and add yogurt; puree until smooth. Season to taste with salt and pepper if desired. Reheat if needed; ladle into shallow bowls; garnish with mint.

What's in it for you?	
Total fat	4.8 g
Saturated fat	1.1 g
Healthy fats	3.5 g
Fiber	2.3 g
Carbohydrates	18.2 g
Sugar	9.5 g
Protein	10 g
Sodium	376 mg
Calcium	84 mg
Magnesium	30.3 mg
Selenium	7.3 mcg
Potassium	466 mg

Lifestyle 180 Avocado and Asparagus Soup

5 servings (about 1 cup each) ❖ *140 calories per serving*

2 avocados, peeled and pitted

2 cups water

2 cups chopped asparagus, woody bottoms removed

2 tablespoons chopped celery

4 teaspoons light soy sauce

2 tablespoons lemon juice

1 teaspoon chopped green onion

1 teaspoon minced garlic

¼ teaspoon dried thyme leaves

1½ teaspoons chopped fresh tarragon, stems removed

¼ cup firmly packed fresh spinach, stems removed

Pinch of cayenne pepper

½ teaspoon salt

Freshly ground black pepper to taste

Optional garnishes: asparagus tips, shaved fennel, radishes in vinegar,
or truffle oil

Combine all ingredients in a tall pot or deep mixing bowl and puree with a vertical stick blender until smooth. Or combine all ingredients in a blender and blend until smooth. (We like the stick blender better.) Pass the mixture through a chinois or other fine-meshed sieve, if desired. Chill. This can be garnished with asparagus tips, shaved fennel, and radishes marinated in vinegar, or truffle oil.

What's in it for you?	
Total fat	11 g
Saturated fat	1.5 g
Healthy fats	8 g
Fiber	6 g
Carbohydrates	10 g
Sugar	2 g
Protein	3 g
Sodium	451 mg
Calcium	46 mg
Magnesium	38 mg
Selenium	1.5 mcg
Potassium	524 mg

Lifestyle 180 Potato-Leek Soup

10 servings (1 cup each) ❖ 100 calories per serving

1 pound sweet onions, diced small

1 tablespoon extra-virgin olive oil

1 tablespoon finely chopped garlic

2 leeks (white parts only), diced

5 cups water

2 tablespoons Minor's vegetable base

1½ pounds Yukon Gold potatoes, peeled and cubed

Sauté onions in extra-virgin olive oil until transparent, add garlic, and sauté 4 minutes without browning, stirring frequently. Add diced leeks and sauté 4 minutes. Add water and vegetable base, bring to a simmer, then add potatoes and simmer until potatoes are fully cooked. Turn off heat and blend with a vertical stick blender until completely pureed. Garnish with chopped parsley or cut chives and serve.

What's in it for you?	
Total fat	1.5 g
Saturated fat	0 g
Healthy fats	1 g
Fiber	3 g
Carbohydrates	20 g
Sugar	5 g
Protein	2 g
Sodium	220 mg
Calcium	51 mg
Magnesium	32 mg
Selenium	1 mcg
Potassium	348 mg

Lifestyle 180 Butternut Squash, Carrot and Ginger Soup

18 servings (1 cup each) ❖ 70 calories per serving

1 cup chopped white onion

2 tablespoons extra-virgin olive oil

2 cups carrots, chopped

1 teaspoon fresh ginger, minced

9 cups butternut squash, cubed

10 cups water

6 tablespoons low-sodium vegetarian vegetable base without MSG

In a stock pot, sauté onion in olive oil over low heat until transparent. Add carrots and sauté 10 minutes. Add ginger and sauté two minutes. Add butternut squash, water, and vegetable base and bring to a boil. Turn heat to medium low and simmer for 45 minutes. Puree with a handheld vertical blender until smooth and serve.

What's in it for you?	
Total fat	2 g
Saturated fat	0 g
Healthy fats	0 g
Fiber	2 g
Carbohydrates	13 g
Sugar	3 g
Protein	1 g
Sodium	160 mg
Calcium	45 mg
Magnesium	28 mg
Selenium	0.43 mcg
Potassium	319 mg

Lifestyle 180 Chicken Soup

20 servings (about 1 cup each) ❖ 170 calories per serving

1½ quarts water

2½ tablespoons chicken base without MSG

3 pounds chicken backs and necks

1 large onion, unpeeled, cut into wedges

4 stalks celery, thickly sliced

1 bunch fresh parsley stems (about ½ cup)

½ cup low-salt vegetable juice cocktail

3 pounds bone-in chicken breasts

1 small (8 ounces) rutabaga, peeled and cut into ½-inch chunks

3 large carrots, sliced

1 pound Yukon Gold potatoes, scrubbed and cut into ½-inch chunks

Salt and freshly ground black pepper (optional)

Combine water and chicken base in an 8-quart Dutch oven; place over high heat. Add chicken backs and necks, onion, celery, parsley stems, and vegetable juice; bring to a boil. Arrange chicken breasts over mixture. Cover; reduce heat to medium low and simmer 20 to 25 minutes or until internal temperature of chicken breasts reaches 160°F. Remove chicken breasts to a plate; let stand until cool. Discard skin and bones and refrigerate for Chicken Salad Véronique (page 325) or for another use. If desired, some of the chicken may be returned to the soup. Meanwhile, continue simmering soup, covered, for 1 hour. Strain the mixture well; discard the solids (see soup tip on the next page). Return broth to Dutch oven. Spoon off and discard fat from broth. Add rutabaga and carrots; simmer 10 minutes. Add potatoes; simmer 10 minutes or until vegetables are tender. Add salt and pepper to taste if desired.

What's in it for you?	
Total fat	5 g
Saturated fat	1.5 g
Healthy fats	2 g
Fiber	1 g
Carbohydrates	7 g
Sugar	1 g
Protein	24 g
Sodium	160 mg
Calcium	34 mg
Magnesium	31 mg
Selenium	17 mcg
Potassium	331 mg

Note: 1 quart low-salt chicken broth plus 2 cups water may be substituted for chicken base.

Tips: Eliminate excess saturated fat by refrigerating strained broth and removing the solidified fat. There are small pieces of chicken meat on the cooked backs that may be removed from the bones and added back to the soup if desired. For an Asian flavor, season the broth with fresh ginger, rice wine, and green onions. For chicken noodle soup, omit the potatoes and add cooked whole grain egg noodles or no-yolk egg noodles.

Lifestyle 180 Jim's Vegan Vegetable and Chia Soup

50 servings (about 1 cup each) ❖ 80 calories per serving

2 pounds sweet onions, finely diced

4 tablespoons extra-virgin olive oil

2 leeks, finely diced

1 cup finely diced celery

6 quarts (24 cups) water

8 tablespoons Minor's vegetable base

2 teaspoons chia seeds

7 cups (2½ pounds) rutabagas, diced

½ cup low-salt vegetable juice cocktail

2 teaspoons Cholula brand hot sauce

16 ounces V8 juice

3 cups diced carrots

44 ounces potatoes, diced

3 cups diced white turnips

1 pound fresh green beans, cut into ¾-inch pieces

12 ounces frozen lima beans

12 ounces frozen peas

In a large soup pot, sauté onions in extra-virgin olive oil until transparent. Add leeks and celery and sauté until tender. Add water, vegetable base, and chia seeds and bring to a simmer. Add rutabagas and simmer until tender. Add tomato soup, Cholula hot sauce, V8, and carrots, and simmer until crisp-tender. Add potatoes, white turnips, green beans, and lima beans and simmer until tender. Add frozen peas and turn off flame. Let sit 15 minutes and serve.

What's in it for you?	
Total fat	1.5 g
Saturated fat	0 g
Healthy fats	1 g
Fiber	3 g
Carbohydrates	14 g
Sugar	3 g
Protein	3 g
Sodium	290 mg
Calcium	37 mg
Magnesium	20 mg
Selenium	0.6 mcg
Potassium	283 mg

Lifestyle 180 Vegetable and Chia Chili

12 servings ❖ 100 calories per serving

4 cups peeled, finely diced eggplant (about one 1½ pounds)

1 cup diced onion

2 tablespoons canola oil

2 tablespoons chopped garlic

3 cups diced zucchini (about three small zucchini)

46 ounces organic V8 juice

2 tablespoons chia seeds

1½ packages McCormick Chili seasoning mix (1.48-ounce packages)
    or other sugar-free brand

2 cups one-inch cut cooked green beans, al dente

8 ounces precooked lima beans

2 teaspoons (or to taste) Cholula brand hot sauce

In a hot, preheated dry nonstick sauté pan add diced eggplant and sauté until golden and tender, remove, and set aside. In a large stockpot sauté onions in canola oil until transparent. Add garlic, sauté two minutes and add zucchini and sauté until crisp-tender. Now add eggplant, V8 juice, chia seed, cooked green beans, cooked lima beans, chili mix, and Cholula hot sauce. Simmer 10 minutes and serve over brown rice.

What's in it for you?	
Fat	3 g
Saturated fat	0 g
Healthy fats	3 g
Fiber	4 g
Carbohydrates	15 g
Sugar	6 g
Protein	4 g
Sodium	330 mg
Calcium	60 mg
Magnesium	9 mg
Selenium	0.3 mcg
Potassium	345 mg

Lifestyle 180 Chia Lentils

19 servings (about ½ cup each) ❖ 110 calories per serving

2 tablespoons extra-virgin olive oil

1 large white onion, chopped (8 oz.)

1 teaspoon minced garlic

2 tablespoons minced fresh ginger

2 teaspoons turmeric

1 teaspoon cumin seeds

1 tablespoon fresh jalapeño, peeled, seeded, and minced

¼ teaspoon ground cardamom

1 tablespoon chia seeds

4 cups water

3 tablespoons vegetable base without MSG or 3½ cups organic
    vegetable broth

2 cups red lentils

2½ cups fire-roasted crushed tomatoes, undrained

4 tablespoons chopped cilantro

Heat oil in large saucepan. Add onions and sauté until lightly carmelized. Add cumin seeds, cardamom, garlic, and sauté two minutes. Add remaining ingredients, bring to a boil, reduce heat to low, cover, simmer, stirring often, until all lentils are tender, about 15 minutes.

What's in it for you?	
Total fat	2 g
Saturated fat	0 g
Healthy fats	1.3 g
Fiber	4 g
Carbohydrates	16 g
Sugar	2 g
Protein	7 g
Sodium	370 mg
Calcium	25 mg
Magnesium	3 mg
Selenium	0 mcg
Potassium	204 mg

Japanese Ginger Salad with Pumpkin Seeds and Sprouts

8 servings ❖ *230 calories per serving*

Dressing Ingredients

½ cup extra-virgin olive oil

½ cup rice vinegar

1 small sweet onion, quartered

1 large carrot, chopped

1 tablespoon orange juice

1 tablespoon grated fresh ginger

¼ teaspoon soy sauce

Salt and freshly ground black pepper (optional)

Salad Ingredients

2 large heads romaine lettuce, torn

½ cup fresh bean sprouts

¼ cup pumpkin seeds

Combine all dressing ingredients except salt and pepper in blender or food processor; puree until smooth. Season to taste with salt and pepper if desired. Toss lettuce with dressing; top with sprouts and seeds.

What's in it for you?	
Total fat	22 g
Saturated fat	1.78 g
Healthy fats	12.1 g
Fiber	6 g
Carbohydrates	16.8 g
Sugar	4 g
Protein	6.4 g
Sodium	53 mg
Calcium	79 mg
Magnesium	74 mg
Selenium	2 mcg
Potassium	499 mg

I LOST MY TOP!

I BLEW MY TOP!

I JUST LIKE GOING TOPLESS!

THAT SHAMELESS CARROT BUNCH

Spinach-Walnut-Citrus Salad

2 servings ❖ 246 calories per serving

Dressing Ingredients

1 tablespoon extra-virgin olive oil

1 tablespoon white wine vinegar

1 teaspoon honey

Dash of cayenne pepper

Salt and freshly ground black pepper (optional)

Salad Ingredients

1 large bunch spinach, washed and trimmed

¼ cup walnut halves, raw or pan-roasted (beware of smoke-detector
   sounds if you do this like Dr. Mike and answer the phone when it
   rings only to forget what is in the pan roasting)

½ orange, cut into segments

½ grapefruit, cut into segments

2 green onions, chopped

Combine oil, vinegar, honey, and cayenne pepper; mix well. Season to taste with salt and pepper if desired. Toss spinach with dressing and walnuts. Arrange orange and grapefruit sections on top and garnish with green onions.

What's in it for you?	
Total fat	17 g
Saturated fat	1.9 g
Healthy fats	14.4 g
Fiber	6.8 g
Carbohydrates	21 g
Sugar	7.6 g
Protein	8 g
Sodium	138 mg
Calcium	218 mg
Magnesium	169 mg
Selenium	3.6 mcg
Potassium	1,203 mg

Cranberries, Walnuts, and Crumbled Cheese Over Greens

2 servings ❖ 304 calories per serving

Dressing Ingredients

1 tablespoon extra-virgin olive oil

1 tablespoon balsamic vinegar

½ teaspoon Dijon mustard

1 garlic clove, minced

¼ teaspoon soy sauce

Salt and freshly ground black pepper (optional)

Salad Ingredients

3 cups packed mixed mesclun or spring greens

¼ cup dried cranberries

¼ cup walnut halves, raw or pan-roasted

¼ cup (1 ounce) crumbled farmer cheese

Combine oil, vinegar, mustard, garlic, and soy sauce; mix well. Season to taste with salt and pepper if desired. Toss greens with dressing, cranberries, and walnuts. Arrange on serving plates; top with cheese.

What's in it for you?	
Total fat	19.7 g
Saturated fat	3 g
Healthy fats	15.6 g
Fiber	4.7 g
Carbohydrates	19.6 g
Sugar	11.9 g
Protein	10 g
Sodium	183 mg
Calcium	146 mg
Magnesium	57 mg
Selenium	3 mcg
Potassium	391 mg

Arugula, Watermelon, and Feta Salad

2 servings ❖ *190 calories per serving*

Dressing Ingredients

1 tablespoon extra-virgin olive oil

1 tablespoon balsamic vinegar

1 small shallot, minced

Salt and freshly ground black pepper (optional)

Salad Ingredients

1 large bunch of arugula (3 cups packed), washed and dried

1 cup cubed seedless watermelon

⅓ cup (1.3 ounces) crumbled low-fat feta cheese

Combine oil, vinegar, and shallot; mix well. Season to taste with salt and pepper if desired; let stand 5 minutes. Arrange arugula on two serving plates. Arrange watermelon and cheese on top of arugula; drizzle with dressing.

What's in it for you?	
Total fat	11.7 g
Saturated fat	3.6 g
Healthy fats	7.3 g
Fiber	1.1 g
Carbohydrates	13 g
Sugar	6.9 g
Protein	6.4 g
Sodium	334 mg
Calcium	235 mg
Magnesium	41.8 mg
Selenium	5 mcg
Potassium	377 mg

IT'S CURLY LETTUCE!

Greek Feta Salad with Peppers and Olives

2 servings ❖ 305 calories per serving

Dressing Ingredients

1 tablespoon extra-virgin olive oil

1 tablespoon red wine vinegar

1 tablespoon lemon juice

½ teaspoon dried oregano

1 garlic clove, minced

½ teaspoon honey

Salt and freshly ground black pepper (optional)

Salad Ingredients

1 head romaine lettuce, torn

1 tomato, quartered

4 pepperoncini peppers

1 small cucumber, sliced

¼ cup (1 ounce) crumbled low-fat feta cheese

Several sprigs fresh dill, chopped

½ green bell pepper, sliced into rings

8 kalamata olives

Combine all dressing ingredients except salt and pepper; mix well. Season to taste with salt and pepper if desired; let stand 5 minutes. Combine all salad ingredients in large bowl; toss with dressing.

What's in it for you?	
Total fat	13.1 g
Saturated fat	2.8 g
Healthy fats	9.6 g
Fiber	10.9 g
Carbohydrates	35.8 g
Sugar	17.9 g
Protein	12 g
Sodium	510 mg
Calcium	324 mg
Magnesium	108 mg
Selenium	619 mcg
Potassium	1.6 mg

Turkish Shepherd Salad

2 servings ❖ 153 calories per serving

1 small cucumber

1 tomato

1 small sweet onion

1 teaspoon extra-virgin olive oil

1 tablespoon red wine vinegar

Salt and freshly ground black pepper (optional)

¼ cup (1 ounce) crumbled low-fat feta cheese

Coarsely chop cucumber, tomato, and onion; transfer to a bowl. Add oil and vinegar; toss well. Season to taste with salt and pepper if desired. Transfer to serving plates; top with cheese.

What's in it for you?	
Total fat	6 g
Saturated fat	4.6 g
Healthy fats	2 g
Fiber	2.2 g
Carbohydrates	14.7 g
Sugar	9 g
Protein	6.1 g
Sodium	329 mg
Calcium	186 mg
Magnesium	39 mg
Selenium	5.1 mcg
Potassium	479 mg

Orient Express Salad with Chopped Peanuts

2 servings ❖ 200 calories per serving

Dressing Ingredients

1 tablespoon extra-virgin olive oil

2 tablespoons orange juice

1 tablespoon rice wine vinegar

1 teaspoon grated fresh ginger

1 teaspoon soy sauce

½ teaspoon toasted sesame oil

Salt and freshly ground black pepper (optional)

Salad Ingredients

2 small heads Boston lettuce, torn

1 small cucumber, sliced

1 small bunch cilantro, coarsely chopped

1 carrot, shredded

2 tablespoons chopped peanuts

2 green onions, chopped

Combine all dressing ingredients except salt and pepper; mix well. Season to taste with salt and pepper if desired. Toss lettuce, cucumber, cilantro, and carrot with the dressing. Transfer to serving plates; top with peanuts and green onions.

What's in it for you?	
Total fat	13.1 g
Saturated fat	1.8 g
Healthy fats	10.6 g
Fiber	5.1 g
Carbohydrates	17.7 g
Sugar	7.9 g
Protein	7.1 g
Sodium	458 mg
Calcium	121 mg
Magnesium	72 mg
Selenium	2.3 mcg
Potassium	936 mg

Mediterranean Cauliflower Salad

4 servings ❖ 94 calories per serving

1 head cauliflower, blanched for 5 minutes

1 small can anchovies, drained, chopped (optional)

1 tablespoon drained capers

2 tablespoons fresh lemon juice

1 tablespoon extra-virgin olive oil

1 garlic clove, pressed or minced

1 tablespoon chopped fresh oregano or 1 teaspoon dried

Drain cauliflower and break into small pieces. Combine cauliflower, anchovies if desired, and capers in a medium bowl. Combine remaining ingredients; toss with cauliflower mixture.

What's in it for you?	
Total fat	4.6 g
Saturated fat	0.7 g
Healthy fats	3.7 g
Fiber	3.8 g
Carbohydrates	8.8 g
Sugar	3.7 g
Protein	6.2 g
Sodium	519 mg
Calcium	63 mg
Magnesium	31 mg
Selenium	8.7 mcg
Potassium	514 mg

Sweet Beet and Gorgonzola Salad

4 servings ❖ 106 calories per serving

6 medium beets, trimmed

1 tablespoon extra-virgin olive oil

1 tablespoon balsamic vinegar

1 teaspoon honey

1 garlic clove, pressed or minced

½ teaspoon soy sauce

½ bunch of chives, finely chopped

2 tablespoons crumbled gorgonzola cheese

In large saucepan, simmer beets in water covered until tender but still firm, about 30 minutes. Drain, cool, and remove skin. Meanwhile, combine oil, vinegar, honey, garlic, and soy sauce in a medium bowl. Cut beets into 1-inch cubes; add to bowl. Toss with dressing and chives. Transfer to serving plates; top with cheese.

What's in it for you?	
Total fat	4.8 g
Saturated fat	1.3 g
Healthy fats	3.3 g
Fiber	3.5 g
Carbohydrates	13.7 g
Sugar	9.8 g
Protein	3.1 g
Sodium	239 mg
Calcium	45 mg
Magnesium	31 mg
Selenium	1.6 mcg
Potassium	424 mg

Hearts of Palm Salad with Tomato and Mushrooms

2 servings ❖ 132 calories per serving

1 can (16 ounces) hearts of palm, drained

1 tomato, chopped

1 shallot, chopped

6 button mushrooms, sliced

1 small bunch parsley, chopped

2 tablespoons red wine vinegar

1 tablespoon extra-virgin olive oil

Salt and freshly ground black pepper (optional)

Slice hearts of palm in half lengthwise; arrange on a serving platter. Combine remaining ingredients except salt and pepper; mix well. Season to taste with salt and pepper if desired. Spoon mixture over hearts of palm.

What's in it for you?	
Total fat	8 g
Saturated fat	1.2 g
Healthy fats	6.2 g
Fiber	5 g
Carbohydrates	12.2 g
Sugar	2.6 g
Protein	6.2 g
Sodium	632 mg
Calcium	102 mg
Magnesium	72 mg
Selenium	6 mcg
Potassium	632 mg

Carrot, Raisin, and Yogurt Slaw

2 servings ❖ 193 calories per serving

4 carrots, shredded

1 small bunch cilantro, chopped

1 cup low-fat Greek-style yogurt

¼ cup golden raisins

1 garlic clove, minced

1 teaspoon lemon juice

Dash of Worcestershire sauce

Salt and freshly ground black pepper (optional)

Combine all ingredients except salt and pepper in a bowl; mix well. Season to taste with salt and pepper if desired.

What's in it for you?	
Total fat	4.5 g
Saturated fat	2.7 g
Healthy fats	1.4 g
Fiber	5.1 g
Carbohydrates	35 g
Sugar	23 g
Protein	6.5 g
Sodium	166 mg
Calcium	2.5 mg
Magnesium	41 mg
Selenium	3.3 mcg
Potassium	850 mg

Sesame Cucumber Salad

2 servings ❖ 187 calories per serving

1 tablespoon rice wine vinegar

1 teaspoon extra-virgin olive oil

½ teaspoon toasted sesame oil

½ teaspoon soy sauce

Dash cayenne pepper

2 cucumbers, cut into ¼-inch-thick slices

½ bunch chives, minced

1 teaspoon sesame seeds

Combine vinegar, olive oil, sesame oil, soy sauce, and cayenne pepper in a medium bowl; mix well. Add cucumbers, chives, and sesame seeds; mix well.

What's in it for you?

Total fat	6.8 g
Saturated fat	1 g
Healthy fats	5.3 g
Fiber	3.2 g
Carbohydrates	29 g
Sugar	8.2 g
Protein	6.2 g
Sodium	180 mg
Calcium	90 mg
Magnesium	85 mg
Selenium	18.1 mcg
Potassium	750 mg

Lifestyle 180 Apple Pear Jicama Waldorf Salad

25 servings ❖ 190 calories per serving

1 pound jicama

2 cups unsweetened pineapple juice

3 Fuji apples

3 pears (variety of colors)

½ cup raisins, red or yellow

½ cup almonds, sliced and toasted

½ cup chopped toasted walnuts

2 cups red grapes

½ cup unsalted sunflower seeds

12 ounces grapeseed oil Vegenaise

Peel the jicama; as you dice the jicama, place it in a bowl with pineapple juice to prevent browning for about 2 minutes. Drain the jicama, reserving the liquid to be used for the other fruit. Wash and dice the apples, placing them in a bowl with the reserved pineapple juice to prevent browning about 2 minutes. Drain the apples, reserving the liquid. Wash and dice the pears, placing them in a bowl with the reserved pineapple juice to prevent browning. Let the pears soak in the pineapple juice while you wash and cut the grapes in half. Drain the pears, reserving the liquid. In a large bowl, combine and mix all the ingredients and toss with Vegenaise.

What's in it for you?	
Total fat	13 g
Saturated fat	2 g
Healthy fats	3 g
Fiber	3 g
Carbohydrates	17 g
Sugar	11 g
Protein	2 g
Sodium	80 mg
Calcium	20 mg
Magnesium	17 mg
Selenium	2 mcg
Potassium	190 mg

Tips: The reserved pineapple juice can be frozen for latter use; cover, date, and label. Pears need to soak the longest to prevent browning, and jicama the shortest time. If more sweetness is desired, you can add 2 tablespoons agave nectar to the Vegenaise.

Lifestyle 180 Chicken Salad Véronique

8 servings (½ cup each) ❖ 220 calories per serving

½ cup Vegenaise

2 tablespoons Dijon mustard

1 tablespoon chopped fresh parsley

½ teaspoon salt

¼ teaspoon freshly ground black pepper

1 pound (2½ cups) diced cooked chicken breast

1 cup halved seedless grapes

⅓ cup finely chopped celery

⅓ cup chopped pecans, walnuts, or almonds, toasted if desired

⅓ cup finely chopped onion

2 hard-cooked egg whites, chopped (about ½ cup)

Combine dressing, mustard, parsley, salt, and pepper in a medium bowl; mix well. Add remaining ingredients; mix well. Cover; chill at least 30 minutes or up to 2 days before serving.

What's in it for you?

Total fat	14 g
Saturated fat	2 g
Healthy fats	0 g
Fiber	1 g
Carbohydrates	7 g
Sugar	4 g
Protein	14 g
Sodium	500 mg
Calcium	15 mg
Magnesium	11 mg
Selenium	0.3 mcg
Potassium	83 mg

Lifestyle 180 "Your Choice" Legume Salad

12 servings (½ cup each) ❖ 90 calories per serving

2 tablespoons extra-virgin olive oil

2 tablespoons balsamic vinegar

2 tablespoons whole grain mustard

¼ cup chopped fresh herbs, such as parsley, basil, cilantro,
    and tarragon

¼ cup chopped green onions

1 tablespoon sherry

1 tablespoon fresh lemon juice

1 tablespoon agave nectar

2 teaspoons minced roasted jalapeños (see chile preparation note,
    page 378)

1 teaspoon minced garlic

1 can (15 to 16 ounces) pinto, kidney, or red beans, drained and rinsed

1 can (15 to 16 ounces) great northern, navy, or cannellini beans,
    drained and rinsed

1½ cups diced seeded beefsteak tomatoes

In a large bowl, combine all ingredients except beans and tomatoes; mix well. Add beans and tomatoes; mix well. Serve as a side salad or over cooked basmati rice.

What's in it for you?	
Total fat	2.5 g
Saturated fat	0 g
Healthy fats	2 g
Fiber	4 g
Carbohydrates	14 g
Sugar	5 g
Protein	4 g
Sodium	280 mg
Calcium	41 mg
Magnesium	1 mg
Selenium	0 mcg
Potassium	116 mg

Lifestyle 180 Navy Bean Salad

6 servings (½ cup each) ❖ 150 calories per serving

½ pound dried navy beans

½ cup finely diced celery

½ cup finely diced red or green bell pepper

¼ cup finely diced red or sweet onion

¼ cup red wine vinegar

2 tablespoons canola oil

2 tablespoons chopped fresh parsley

2 teaspoons agave nectar

1 teaspoon minced garlic

½ teaspoon kosher or sea salt

¼ teaspoon freshly ground black pepper

¼ teaspoon dry mustard

¼ teaspoon paprika or smoked paprika

Soak beans overnight in refrigerator. Drain, rinse, place in soup pot, cover with clean water, and simmer until tender (about 1 hour). Drain, cool, add remaining ingredients, and mix well. Label, date, and refrigerate. Chill for about 2 hours before serving cold.

Before serving, combine all remaining ingredients in a large bowl and mix with the beans.

What's in it for you?	
Total fat	4.5 g
Saturated fat	0 g
Healthy fats	4.5 g
Fiber	8 g
Carbohydrates	22 g
Sugar	2 g
Protein	6 g
Sodium	140 mg
Calcium	59 mg
Magnesium	43 mg
Selenium	2 mcg
Potassium	344 mg

Lifestyle 180 Vegetable and Country Dijon Potato Salad

14 servings ❖ 120 calories per serving

This summer recipe is a good way to include vegetables and reduce the fat normally found in this popular salad. You can substitute asparagus for the green beans, use both, or add any of your favorite vegetables, as this dressing will complement most vegetables.

1 pound (4 cups, loosely packed) fresh green beans,
    cut into ¾-inch pieces

3 pounds new red potatoes, cubed

½ cup Country Dijon mustard

3 tablespoons extra-virgin olive oil

1 tablespoon lemon juice

¼ cup Sutter Home Non-Alcoholic White Zinfandel
    (champagne or rice wine vinegar could be substituted)

1 teaspoon finely minced garlic

2 tablespoons chopped fresh parsley

1 teaspoon salt

¼ teaspoon black pepper

1 cup diced red peppers

1 cup diced red onion (about ½ small onion)

Cook the beans and potatoes separately until tender and set aside to cool. In a large mixing bowl, combine Country Dijon mustard, extra-virgin olive oil, lemon juice, Zinfandel, garlic, parsley, salt, and pepper, and whisk until well blended. Add potatoes, green beans, red peppers, and red onion and gently toss until well coated.

Tips: For a little sweetness, you can add 1 tablespoon agave nectar to the wet ingredients. The Sutter Home Non-Alcoholic White Zinfandel provides a pleasant, light flavor and is widely available in supermarkets.

What's in it for you?	
Total fat	3 g
Saturated fat	0 g
Healthy fats	3 g
Fiber	3 g
Carbohydrates	20 g
Sugar	2 g
Protein	2 g
Sodium	380 mg
Calcium	20 mg
Magnesium	14 mg
Selenium	0.5 mcg
Potassium	470 mg

Asian Salmon with Brown Rice Pilaf

4 servings ❖ 674 calories per serving

Brown Rice

1 tablespoon extra-virgin olive oil

½ onion, chopped

½ red bell pepper, chopped

2 cups water

1 cup uncooked short-grain brown rice

¼ cup finely chopped parsley

Salt and freshly ground black pepper (optional)

Salmon Ingredients

4 skinless salmon fillets (about 4 ounces each)

1 tablespoon extra-virgin olive oil

1 garlic clove, pressed or minced

1 tablespoon grated fresh ginger

1 teaspoon soy sauce

1 teaspoon maple syrup

2 green onions, chopped

To make the rice, heat oil in a medium saucepan. Add onion and bell pepper; cook 3 minutes. Add water and rice; bring to a boil. Reduce heat; cover and simmer 50 minutes, or until rice is tender and liquid is absorbed. Fluff with a fork; stir in parsley. Season with salt and pepper if desired. Meanwhile, place salmon in a pie plate or shallow dish. Combine remaining salmon ingredients; mix well. Pour marinade over salmon; let stand 15 to 20 minutes. Heat a ridged grill pan over medium heat until hot. Add salmon, discarding marinade; cook 3 to 4 minutes per side, or until salmon is opaque and firm to the touch. Serve with brown rice.

What's in it for you?

Total fat	20.5 g
Saturated fat	3.4 g
Healthy fats	15 g
Fiber	2.6 g
Carbohydrates	45.9 g
Sugar	4.9 g
Protein	71 g
Sodium	411 mg
Calcium	81 mg
Magnesium	165 mg
Selenium	145 mcg
Potassium	1.4 mg

Spicy Chili

4 servings ❖ 390 calories per serving

1 tablespoon extra-virgin olive oil

½ pound ground turkey or ground meat substitute
   (such as Boca Crumbles)

½ onion, chopped

2 garlic cloves, minced

1 can (28 ounces) crushed tomatoes, undrained

1 can (16 ounces) kidney beans, drained

½ teaspoon chili powder

Pinch of cayenne pepper

1 teaspoon maple syrup

1 teaspoon wine vinegar

½ teaspoon ground coriander

½ teaspoon turmeric

Brown Rice Pilaf (recipe on page 329)

Heat oil in a large saucepan. Add turkey, onion, and garlic; cook 5 minutes, stirring frequently. Add remaining ingredients; simmer uncovered 25 minutes. Serve over Brown Rice Pilaf.

What's in it for you?	
Total fat	8.9 g
Saturated fat	1.9 g
Healthy fats	6.2 g
Fiber	10.7 g
Carbohydrates	31.5 g
Sugar	2.2 g
Protein	18.8 g
Sodium	646 mg
Calcium	86 mg
Magnesium	73 mg
Selenium	13.3 mcg
Potassium	838 mg

TRUST CRUST

When baking your own whole wheat pizza crust, plan on 25 to 70 extra minutes from start to finish, including time for yeast to do its thing. In a small bowl, combine about 1 tablespoon of dry yeast and ⅛ teaspoon of sugar with 1½ cups of warm water. Let that sit for 10 minutes. In a separate large bowl, combine 1½ cups 100 percent whole wheat flour and 1½ cups all-purpose (enriched) flour. (After you've tried this on your family several times, you can gradually increase in ½-cup lots the ratio of whole wheat to all-purpose flour to 2½ cups whole wheat to ½ cup all-purpose.) Add 1 teaspoon ground kosher salt to this. Mix well. Then add the yeast mixture and mix by hand thoroughly. Add 1 tablespoon olive oil. Knead for about 2 minutes until dough is smooth. Cover bowl and let rise in warm area until dough has doubled in size (20 to 60 minutes). Punch down dough with your fist and knead for 1 to 2 minutes. Divide into 4 equal portions (extra portions can be stored in your refrigerator). Roll into balls and preheat oven to 450°F. Lightly coat a baking sheet with olive oil. With a rolling pin, roll one of the dough balls on rolling board or on baking sheet (add flour if dough sticks to pin too much) and flatten into 10- to 12-inch pizza crust circle. Poke with a fork 4 to 6 times. Bake for 5 minutes. Remove from oven, then add ingredients.

Stuffed Whole Wheat Pizza

4 servings (2 slices per serving);
for the first two weeks, you can have up to half of the pizza,
but most will not need that much to be full ❖ 322 calories per serving

Cooking oil spray
1 pound fresh stir-fry vegetables such as asparagus, broccoli,
   cauliflower, mushrooms, multicolored bell peppers, red and white
   onions, and zucchini, cut up
2 garlic cloves, minced
Salt and freshly ground black pepper (optional)
1 cup pizza sauce or tomato sauce
2 tablespoons olive relish or tapenade
2 tablespoons sundried-tomato bits
One 12-inch or 10-ounce prepared thin whole wheat pizza crust
½ cup (2 ounces) finely shredded part-skim mozzarella cheese

Heat oven to 425°F. Heat a large nonstick skillet over medium-high heat until hot; coat with cooking spray. Add vegetables and garlic; stir-fry (really sauté) 2 to 5 minutes, or until vegetables are crisp-tender. Season to taste with salt and pepper if desired. Combine pizza sauce, olive relish, and sundried-tomato bits. Spread over pizza crust; top with cooked vegetables and cheese. Bake pizza directly on oven rack 10 to 15 minutes, or until crust is golden brown and cheese is melted. Cut pizza into 8 wedges.

What's in it for you?

Total fat	11.5 g
Saturated fat	3.5 g
Healthy fats	7.9 g
Fiber	5.7 g
Carbohydrates	44.2 g
Sugar	3.5 g
Protein	12.2 g
Sodium	682 mg
Calcium	151 mg
Magnesium	44 mg
Selenium	2.9 mcg
Potassium	481 mg

Mediterranean Chicken with Tomatoes, Olives, and Herbed White Beans

2 servings ❖ 567 calories per serving

Chicken Ingredients

2 bone-in chicken thighs without skin

1 tomato, chopped

½ onion, chopped

8 pitted kalamata olives, halved

1 tablespoon extra-virgin olive oil

1 teaspoon wine vinegar or balsamic vinegar

1 small bunch fresh basil, chopped

Bean Ingredients

1 tablespoon extra-virgin olive oil

2 garlic cloves, minced

1 can (15 or 16 ounces) white beans, rinsed and drained

1 tomato, chopped

¼ cup chopped fresh mixed herbs

1 teaspoon red wine vinegar or balsamic vinegar

Salt and freshly ground black pepper (optional)

To make the chicken, heat oven to 375°F. Place each chicken thigh on a large square of aluminum foil. Combine remaining chicken ingredients; spoon over chicken. Fold foil up and over chicken, sealing edges and forming a packet. Bake 25 minutes, or until chicken is cooked through. Meanwhile, to prepare the beans, heat oil in a medium saucepan over medium heat. Add garlic; cook 2 minutes. Add remaining bean ingredients; cook 5 minutes, or until heated through. Carefully open chicken packets and transfer mixture to two serving plates; serve beans alongside chicken.

What's in it for you?	
Total fat	19.2 g
Saturated fat	3.1 g
Healthy fats	15 g
Fiber	15.2 g
Carbohydrates	67.4 g
Sugar	5.1 g
Protein	34.4 g
Sodium	313 mg
Calcium	243 mg
Magnesium	171 mg
Selenium	14.3 mcg
Potassium	1,715 mg

Royal Pasta Primavera Provençale

2 servings ❖ 451 calories per serving

6 ounces whole wheat rigatoni or linguine pasta

1 small dried ancho or pasilla chili pepper

1 cup (4 ounces) diced (½-inch cubes) unpeeled eggplant

1 teaspoon extra-virgin olive oil

1 small yellow onion, coarsely chopped

1 yellow or orange bell pepper, coarsely chopped

3 garlic cloves, sliced

2 cans (14 ½ ounces each) stewed tomatoes, undrained, coarsely chopped

1 cup packed mesclun or mixed spring salad greens

1 teaspoon chopped fresh thyme or lemon thyme

Salt and freshly ground black pepper (optional)

Cook pasta according to package directions, omitting salt and fat. Meanwhile, heat a large, deep skillet over medium heat until hot. Add the chili pepper; cook, turning occasionally until fragrant and toasted, about 2 minutes. When the chili pepper is cool enough to handle, discard its stem and set the seeds aside for a garnish. Chop the chili pepper. Add eggplant to hot skillet; cook until browned, about 4 minutes, stirring frequently. Add oil, then chopped onion, bell pepper, and garlic; cook 3 minutes, stirring occasionally. Add tomatoes and chopped chili pepper. Reduce heat; simmer uncovered 10 minutes, or until vegetables are tender and sauce thickens. Remove from heat; stir in salad greens and thyme. Season to taste with salt and pepper if desired. Drain pasta; transfer to two serving plates and top with sauce.

What's in it for you?	
Total fat	4.3 g
Saturated fat	0.6 g
Healthy fats	2.9 g
Fiber	6.3 g
Carbohydrates	95.2 g
Sugar	15.4 g
Protein	17.6 g
Sodium	533 mg
Calcium	179 mg
Magnesium	183 mg
Selenium	65.5 mcg
Potassium	1,163 mg

Apricot Chicken and Green Beans with Almond Slivers

2 servings ❖ 430 calories per serving

Chicken Ingredients

2 skinless, boneless chicken breast halves (about 4 ounces each)
   (or substitute pork)

4 dried apricots, chopped

2 tablespoons white wine

2 shallots, chopped

1 tablespoon extra-virgin olive oil

⅛ teaspoon ground cinnamon

Green Bean Ingredients

1 cup thin green beans

3 shallots, thinly sliced

1 tablespoon extra-virgin olive oil

1 teaspoon wine vinegar

1 teaspoon maple syrup

¼ cup slivered almonds

Salt and freshly ground black pepper (optional)

To make the chicken, heat oven to 375°F. Place chicken in a glass baking dish. Sauté remaining chicken ingredients together until tender; transfer to blender or food processor and puree. Spoon over chicken and bake until chicken is cooked through, 15 to 20 minutes. Meanwhile, to prepare the beans, steam or blanch beans until tender but still firm and bright green. Sauté shallots in olive oil, vinegar, and maple syrup until translucent. Add almonds and brown slightly; toss with beans. Season to taste with salt and pepper if desired. Serve alongside chicken.

What's in it for you?	
Total fat	22 g
Saturated fat	2.8 g
Healthy fats	18.1 g
Fiber	4.6 g
Carbohydrates	25 g
Sugar	3.5 g
Protein	32.7 g
Sodium	89 mg
Calcium	95 mg
Magnesium	100 mg
Selenium	22.4 mcg
Potassium	813 mg

Turkey Tortilla Wraps with Red Baked Potato

2 servings ❖ 497 calories per serving

Red Potato Ingredients

1 large russet baking potato, washed, pierced with tip of knife

2 tablespoons marinara sauce or other red tomato sauce

Turkey Wrap Ingredients

Two 6-inch whole wheat flour tortillas

4 slices deli roast turkey breast

4 romaine lettuce leaves

4 slices tomato

2 thin slices red or yellow onion

Mustard or hot peppers (optional)

To make the red potato, cook in microwave on high power 8 to 9 minutes or until fork-tender. Slice lengthwise in half; spoon 1 tablespoon sauce over each half. Meanwhile, to prepare the turkey wraps, layer all turkey wrap ingredients on tortillas; roll up.

What's in it for you?	
Total fat	14.5 g
Saturated fat	4.5 g
Healthy fats	10 g
Fiber	7 g
Carbohydrates	64 g
Sugar	6.5 g
Protein	28.5 g
Sodium	1,654 mg
Calcium	180 mg
Magnesium	71 mg
Selenium	11.3 mcg
Potassium	1,596 mg

Broiled Trout, Orata, or Branzini with Rosemary and Lemon

2 servings ❖ 182 calories per serving

8 ounces whole fish (trout, orata, or branzini)
Salt and freshly ground black pepper (optional)
2 garlic cloves, sliced
4 sprigs of fresh rosemary
1 lemon, sliced

Preheat broiler. Open fish like a book; season to taste with salt and pepper if desired. Arrange garlic, rosemary, and lemon slices on one side of each fish; close other side and transfer fish to greased rack of broiler pan. Broil 5 to 6 inches from heat source 5 minutes. Turn fish over; continue to broil 4 to 5 minutes, or until fish is opaque throughout. (An alternative for those who like fast and easy: Fish can be cooked in a sort of double boiler in the microwave by filling a Pyrex bowl with water and placing the fish in a smaller microwave-safe bowl inside it.)

What's in it for you?

Total fat	7.3 g
Saturated fat	1 g
Healthy fat	4.9 g
Fiber	2.7 g
Carbohydrates	10.3 g
Sugar	4.9 g
Protein	15.8 g
Sodium	126 mg
Calcium	76 mg
Magnesium	43 mg
Selenium	10.7 mcg
Potassium	688 mg

FACTOID

Only trout and salmon must be picky enough eaters to avoid corn and soybean meals. Yup, trout and salmon are the only two fish categories that still have omega-3s in them. The rest have omega-6s, a big change from even five years ago.

Chicken Kabobs with Tabbouleh

2 servings ❖ 397 calories per serving

Chicken Ingredients

2 skinless, boneless chicken breast halves (about 4 ounces each),
    cut into 1-inch cubes

1 teaspoon dried oregano

½ teaspoon dried sage

1 red chili pepper, crushed (optional)

1 onion, quartered

1 tomato, quartered

1 bell pepper, seeded, stemmed, quartered

4 button mushrooms

Tabbouleh Ingredients

¾ cup bulgur wheat

1½ cups boiling water

1 tomato, chopped

1 bunch green onions, chopped

1 large bunch parsley, finely chopped

1 small bunch fresh mint leaves, finely chopped

2 tablespoons lemon juice

1 tablespoon extra-virgin olive oil

Salt and freshly ground black pepper (optional)

To make the chicken, prepare grill. Toss chicken with oregano, sage, and, if desired, chili pepper. Alternately thread chicken, onion, tomato, bell pepper, and mushrooms onto metal skewers. Cook on covered grill 3 to 4 minutes per side, or until chicken is cooked through and vegetables are tender. Meanwhile, to prepare the tabbouleh, place bulgur wheat in medium bowl; add boiling water and mix well. Let stand until all water is absorbed, about 30 minutes. (Pour off any excess water.) Add remaining ingredients except salt and pepper; mix well. Season with salt and pepper if desired. Serve tabbouleh with grilled chicken and vegetables.

What's in it for you?	
Total fat	9.4 g
Saturated fat	1.5 g
Healthy fats	7.1 g
Fiber	5.6 g
Carbohydrates	72.1 g
Sugar	12.1 g
Protein	14.2 g
Sodium	22.4 mg
Calcium	93 mg
Magnesium	148 mg
Selenium	68 mcg
Potassium	1,121 mg

SLIGHTLY
TIPSY

Lemon Caper Chicken with Sweet Potato Puree

2 servings ❖ *273 calories per serving*

Chicken Ingredients

2 skinless, boneless chicken thighs (about 4 ounces each)

Juice of 1 lemon

1 tablespoon extra-virgin olive oil

2 shallots, minced

1 tablespoon capers, drained

1 teaspoon Dijon mustard

Sweet Potato Ingredients

2 sweet potatoes, microwaved or baked

2 tablespoons orange juice

¼ cup golden raisins

½ teaspoon ground cinnamon

Salt and freshly ground black pepper (optional)

To make the chicken, preheat broiler. Place chicken in a shallow roasting pan. Combine remaining chicken ingredients and pour over chicken. Broil 6 inches from heat source 12 to 15 minutes, or until chicken is cooked through. To prepare the potatoes, scoop hot sweet potato pulp into bowl. Add remaining sweet potato ingredients except salt and pepper; mix well. Season to taste with salt and pepper if desired. Serve with chicken.

What's in it for you?	
Total fat	10.9 g
Saturated fat	2 g
Healthy fats	7.9 g
Fiber	1.4 g
Carbohydrates	20.6 g
Sugar	12.7 g
Protein	24.7 g
Sodium	336 mg
Calcium	39.5 mg
Magnesium	41 mg
Selenium	16.5 mcg
Potassium	494 mg

Hot Wild Salmon

2 servings ❖ *384 calories per serving*

2 wild salmon fillets with skin (about 4 ounces each) or salmon
     steaks (preferably line-caught)
2 tablespoons finely chopped fresh ginger
1 tablespoon wasabi paste
¼ teaspoon turmeric
Rock Asparagus (recipe on page 357)

Prepare grill or preheat broiler. Brush skinless side of salmon with combined ginger, wasabi paste, and turmeric. Grill or broil 4 to 6 inches from heat source 10 to 12 minutes without turning, or until salmon is opaque in center. Serve with Rock Asparagus.

What's in it for you?

Total fat	14.5 g
Saturated fat	2.3 g
Healthy fats	10.6 g
Fiber	0.4 g
Carbohydrates	2.7 g
Sugar	0.2 g
Protein	45.2 g
Sodium	11 mg
Calcium	31 mg
Magnesium	73 mg
Selenium	82.5 mcg
Potassium	1,176 mcg

Grilled Peanut Shrimp with Sesame Snow Peas

2 servings ❖ 163 calories per serving

Peanut Sauce Ingredients

1 tablespoon natural peanut butter

1 tablespoon canned light coconut milk

1 teaspoon fresh lime juice

Pinch of cayenne pepper

1 teaspoon honey

¼ teaspoon soy sauce

¼ cup water

1 garlic clove, peeled

10 medium uncooked shrimp, peeled and deveined

Snow Peas Ingredients

1 cup fresh snow peas

1 garlic clove, minced

1 teaspoon sesame seeds

1 teaspoon extra-virgin olive oil

½ teaspoon toasted sesame oil

Prepare grill. Place all ingredients for peanut sauce except shrimp in blender or food processor; puree. Pour mixture over shrimp; let stand 15 minutes. Thread shrimp onto skewers; discard any excess marinade not clinging to shrimp. Grill 2 to 3 minutes per side, or until shrimp are opaque. Meanwhile, blanch snow peas in boiling water 2 minutes; drain and rinse with cold water. Cook garlic and sesame seeds in olive and sesame oils 2 minutes. Add drained snow peas; heat through, tossing well. Serve with shrimp.

What's in it for you?	
Total fat	10.5 g
Saturated fat	2.9 g
Healthy fats	7 g
Fiber	1.9 g
Carbohydrates	8.8 g
Sugar	5.1 g
Protein	9.5 g
Sodium	128 mg
Calcium	51.5 mg
Magnesium	40.6 mg
Selenium	13.1 mcg
Potassium	220 mg

Vegetable Tofu Stir-fry

2 servings ❖ 602 calories per serving

1 tablespoon extra-virgin olive oil

½ teaspoon toasted sesame oil

¼ teaspoon crushed red pepper flakes

½ onion, sliced

2 garlic cloves, sliced

1 cup broccoli florets

½ red bell pepper, sliced

6 large button mushrooms, halved

1 teaspoon soy sauce

4 small 2-ounce blocks baked tofu, cubed

2 green onions, chopped

1 small bunch cilantro, chopped

1 teaspoon sesame seeds

In wok or large skillet, heat olive and sesame oils and pepper flakes over medium-high heat. Add onion and garlic; stir-fry 2 minutes. Add broccoli, bell pepper, mushrooms, and soy sauce; stir-fry until vegetables are crisp-tender, 2 to 3 minutes. Add tofu, green onions, cilantro, and sesame seeds; stir-fry until heated through.

What's in it for you?

Total fat	23 g
Saturated fat	3.3 g
Healthy fats	18.9 g
Fiber	11.1 g
Carbohydrates	43 g
Sugar	16.4 g
Protein	62.2 g
Sodium	873 mg
Calcium	400 mg
Magnesium	273 mg
Selenium	13.5 mcg
Potassium	2,403 mg

Tofu or Turkey Dogs with Sauerkraut

2 Servings ❖ 298 calories per serving

4 tofu (meatless) or turkey hot dogs

1 cup sauerkraut

Whole wheat buns (optional)

2 tablespoons inexpensive mustard, such as spicy brown
    or coarse-grained

Simmer hot dogs in water with sauerkraut until heated through, about 5 minutes. Drain; serve with mustard (with or without buns).

(Note: There's a lot of saturated fat here, so we recommend it only as a last-ditch resort.)

What's in it for you?	
Total fat	26 g
Saturated fat	9 g
Healthy fats	15.4 g
Fiber	0.7 g
Carbohydrates	3.8 g
Sugar	2.1 g
Protein	11.2 g
Sodium	1,219 mg
Calcium	158 mg
Magnesium	27 mg
Selenium	1.9 mcg
Potassium	160 mg

Lifestyle 180 Chia Sausage or Meatballs

12 servings ❖ 130 calories per serving

¾ cup nonalcoholic red wine

2 tablespoons finely minced garlic

2 tablespoons ground chia seeds

1 tablespoon fennel seed

½ teaspoon dried basil

¼ teaspoon dried oregano

¼ teaspoon dried thyme

¼ teaspoon freshly ground black pepper

2 teaspoons seasoned salt

½ teaspoon crushed red pepper flakes

¼ cup chopped fresh parsley

2 pounds ground turkey breast

In large bowl combine nonalcoholic red wine, garlic, and chia seeds. Set aside and allow chia seeds to swell for 30 minutes. Add remaining ingredients except for turkey and mix well. Add turkey and mix until well blended. In a large nonstick pan, cook sausage in either patty form or bulk form until slightly brown and stir to crumble. Drain and serve or cool and refrigerate.

Recipe Variation: Makes great Italian meatballs for sandwiches or to go with pasta by adding 2 egg whites and ½ cup breadcrumbs to the wine. Scoop or roll into 1-ounce meatballs and place in a shallow baking pan. Bake in a 375°F oven for 20 minutes or to an internal temperature of 165°F. Remove and serve or cool and refrigerate. Yields 40 1-ounce meatballs.

Tips: Use crumbled Italian sausage for pizza toppings, or mix with pasta and your choice of sauce. Milk, broth, V8 juice, or water can be substituted for wine, if desired.

What's in it for you?

Total fat	2 g
Saturated fat	0 g
Healthy fats	1 g
Fiber	2 g
Carbohydrates	3 g
Sugar	0 g
Protein	22 g
Sodium	320 mg
Calcium	38 mg
Magnesium	7.5 mg
Selenium	2 mcg
Potassium	55 mg

Lifestyle 180 Piccata-Style Chicken Scaloppini

2 servings (4 ounces each) ❖ 150 calories per serving

Sauce base

1¼ cups water

1 teaspoon Minor's chicken base

½ teaspoon Minor's vegetable base

2 teaspoons arrowroot

2 teaspoons cold water

In small sauce pan bring 1¼ cups water to a simmer and then add both chicken and vegetable bases to make a stock. In a small bowl combine arrowroot and cold water to make a slurry and whisk into boiling stock until it begins to lightly thicken and remove from heat.

Chicken

2 5-ounce skinless, boneless chicken breasts

½ teaspoon kosher salt

¼ teaspoon coarsely ground black pepper

2 tablespoons extra-virgin olive oil

½ cup 100% whole wheat flour

1 teaspoon finely chopped garlic

1 teaspoon extra-virgin olive oil

1 teaspoon finely chopped fresh parsley

1 teaspoon capers

1 tablespoon lemon juice

1 cup sauce base

Trim away any visible fat, sliver skin, and cut each chicken breast into three equal pieces. Then place the chicken between cellophane and lightly pound with mallet to about a ⅓-inch thickness. Season chicken with salt and pepper and set aside.

In a 12-inch nonstick sauté pan add and heat oil. Dredge or lightly coat chicken with flour and place into heated oil and sauté over medium heat until juices begin to rise to top of chicken, about 2 minutes. Turn over with spatula and sauté on other side about 1 minute. Then add garlic and one teaspoon olive oil. Sauté until garlic begins to turn light golden in color. While garlic is sautéing add parsley and capers. Then add lemon juice and sauce base right at the time the garlic begins to color. Shake pan and allow all the ingredients to mix, deglazing bottom of pan for no more then 30 seconds as further cooking in the sauce will toughen and dry out the chicken. After the 30 seconds, remove the chicken to a side plate and continue to simmer the sauce to reduce until desired consistency. Remove pan from heat, add chicken back to pan to warm, then place chicken on plate and pour sauce over it and serve with Lifestyle 180 Vegetable Rice (recipe on page 351) or your favorite side dish.

What's in it for you?	
Total fat	6 g
Saturated fat	1 g
Healthy fats	4.5 g
Fiber	1 g
Carbohydrates	9 g
Sugar	0 g
Protein	13 g
Sodium	330 mg
Calcium	12 mg
Magnesium	30 mg
Selenium	17 mcg
Potassium	181 mg

Lifestyle 180 Curried Vegetable Ragout

5 servings ❖ *160 calories per serving*

1 medium eggplant, peeled and cut into ½-inch chunks

1 tablespoon grapeseed or extra-virgin olive oil

½ cup chopped red onion

1½ teaspoons minced garlic

2 small zucchini, cut into ½-inch chunks

1 cup cut green beans (½-inch pieces)

¾ cup orange juice or vegetable broth

½ cup chopped fresh tomato

¼ cup golden raisins

1 tablespoon balsamic vinegar

½ teaspoon drained capers

2 teaspoons agave nectar

1½ teaspoons curry powder

½ teaspoon minced fresh ginger

¼ teaspoon red pepper flakes

2 tablespoons chopped fresh basil

2 tablespoons chopped fresh parsley

1 tablespoon chopped fresh cilantro

Sauté eggplant in a nonstick skillet coated with cooking spray over medium heat until golden brown, about 5 minutes. Heat oil in a large saucepan over medium heat. Add onion and garlic; sauté 4 minutes. Add zucchini, green beans, browned eggplant, orange juice, tomato, raisins, balsamic vinegar, capers, agave nectar, balsamic vinegar, curry powder, ginger, and pepper flakes; bring to a gentle simmer. Simmer 20 minutes or until vegetables are tender. Stir in basil, parsley, and cilantro. Serve over hot cooked brown rice or as an accompaniment to seafood.

What's in it for you?

Total fat	3.5 g
Saturated fat	0 g
Healthy fats	2.5 g
Fiber	8 g
Carbohydrates	29 g
Sugar	15 g
Protein	5 g
Sodium	75 mg
Calcium	83 mg
Magnesium	47 mg
Selenium	1.5 mcg
Potassium	560 mg

Lifestyle 180 Italian Sausage Meatballs and Whole Wheat Penne

8 servings (1 cup each) ❖ 180 calories per serving

2 tablespoons extra-virgin olive oil

4 garlic cloves, slivered lengthwise

2 cups zucchini, halved and sliced into ¼-inch slices

½ teaspoon salt

¼ teaspoon pepper

2 cups broccoli florets

12 ounces 100% whole wheat penne

1 can (26-ounce) tomato sauce, sugar-free, corn-syrup-free

12 Lifestyle 180 Meatballs (page 345)

Heat olive oil in large pot. Add the garlic and sauté over medium heat until golden, remove, and set aside. Add zucchini, season with salt and pepper, and sauté until tender, remove, and set aside. Add water to pot and bring to a boil. Lightly salt water, add broccoli florets, and blanch for about 3 minutes or until just tender. Remove broccoli with a slotted spoon, drain well, place on a flat baking tray, and allow to cool.

Cook penne in the broccoli water until tender and drain. Add the tomato sauce to the penne and stir until mixed. Add the cooked meatballs (see Lifestyle 180 Chia Sausage, page 345), zucchini, and broccoli florets, mix well and serve garnished with the slivered garlic.

What's in it for you?	
Total fat	6 g
Saturated fat	0.5 g
Healthy fats	3.5 g
Fiber	5 g
Carbohydrates	20 g
Sugar	5 g
Protein	13 g
Sodium	540 mg
Calcium	69 mg
Magnesium	27 mg
Selenium	13 mcg
Potassium	182 mg

Lifestyle 180 Spaghetti Squash

19 servings ❖ 15 calories per serving

1 two-pound spaghetti squash
6 cups water
2 tablespoons vegetable base without MSG
½ teaspoon grated lemon zest
Salt (optional)
Freshly ground black pepper (optional)

Cut the top and bottom off the squash. Stand squash up on a carving board. Trim off and discard the skin and cream-colored rind. Cut squash in half lengthwise; scrape out and discard seeds. Lay the flat side down; cut crosswise into ¾-inch slices.

Combine water and vegetable base in a large deep sauté pan or saucepan; bring to a boil over high heat. Add squash; cover and simmer 6 to 8 minutes, or until squash is tender. Remove to a large bowl with a slotted spoon. While warm, use two forks or fingers to pull squash into "strands of spaghetti." Season with lemon zest, salt, and freshly ground black pepper to taste. Strain the vegetable broth and refrigerate or freeze to use another time.

What's in it for you?	
Total fat	0 g
Saturated fat	0 g
Healthy fats	0 g
Fiber	1 g
Carbohydrates	3 g
Sugar	1 g
Protein	0 g
Sodium	29 mg
Calcium	11 mg
Magnesium	5 mg
Selenium	0.1 mcg
Potassium	48 mg

Lifestyle 180 Vegetable Rice

4 servings ❖ 160 calories per serving

½ cup finely diced sweet onion

2 tablespoons extra-virgin olive oil

¼ cup thinly sliced shiitake mushrooms

1 tablespoon finely chopped garlic

¼ cup finely diced red pepper

¼ cup finely diced yellow pepper

½ cup finely diced zucchini

½ cup blanched green beans, crosscut to fine-dice size

½ teaspoon kosher salt

¼ teaspoon coarsely ground black pepper

1 cup cooked brown rice

Zest of 1 lemon

In a 12-inch sauté pan, sauté the onions in oil, until they are translucent, about 5 minutes. Add shiitake mushrooms and sauté until they are golden brown to bring out their flavor. Add garlic and sauté 1 minute, then add peppers and zucchini and sauté until just tender. Add green beans, salt, and pepper, and stir well. Add brown rice and lemon zest, stir well again, sauté until thoroughly heated, and serve.

What's in it for you?

Total fat	8 g
Saturated fat	1 g
Healthy fats	6 g
Fiber	3 g
Carbohydrates	17 g
Sugar	2 g
Protein	2 g
Sodium	250 mg
Calcium	22 mg
Magnesium	28 mg
Selenium	7 mcg
Potassium	125 mg

Pork Tenderloin with Broccoli and Szechuan Noodles

6 servings (1 cup each) ❖ 330 calories per serving

Szechuan Noodles

1 pound 100% whole wheat spaghetti

3½ tablespoons dark toasted sesame oil

3½ tablespoons soy sauce

1½ tablespoons balsamic vinegar

2 teaspoons agave nectar

1 tablespoon hot chile toasted sesame oil

½ teaspoon finely chopped garlic

⅓ cup sliced scallions

Cook spaghetti as directed on package, drain, and rinse to cool. In a separate bowl, combine the other ingredients and mix well. Toss with spaghetti, cover, and refrigerate.

Broccoli

3 cups broccoli florets

Add water to a large pot and bring to boil. Lightly salt water and add broccoli florets and blanch for about 3 minutes or until just tender. Remove broccoli with slotted spoon, drain well, place on a flat baking tray, and allow to cool.

Pork Tenderloin

3 tablespoons agave nectar

1 tablespoon balsamic vinegar

1 teaspoon grated fresh ginger

1 teaspoon finely minced garlic

2 tablespoons rice wine vinegar

12 ounces pork tenderloin cut into two 6-ounce pieces

Combine agave nectar, balsamic vinegar, tamari sauce, ginger, garlic, and rice wine vinegar in a bowl and marinate pork in the refrigerator for 30 minutes. Set pork tenderloin on rimmed baking sheet and preheat oven to 375°F. Add marinade to small saucepan and bring to a simmer. Cook until reduced by half (3 tablespoons) and allow to cool 5 minutes to a glaze consistency. Coat pork tenderloin with marinade glaze and roast in oven for about 25 minutes or until an instant read thermometer inserted in the thickest part reads 150°F internal temperature.

Allow to rest 10 minutes, slice into six 2-ounce pieces, and serve each piece with ½ cup broccoli and ½ cup Szechuan noodles.

What's in it for you?	
Total fat	14 g
Saturated fat	2.5 g
Healthy fats	1 g
Fiber	3 g
Carbohydrates	35 g
Sugar	12 g
Protein	20 g
Sodium	600 mg
Calcium	39 mg
Magnesium	51 mg
Selenium	44 mcg
Potassium	417 mg

Lifestyle 180 Rutabaga, Carrot, and Potato Mash

12 servings ❖ 70 calories per serving

1 small (¾ pound) rutabaga, peeled and cut into 1½-inch cubes

32 ounces vegetable broth

1 pound carrots, thinly sliced

½ pound red potatoes, peeled and cut into ½-inch cubes

2 teaspoons canola oil

2 teaspoons minced garlic

¼ teaspoon kosher or sea salt

¼ teaspoon freshly ground black pepper

Combine rutabaga and broth in a large saucepan; bring to a boil over high heat. Reduce heat; simmer 10 minutes. Add carrots and potatoes; cover and simmer 18 to 20 minutes, or until vegetables are very tender. Drain vegetables, reserving broth. Heat oil in the same saucepan. Add garlic; cook 1 minute. Add reserved broth; cook over medium-high heat until mixture is reduced to ⅓ to ½ cup. Add drained vegetables, salt, and pepper; mash with a potato masher or handheld blender to desired consistency.

What's in it for you?	
Total fat	1.5 g
Saturated fat	0 g
Healthy fats	1 g
Fiber	3 g
Carbohydrates	14 g
Sugar	6 g
Protein	2 g
Sodium	230 mg
Calcium	47 mg
Magnesium	22 mg
Selenium	0.5 mcg
Potassium	228 mg

Vegetables with Chicken and Brown Rice

7 servings ❖ 160 calories per serving

1 cup long-grain brown rice

2 cups broccoli florets

1 cup thinly sliced or matchstick-cut carrots

1 cup sliced green beans (½-inch pieces)

1 cup frozen baby lima beans, thawed

1 cup chopped red bell pepper

1 small zucchini squash, thinly sliced

1¼ cups Lifestyle 180 Ginger Sweet-and-Sour Sauce (page 380)

¾ pound chopped cooked chicken breast

Cook rice according to package directions. Meanwhile, combine all vegetables in a steamer or microwave-safe casserole dish (add 1 tablespoon water to the dish). Cover; steam over simmering water or cook at high power in microwave oven 4 to 5 minutes, or until vegetables are tender-crisp.

Combine Ginger Sweet-and-Sour Sauce and drained vegetables in a medium saucepan. Cook over medium-high heat until vegetables are heated through. Stir in chicken; heat through. Serve over hot cooked brown rice.

What's in it for you?	
Total fat	1.5 g
Saturated fat	0 g
Healthy fats	0.5 g
Fiber	6 g
Carbohydrates	22 g
Sugar	6 g
Protein	14 g
Sodium	370 mg
Calcium	38 mg
Magnesium	48 mg
Selenium	5 mcg
Potassium	400 mg

Lifestyle 180 Vegan Vegetable Stuffing

8 servings ❖ 130 calories per serving

⅓ cup finely diced white button mushrooms

1 teaspoon extra-virgin olive oil

1⅓ cups zucchini

4 tablespoons vegenaise

1 teaspoon Cholula hot sauce

3 teaspoons chopped parsley

⅓ cup finely diced red pepper

⅓ cup finely diced orange pepper

3 tablespoons finely diced red onion

⅔ cup finely chopped sundried tomato, reconstituted

½ cup whole wheat panko bread crumbs

Sauté the diced mushrooms in olive oil in a sauté pan until slightly browned, add zucchini and sauté about 2 minutes until zucchini just becomes tender but still crisp. Remove from pan, place in bowl, and refrigerate until cool. In a medium-size bowl, combine Vegenaise, Cholula hot sauce, and parsley and mix. Add remaining ingredients except for panko and mix. Add panko crumbs and mix until all the ingredients are moistened.

What's in it for you?

Total fat	5 g
Saturated fat	1 g
Healthy fats	0.5 g
Fiber	1 g
Carbohydrates	18 g
Sugar	3 g
Protein	2 g
Sodium	180 mg
Calcium	13 mg
Magnesium	15 mg
Selenium	1 mcg
Potassium	256 mg

Rock Asparagus

4 servings ❖ 38 calories per serving

1 pound asparagus spears, trimmed

1 teaspoon extra-virgin olive oil

Kosher salt, to taste (optional)

¼ teaspoon *each:* dried thyme, oregano, basil, and black pepper

Optional garnish: diced tomato

Heat oven to 350°F. Toss the asparagus in a 13 x 9-inch baking dish or a shallow 3-quart casserole pan with the olive oil, kosher salt if desired, thyme, oregano, basil, and black pepper. Arrange asparagus in a single layer in the dish. Bake uncovered 12 to 13 minutes for thin asparagus or 15 to 18 minutes for thick asparagus, or until crisp-tender. Garnish with tomato if desired.

What's in it for you?	
Total fat	1.5 g
Saturated fat	0.2 g
Healthy fats	1.1 g
Fiber	1.4 g
Carbohydrates	5 g
Sugar	1.8 g
Protein	2.9 g
Sodium	5 mg
Calcium	27 mg
Magnesium	22 mg
Selenium	4 mcg
Potassium	352 mg

Tomato-Avocado Salsamole

2 servings ❖ 90 calories per serving

¼ cup finely chopped red onion

1 teaspoon minced jalapeño, or more to taste

1 tablespoon lime juice

1 tablespoon cider vinegar

1 teaspoon minced garlic

¼ teaspoon salt

1 ripe avocado (preferably Hass), peeled, pitted, and coarsely mashed

1 medium tomato, chopped

¼ cup chopped cilantro

Combine onion, jalapeño, lime juice, vinegar, garlic, and salt in bowl. Add avocado, tomato, and cilantro; stir well. Serve immediately or, to store, reserve avocado pit, add to mixture to prevent browning, cover tightly with plastic wrap, and refrigerate. Serve with lightly toasted whole wheat pita cut into triangles.

What's in it for you?

Total fat	8 g
Saturated fat	2.1 g
Healthy fats	5.3 g
Fiber	3.1 g
Carbohydrates	8 g
Sugar	2 g
Protein	2 g
Sodium	25 mg
Calcium	20 mg
Magnesium	54 mg
Selenium	0 mcg
Potassium	805 mg

Lifestyle 180 Chia Cole Slaw

6 servings ❖ 180 calories per serving

½ cup Vegenaise

1½ tablespoons fresh lemon juice

1½ tablespoons rice wine vinegar

1 tablespoon chopped fresh parsley

2 teaspoons agave nectar

2 teaspoons chia seeds

1 garlic clove, minced

½ teaspoon salt

¼ teaspoon freshly ground black pepper

4½ cups (1 pound) finely chopped or shredded green cabbage

2¼ cups (½ pound) finely chopped or shredded red cabbage

1 cup shredded carrots

⅓ cup grated or finely chopped sweet onion

In a large bowl, whisk together Vegenaise, lemon juice, vinegar, parsley, agave nectar, chia seeds, garlic, salt, and pepper. Refrigerate 20 minutes to allow the chia seeds to swell. Add cabbages, carrots, and onion; toss well. Cover; refrigerate up to 2 days.

What's in it for you?	
Total fat	12 g
Saturated fat	2 g
Healthy fats	0 g
Fiber	4 g
Carbohydrates	15 g
Sugar	8 g
Protein	2 g
Sodium	320 mg
Calcium	70 mg
Magnesium	8.5 mg
Selenium	0.3 mcg
Potassium	273 mg

Lifestyle 180 Quinoa Tabouli

7 servings ❖ 110 calories per serving

½ cup bulgar

½ cup cold water

⅓ cup lemon juice

¼ cup extra-virgin olive oil

¼ cup chopped fresh mint leaves

1 cup chopped fresh parsley

¼ cup finely diced red onion

1 teaspoon finely chopped garlic

½ teaspoon freshly ground black pepper

½ teaspoon salt

2 cups finely diced tomato

2 cups peeled, seeded, and diced cucumber

1 cup cooked quinoa

In a mixing bowl, combine bulgar with water, lemon juice, and 2 table-spoons of olive oil and toss until well mixed. Set aside for 30 minutes at room temperature until liquid is absorbed. Add remaining olive oil along with rest of ingredients. Let stand for 10 minutes to allow the flavors to mingle, and serve.

What's in it for you?	
Total fat	7 g
Saturated fat	1 g
Healthy fats	5.3 g
Fiber	2 g
Carbohydrates	10 g
Sugar	2 g
Protein	2 g
Sodium	140 mg
Calcium	29 mg
Magnesium	30 mg
Selenium	0.7 mcg
Potassium	241 mg

Note: Cook the quinoa according to directions on package. The saponin coating on some organic brands is removed by rubbing. Others are removed by washing in water, which can reduce flavor and nutrients. Therefore these organic brands should only be rinsed in cold water before cooking.

Lifestyle 180 Olive, Toasted Walnut, and Sundried Tomato Tapenade

19 servings ❖ 40 calories per serving

1 cup hot water

½ cup sundried tomatoes (not oil packed)

2 large garlic cloves

1 jar (6 ounces) pitted kalamata olives, drained

½ cup walnuts, toasted

2 tablespoons drained capers

1 tablespoon extra-virgin olive oil

1 tablespoon coarsely chopped fresh parsley

1 tablespoon coarsely chopped fresh basil

1 teaspoon anchovy paste

1 teaspoon Dijon mustard

Combine water and tomatoes; set aside for 30 minutes. Drop the garlic through the feed tube of a food processor with the motor running; process until minced. Drain tomatoes, discarding the liquid (or reserve it for another use). Add the tomatoes to food processor. Pulse several times to chop tomatoes. Add remaining ingredients; process until olives are minced and mixture is well blended. Serve as a spread on toasted whole grain crostini or as a stuffing for cherry tomatoes, or stir into tomato soup or mix with Vegenaise for a vegetable dip.

What's in it for you?	
Total fat	4 g
Saturated fat	0 g
Healthy fats	3 g
Fiber	1 g
Carbohydrates	2 g
Sugar	1 g
Protein	1 g
Sodium	140 mg
Calcium	17 mg
Magnesium	9 mg
Selenium	0.4 mcg
Potassium	73 mg

Note: As a condiment, this exceeds Lifestyle 180 criteria for sodium at less than 75 mg per serving.

Lifestyle 180 Cannellini Cilantro Hummus

8 servings ❖ 80 calories per serving

1 teaspoon finely minced garlic

1 can (15 ounces) cannellini beans, drained

2 tablespoons lemon juice

2 tablespoons extra-virgin olive oil

1 teaspoon ground cumin

½ teaspoon chili powder

½ teaspoon kosher salt

¼ teaspoon freshly ground black pepper

3 tablespoons chopped fresh cilantro

1 teaspoon chopped fresh cilantro, for garnish.

In a food processor combine garlic and cannellini beans with lemon juice and process until smooth. Mix in oil, cumin, chili powder, salt and pepper and process until blended. Add 3 tablespoons cilantro and pulse until mixed. Place in bowl and garnish with cilantro.

What's in it for you?	
Total fat	3.5 g
Saturated fat	0.5 g
Healthy fats	3 g
Fiber	3 g
Carbohydrates	9 g
Sugar	1 g
Protein	3 g
Sodium	260 mg
Calcium	28 mg
Magnesium	0.6 mg
Selenium	0 mcg
Potassium	9 mg

Lifestyle 180 Roasted Red Pepper Hummus

5 servings ❖ 110 calories per serving

2 garlic cloves

1 can (15 ounces) garbanzo beans, drained

½ cup (4 ounces) drained bottled roasted red peppers

3 tablespoons lemon juice

½ teaspoon ground cumin

¼ to ½ teaspoon cayenne pepper, to taste

¼ teaspoon salt

1 tablespoon chopped fresh parsley

Drop the garlic through the feed tube of a food processor with the motor running; process until minced. Add remaining ingredients except parsley. Process until fairly smooth. Transfer to a serving bowl and refrigerate for at least 1 hour. Garnish with parsley just before serving.

What's in it for you?

Total fat	1.5 g
Saturated fat	0 g
Healthy fats	0 g
Fiber	4 g
Carbohydrates	18 g
Sugar	2 g
Protein	6 g
Sodium	210 mg
Calcium	49 mg
Magnesium	25 mg
Selenium	0 mcg
Potassium	164 mg

Lifestyle 180 Roasted Garlic Baba Ghanoush

10 servings ❖ 110 calories per serving

2 eggplants (1 pound each)

½ cup tahini

½ cup chopped fresh parsley

4 tablespoons fresh lemon juice

8 garlic cloves, roasted

¾ teaspoon salt

⅛ teaspoon cayenne pepper

Heat oven to 450°F. Place the whole eggplants on a baking sheet; prick in several places with a fork. Bake 25 to 30 minutes or until eggplants are very soft. Cool, cut in half lengthwise, and scoop pulp onto a carving board. Drain off excess liquid, coarsely chop pulp, and place in food processor. Process until finely chopped. Add remaining ingredients; process until fairly smooth. Transfer to a serving dish; garnish with additional parsley and serve with pita or other flatbread.

What's in it for you?	
Total fat	8 g
Saturated fat	1 g
Healthy fats	0 g
Fiber	4 g
Carbohydrates	8 g
Sugar	3 g
Protein	4 g
Sodium	180 mg
Calcium	31 mg
Magnesium	12 mg
Selenium	0.4 mcg
Potassium	144 mg

Note: To roast garlic, toss 8 garlic cloves with ½ teaspoon extra-virgin olive oil on a sheet of aluminum foil. Wrap foil loosely around the garlic and crimp the edges to seal. Bake in a 350°F oven or toaster oven about 20 to 25 minutes or until golden brown.

Lifestyle 180 Spicy Broccoli

7 servings ❖ 45 calories per serving

2 teaspoons extra-virgin olive oil

3 garlic cloves, minced

½ teaspoon red pepper flakes

6 cups coarsely chopped broccoli (1 large bunch with stems)

1 can (14½ ounces) crushed fire-roasted tomatoes, undrained

Heat oil in a large, deep sauté pan over medium heat. Add garlic and red pepper flakes; sauté 2 minutes. Add broccoli and tomatoes with their liquid bring to a boil. Reduce heat to medium low. Cover and simmer until broccoli is crisp-tender, 6 to 8 minutes.

What's in it for you?	
Total fat	1.5 g
Saturated fat	0 g
Healthy fats	1 g
Fiber	3 g
Carbohydrates	7 g
Sugar	0 g
Protein	3 g
Sodium	90 mg
Calcium	48 mg
Magnesium	26 mg
Selenium	2 mcg
Potassium	352 mg

Lifestyle 180 Pomegranate and Chia Tabouli

14 servings ❖ 70 calories per serving

1 cup cracked wheat (fine or medium grade)

2 cups warm water

1 tablespoon chia seeds

¼ cup cold water

2 cups chopped green onions

2 cups chopped seeded tomatoes

3 cups chopped fresh parsley

½ cup pomegranate seeds

¼ cup fresh lemon juice

½ teaspoon kosher or sea salt

¼ teaspoon freshly ground black pepper

Soak cracked wheat in warm water until tender, 45 to 55 minutes; drain. Meanwhile, in a large bowl, combine chia seeds and cold water; let stand 5 minutes. Add remaining ingredients; mix well. Drain wheat; add to salad and toss well. Serve at room temperature, or cover and chill up to 2 days before serving.

What's in it for you?

Total fat	0.5 g
Saturated fat	0 g
Healthy fats	0.5 g
Fiber	3 g
Carbohydrates	13 g
Sugar	2 g
Protein	3 g
Sodium	80 mg
Calcium	39 mg
Magnesium	15 mg
Selenium	0.1 mcg
Potassium	197 mg

Lifestyle 180 Vegetable Frittata

2 servings ❖ 190 calories per serving

8 egg whites

1 egg yolk

1 tablespoon canola oil

½ cup finely julienned shiitake mushrooms

½ cup finely diced sweet onion

½ cup finely diced red pepper

½ cup finely diced zucchini

Salt and pepper to taste

1 teaspoon turmeric powder

½ teaspoon canola oil (for pan-flip method only)

In a bowl, combine egg whites with egg yolk and whisk with wire whisk until frothy. In a 10-inch nonstick sauté pan, heat the canola oil. When the pan becomes hot, add shiitake mushrooms and stir continuously until they begin to turn light brown. Then add onion, pepper, and zucchini and season to taste with salt and pepper, stirring frequently. As soon as all is stirred and coated with oil, add turmeric and sauté until vegetables are just becoming tender. Add beaten eggs evenly around vegetables and begin to gently fold in sides inward from rim of pan when the eggs begin to cook while tilting the pan in the direction of the fold to allow the loose uncooked eggs to fill that area and cook. Continually tilt the pan in all directions to very quickly cook your eggs, which will begin to create the frittata. At this point you can finish cooking the top of the eggs by putting the pan under a preheated broiler or in a preheated 350°F oven until eggs are done. The brave of heart can do a pan flip to reverse the sides by adding ½ teaspoon of oil around the sides of the pan to help the frittata move easily in the pan and then, with a quick upward motion, flip the frittata. With the pan-flip method correctly done, remove the pan from the heat and allow the residual pan heat to finish the cooking process, which will provide the best chance for not overcooking the eggs. Serve immediately.

Note: You can use any combination of vegetables you like. This is a good way to use leftover cooked broccoli, asparagus, squash, and other vegetables. Just sauté the raw vegetables first and add any previously cooked items after the raw ingredients become tender.

Tips: Cooking the turmeric in the oil with the vegetables increases its benefits. Culinary supply stores also sell double-hinged pans with the same-sized top and bottom, so you can add the top side when ready to flip and then just invert the pan instead of having to flip. Practice pan flipping on a plain, fully cooked open-face omelet.

What's in it for you?	
Total fat	10 g
Saturated fat	1.5 g
Healthy fats	8 g
Fiber	2 g
Carbohydrates	10 g
Sugar	5 g
Protein	16 g
Sodium	500 mg
Calcium	40 mg
Magnesium	31 mg
Selenium	34 mcg
Potassium	529 mg

Lifestyle 180 Oven-Baked Butternut Squash Fries

8 (½ cup) servings ❖ 80 calories per serving

1½ tablespoons canola or extra-virgin olive oil

2 teaspoons minced garlic

1 teaspoon ground cumin

1 teaspoon chili powder

1 teaspoon salt

½ teaspoon freshly ground black pepper

5 cups butternut squash (about 2 pounds), peeled, seeded, and chopped into ½-inch chunks

Preheat oven to 375°F. In a medium bowl, combine oil, garlic, and seasonings; mix well. Add squash; toss until well coated. Spread in a single layer in a 15- x 10-inch jelly roll pan. Bake 15 minutes; toss well. Continue baking 15 minutes, or until squash is tender.

What's in it for you?	
Total fat	3 g
Saturated fat	0 g
Healthy fats	2 g
Fiber	2 g
Carbohydrates	13 g
Sugar	2 g
Protein	1 g
Sodium	290 mg
Calcium	56 mg
Magnesium	38 mg
Selenium	0.6 mcg
Potassium	394 mg

Lifestyle 180 Oven-Baked Sweet Potato Home Fries

8 servings ❖ 120 calories per serving

1½ tablespoons canola or extra-virgin olive oil

2 teaspoons finely minced garlic

2 teaspoons cumin

1 teaspoon salt

½ teaspoon freshly ground black pepper

2 pounds washed and peeled sweet potatoes, cut into ¼-inch cubes

Preheat oven to 375°F. Combine oil with garlic and seasonings. Mix and add potatoes, tossing until well coated. Place on nonstick baking pan and bake about 35 minutes, or until tender.

What's in it for you?

Total fat	3 g
Saturated fat	0 g
Healthy fats	2 g
Fiber	4 g
Carbohydrates	23 g
Sugar	5 g
Protein	2 g
Sodium	340 mg
Calcium	38 mg
Magnesium	28 mg
Selenium	0.7 mcg
Potassium	372 mg

Lifestyle 180 Walnut and Pecan Pesto Green Beans

18 servings ❖ 120 calories per serving

9 cups cooked green beans, drained well

1 teaspoon fine chopped fresh garlic

½ cup fresh parsley leaves

3 ounces toasted and chopped walnuts

3 ounces toasted and chopped pecans

3 ounces extra-virgin olive oil

½ teaspoon salt

¼ teaspoon freshly ground black pepper

½ cup fresh spinach leaves

½ cup fresh basil leaves

Cut green beans into 1½-inch pieces. Place in a medium saucepan; add water to cover. Bring to a boil over high heat. Reduce heat; simmer until green beans are crisp-tender, about 6 minutes. Drain; rinse with cold water to stop the cooking.

Meanwhile, drop garlic through the feed tube of a food processor with motor running; process until minced. Add remaining ingredients; process until nuts and herbs are finely chopped. Toss mixture with green beans. Serve warm or at room temperature for a side dish or chilled as a salad.

What's in it for you?	
Total fat	10 g
Saturated fat	1 g
Healthy fats	5.6 g
Fiber	3 g
Carbohydrates	6 g
Sugar	3 g
Protein	2 g
Sodium	70 mg
Calcium	32 mg
Magnesium	8 mg
Selenium	0 mcg
Potassium	34 mg

Lifestyle 180 Cauliflower Gold

4 servings ❖ 190 calories per serving

1 cauliflower, broken up into small florets

4 tablespoons extra-virgin olive oil

½ teaspoon chili powder

1 teaspoon ground cumin

½ teaspoon tumeric

1 tablespoon garam masala

Pinch of cayenne pepper

1½ cups vegetable stock

3 tablespoons tomato paste

¼ cup ground toasted walnuts

Lightly brown cauliflower in olive oil, agitating frequently (takes about 15 to 20 minutes), and remove from heat. To the hot pan add the spices and toast lightly in pan (about 30 seconds). Add the vegetable stock to prevent spices from overtoasting. Add tomato paste and mix well. Add cauliflower, toss, and sauté 2 minutes. Add ground almonds, mix well, and serve.

What's in it for you?

Total fat	6 g
Saturated fat	2 g
Healthy fats	15 g
Fiber	4 g
Carbohydrates	11 g
Sugar	6 g
Protein	4 g
Sodium	300 mg
Calcium	42 mg
Magnesium	34 mg
Selenium	2 mcg
Potassium	519 mg

Lifestyle 180 Asian Dressing

1 tablespoon ❖ *35 calories per serving*

1 teaspoon agave nectar

1 tablespoon extra-virgin olive oil

1 tablespoon toasted sesame oil

1 teaspoon light soy sauce

1 teaspoon minced garlic

½ teaspoon minced fresh ginger

4 tablespoons rice vinegar or champagne vinegar

Place all the ingredients in a small bowl, whisk while slowly adding the oil.

What's in it for you?	
Total fat	3.5 g
Saturated fat	0.5 g
Healthy fats	1.5 g
Fiber	0 g
Carbohydrates	1 g
Sugar	1 g
Sodium	75 mg
Calcium	0 mg
Magnesium	0 mg
Selenium	0 mcg
Potassium	1 mg

Lifestyle 180 Guacamole

15 servings (about ¼ cup each) ❖ 60 calories per serving

3 ripe avocados, peeled and pitted

2 tablespoons chopped fresh cilantro

2 tablespoons fresh lime juice

2 teaspoons minced fire-roasted or fresh jalapeño chilies
(see chile preparation note, page 378)

1 teaspoon minced garlic

1 teaspoon salt

1½ cups seeded, diced tomatoes

Mash avocados with a fork or potato masher in a medium bowl. Add remaining ingredients except for tomatoes; mix well. Stir in tomatoes; transfer to serving bowl and serve.

What's in it for you?

Total fat	5 g
Saturated fat	0.5 g
Healthy fats	3.6 g
Fiber	2 g
Carbohydrates	4 g
Sugar	1 g
Protein	1 g
Sodium	180 mg
Calcium	8 mg
Magnesium	10 mg
Selenium	0.14 mcg
Potassium	164 mg

Asian-Style BBQ Disease Reversal Sauce

20 servings (about ¼ cup each) ❖ 60 calories per serving

¼ cup sesame oil

1 tablespoon finely minced garlic

3¼ cups organic sugar-free, syrup-free ketchup

½ cup organic soy sauce

½ cup nonalcoholic red wine

¼ cup lemon juice

6 teaspoons agave nectar

1 tablespoon coarsely ground black pepper

In a medium saucepan combine ingredients and bring to a simmer. Remove from heat, cool, label, date, and refrigerate.

What's in it for you?

Total fat	2.5 g
Saturated fat	0 g
Healthy fats	0 g
Carbohydrates	7 g
Sugar	4 g
Sodium	270 mg
Calcium	3 mg
Magnesium	1 mg
Selenium	0 mcg
Potassium	27 mg

Note: This recipe exceeds the sodium criteria for condiments for Lifestyle 180. Consume only if sodium is not an issue for you.

Lifestyle 180 Salsa Verde

12 servings (about 2 tablespoons each) ❖ 50 calories per serving

3 cups loosely packed parsley

2 tablespoons grapeseed oil

2 tablespoons flaxseed oil

3 tablespoons lemon juice

3 garlic cloves, chopped

2 drained anchovy fillets or 2 teaspoons anchovy paste

¼ cup thinly sliced green onions

1 tablespoon whole grain Dijon mustard

½ teaspoon grated lemon zest

Salt and freshly ground pepper

Combine all ingredients in a food processor. Process on pulse mode intermittently until coarse paste forms. Season to taste with salt and pepper. Label, date, and refrigerate.

What's in it for you?

Total fat	4.5 g
Saturated fat	0 g
Healthy fats	5 g
Fiber	1 g
Carbohydrates	2 g
Sugar	2 g
Protein	1 g
Sodium	50 mg
Calcium	24 mg
Magnesium	9 mg
Selenium	0.6 mcg
Potassium	96 mg

Lifestyle 180 Chia Salsa Cruda

8 servings (about ½ cup each)   ❖   50 calories per serving

½ teaspoon chia seeds

4 cups diced fresh tomatoes, drained, reserving any liquid

2 tablespoons extra-virgin olive oil

1 teaspoon minced garlic

¼ teaspoon grated lemon zest

2 teaspoons balsamic vinegar

1 teaspoon fig vinegar

1 teaspoon balsamic vinegar (optional)

½ teaspoon salt

¼ teaspoon freshly ground black pepper

Combine chia seeds and tomato liquid in a small bowl; let stand 10 minutes. In a large bowl, combine oil, garlic, and lemon zest. Whisk in vinegars. Add tomatoes, salt, pepper, and tomato liquid–chia seed mixture; mix well and let stand 15 minutes for flavors to blend. Serve over pasta, fish, lettuce, or chicken, or with whole wheat crostini.

What's in it for you?	
Total fat	4 g
Saturated fat	0.5 g
Healthy fats	3 g
Fiber	1 g
Carbohydrates	4 g
Sugar	4 g
Protein	1 g
Sodium	150 mg
Calcium	12 mg
Magnesium	10 mg
Selenium	0 mcg
Potassium	217 mg

Note: This recipe exceeds the sodium criteria for condiments for Lifestyle 180. Consume only if sodium is not an issue for you.

Lifestyle 180 Roasted Pepper, Tomato, Walnut, Almond, and Ancho Chile Sauce

12 servings (about ¼ cup each) ❖ 70 calories per serving

½ cup finely diced sweet onion

2 tablespoons extra-virgin olive oil

2 teaspoons finely minced garlic

¼ cup toasted walnuts

¼ cup sliced toasted almonds

2 cups peeled and seeded tomatoes

1 cup roasted red peppers

2 tablespoons ancho chile paste

1 teaspoon salt

⅛ teaspoon cayenne pepper

In a saucepan, sauté onion in olive oil over a low flame until onions are translucent, add garlic and sauté until garlic begins to turn a light golden color. Turn off heat and place saucepan over a cold burner on stove.

Place walnuts and almonds in a food processor and pulse until finely chopped. Add tomatoes, roasted peppers, chili paste, salt, and cayenne and puree until mixture is smooth. Pour tomato, pepper, and nut mixture into a saucepan, simmer on very low heat for 15 minutes, and serve.

What's in it for you?	
Total fat	5 g
Saturated fat	0.5 g
Healthy fats	4.5 g
Fiber	2 g
Carbohydrates	5 g
Sugar	2 g
Protein	1 g
Sodium	190 mg
Calcium	14 mg
Magnesium	17 mg
Selenium	0 mcg
Potassium	89 mg

Note: To roast peppers, cut peppers in quarters and remove seeds, white membrane, and stem. Place peppers skin side up under an oven broiler 3 to 4 inches from heat source. Broil the peppers until blistered. Place on a plate blackened side up, cover with plastic wrap, and allow to cool about 5 minutes. Remove plastic wrap and scrape off the blackened skin.

Note: To make ancho chile paste, place a dried ancho chile in a small bowl, cover with water, and set at room temperature until reconstituted and soft. Remove seeds, stem, and tough skin membranes. Finely mince and mash into a paste with the side of a knife.

Lifestyle 180 Basic Tomato Sauce

6 servings (about ¾ cup each) ❖ 130 calories per serving

4 ounces finely diced onion

2 tablespoons extra-virgin olive oil

2 teaspoons minced garlic

6 ounces tomato paste

6 ounces nonalcoholic red wine

1¼ pounds fresh plum tomatoes, flesh only

12 ounces vegetable stock

5 fresh basil leaves

1 teaspoon salt

Freshly ground black pepper, to taste

Sauté onion in oil until transparent, add garlic, and sauté about 2 minutes. Add tomato paste and cook lightly until just beginning to caramelize. Add wine, stock, and basil. Simmer 30 minutes. Blend with stick blender and season with salt and pepper.

What's in it for you?

Total fat	6 g
Saturated fat	1 g
Healthy fats	0 g
Fiber	3 g
Carbohydrates	13 g
Sugar	8 g
Protein	4 g
Sodium	110 mg
Calcium	29 mg
Magnesium	27 mg
Selenium	3 mcg
Potassium	614 mg

Lifestyle 180 Ginger Sweet-and-Sour Sauce

11 servings (about ¼ cup each) ❖ 30 calories per serving

1⅓ cups unsweetened pineapple juice

¼ cup organic, sugar-free, corn-syrup-free ketchup

2 tablespoons light soy sauce

2 tablespoons white wine vinegar

2 tablespoons rice wine vinegar

1 tablespoon plus 1 teaspoon agave nectar

½ teaspoon minced fresh ginger

½ teaspoon minced fire-roasted jalapeño (or use canned)

1 tablespoon arrowroot or cornstarch

Combine all ingredients except arrowroot in a medium saucepan. Bring to a simmer over high heat. Dissolve arrowroot in 3 tablespoons cold water; stir into sauce. Simmer, stirring frequently, for 10 minutes, or until sauce is slightly thickened.

What's in it for you?	
Total fat	0 g
Saturated fat	0 g
Healthy fats	0 g
Fiber	0 g
Carbohydrates	8 g
Sugar	6 g
Protein	0 g
Sodium	220 mg
Calcium	5 mg
Magnesium	0 mg
Selenium	0 mcg
Potassium	43 mg

Cinnamon Baked Apples with Tangerines and Cranberries

4 servings ❖ 146 calories per serving

2 large baking apples, such as McIntosh or Rome Beauty
    (or substitute pears)
1¼ cups unsweetened apple juice, preferably unfiltered organic
½ cup (2 ounces) dried cranberries (or substitute cherries)
¼ teaspoon ground cinnamon
¼ teaspoon ground cloves
2 seedless clementines or tangerines, peeled, separated into segments

Heat oven to 400°F. Cut apples in half lengthwise; cut out and discard cores, seeds, and stems. Place ¼ cup of the apple juice in an 8-inch baking dish or casserole pan. Place apples cut side down in juice. Bake 15 to 18 minutes or until apples are tender. Meanwhile, simmer remaining 1 cup apple juice in a small saucepan over medium-high heat 5 minutes. Add cranberries, cinnamon, and cloves; reduce heat and simmer uncovered 10 minutes, or until cranberries are plumped, stirring occasionally. Remove from heat; stir in clementine sections. Arrange apple halves cut side up on serving dishes. Pour any remaining liquid from dish into cranberry mixture; spoon over apples.

What's in it for you?

Total fat	0.6 g
Saturated fat	0.1 g
Healthy fats	0.3 g
Fiber	4.1 g
Carbohydrates	37.7 g
Sugar	30.4 g
Protein	0.7 g
Sodium	15 mg
Calcium	30 mg
Magnesium	13 mg
Selenium	0.2 mg
Potassium	281 mg

Cinnamon Apple Sauté à la Mode

2 servings ❖ 220 calories per serving

2 small apples, such as Jonagold or Ambrosia

1 tablespoon apple butter

1 tablespoon unsweetened apple juice or cider, preferably organic

½ teaspoon ground cinnamon

6 walnut halves, toasted, coarsely chopped

½ cup nonfat or low-fat vanilla frozen yogurt

Cut apples into quarters; discard stems, cores, and seeds. Cut apple quarters into thin slices. Heat a large nonstick skillet over medium-high heat until hot. Add apples; cook until apples begin to brown, about 4 minutes, tossing occasionally. Stir in apple butter, apple juice, and cinnamon; continue to cook 5 to 8 minutes, or until apples are tender and sauce thickens, tossing frequently. Transfer to serving plates; top with nuts. Serve with frozen yogurt.

What's in it for you?	
Total fat	8.4 g
Saturated fat	0.8 g
Healthy fats	7 g
Fiber	6.7 g
Carbohydrates	38 g
Sugar	27.6 g
Protein	3.6 g
Sodium	23 mg
Calcium	83 mg
Magnesium	35 mg
Selenium	2 mcg
Potassium	346 mg

PROOF AGAINST M.D.s

Roasted Pear with Raspberry Coulis, Chocolate, and Pistachios

2 servings ❖ 184 calories per serving

1 large red pear

½ cup white wine (high-quality)

6 ounces frozen unsweetened raspberries, thawed, or
    1 cup fresh raspberries

1 tablespoon mini semisweet chocolate chips

1½ tablespoons coarsely chopped pistachios, toasted

Heat oven to 400°F. Cut pear in half; remove core with a melon baller or metal measuring teaspoon. Arrange pear halves, cut side down, in a shallow baking dish. Pour wine over pears. Bake 18 to 20 minutes, or until pears are tender when pierced with the tip of a sharp knife. Meanwhile, puree raspberries in food processor; strain and discard seeds. Transfer roasted pears to serving plates, cut side up; sprinkle chocolate chips over the pears (the heat of the pears will melt the chips). Combine pureed raspberries and liquid remaining in baking dish in a small saucepan. Cook over high heat until sauce is slightly thickened. Spoon sauce over and around pears; sprinkle with pistachios. Serve warm or at room temperature.

What's in it for you?	
Total fat	5.2 g
Saturated fat	1.4 g
Healthy fats	3.3 g
Fiber	4.9 g
Carbohydrates	31.8 g
Sugar	24 g
Protein	2.7 g
Sodium	7 mg
Calcium	45 mg
Magnesium	32 mg
Selenium	2 mcg
Potassium	344 mg

Sliced Peaches with Raspberries, Blueberries, and Chocolate Chips

2 servings ❖ 46 calories per serving

2 small ripe peaches, sliced

½ teaspoon ground cinnamon

Pinch of nutmeg

¼ cup (1 ounce) fresh raspberries

¼ cup (1 ounce) fresh blueberries

1½ tablespoons mini semisweet chocolate chips

Combine sliced peaches with cinnamon and nutmeg; transfer to two serving plates. Top peaches with raspberries, blueberries, and chocolate chips.

What's in it for you?	
Total fat	0.4 g
Saturated fat	0.1 g
Healthy fats	0.28 g
Fiber	2.6 g
Carbohydrates	11.5 g
Sugar	8.9 g
Protein	1 g
Sodium	0.5 mg
Calcium	22 mg
Magnesium	11.5 mg
Selenium	0.1 mcg
Potassium	202 mg

I EAT MILK CHOCOLATE FOR BREAKFAST!

Bill's DARK, DARK, DARK Chocolate

Lifestyle 180 Peanut Butter, Chocolate, and Vanilla Tofu Mousse

15 ¼-cup servings ❖ 140 calories per serving

12 ounces extra-firm tofu

2 ounces unsweetened baking chocolate

¾ cup natural creamy peanut butter

2 tablespoons agave nectar

1 tablespoon vanilla extract

6 tablespoons unsweetened cocoa powder

2 medium fresh bananas

Combine chocolate and peanut butter in glass bowl and microwave for 30-second increments stirring each time until chocolate is melted and blended with peanut butter. Add tofu to food processor and process until smooth, scrape down sides of bowl, add agave and vanilla and process until smooth. Add melted chocolate and process until smooth; remove and scrape into individual dishes or large bowl. Cover and refrigerate.

What's in it for you?	
Total fat	10 g
Saturated fat	2 g
Healthy fats	0 g
Fiber	2 g
Carbohydrates	10 g
Sugars	5 g
Protein	5 g
Sodium	45 mg
Calcium	41 mg
Magnesium	4 mg
Selenium	0.15 mcg
Potassium	84 mg

Lifestyle 180 Chocolate Espresso Tofu Mousse

9 servings (3 ounces each) ❖ 120 calories per serving

12 ounces silken extra-firm tofu

2 large ripe bananas, broken into chunks

2 ounces 70% cocoa bittersweet chocolate bar

6 tablespoons unsweetened cocoa powder

1 tablespoon agave nectar

2 tablespoons instant espresso powder

2 teaspoons vanilla extract

Place tofu in food processor; process until creamy. Add bananas; process until smooth. Melt chocolate according to package directions. Add chocolate and remaining ingredients to banana mixture; process until smooth. Transfer to individual dishes or a large bowl; cover and refrigerate at least 30 minutes before serving.

What's in it for you?	
Total fat	8 g
Saturated fat	2 g
Healthy fats	0 g
Fiber	3 g
Carbohydrates	14 g
Sugar	6 g
Protein	5 g
Sodium	0 mg
Calcium	74 mg
Magnesium	10 mg
Selenium	0.3 mcg
Potassium	153 mg

Lifestyle 180 Chia Banana Cake

24 squares ❖ 130 calories per square

1 tablespoon chia seeds

½ cup water

4 very ripe bananas

1 teaspoon vanilla extract

¼ cup canola oil

5 tablespoons agave nectar

1¼ cups water

2 cups whole wheat flour

2 teaspoons baking powder

1 teaspoon baking soda

1 teaspoon salt

1 teaspoon cinnamon

½ cup chopped toasted walnuts

Combine in small mixing bowl the chia seeds and water, mix well, and set at room temperature for 15 minutes to allow chia seeds to swell. While chia seeds are swelling, in another large bowl combine peeled banana, vanilla, canola oil, and agave nectar and mix with electric mixer until the mixture is very smooth with no lumps. Once chia seeds have swelled, add to banana mixture and blend well. Add remaining one cup water and mix with electric mixer until well blended.

In a large bowl, combine whole wheat flour, baking powder, baking soda, salt, and cinnamon and mix with a wire whisk. Slowly add dry ingredients to wet ingredients in one-third increments while mixing with electric mixer until well blended before adding more. After all of the dry ingredients are added and well blended, add walnuts, mix well, and pour into a 9- x 13-inch lined and nonstick sprayed baking pan. Bake in a 350°F oven for 30 minutes or until a toothpick comes out clean. Allow to cool, cut into squares, and serve.

What's in it for you?	
Total fat	6 g
Saturated fat	0.5 g
Healthy fats	5.5 g
Fiber	4 g
Carbohydrates	21 g
Sugar	8 g
Protein	3 g
Sodium	190 mg
Calcium	26 mg
Magnesium	30 mg
Selenium	9 mcg
Potassium	158 mg

"Dive into the Dark Side" Bars

24 bars (1 ounce each) ❖ 110 calories per bar

1 cup toasted walnuts

¾ cup golden raisins

¾ cup unsweetened dried cranberries

5 brown rice rice cakes, broken into chunks

2 tablespoons agave nectar

2 tablespoons orange juice

1 tablespoon vanilla extract

¼ teaspoon cinnamon

5 ounces 70% dark bittersweet chocolate bar, broken into chunks

5 tablespoons fat-free milk or orange juice

1 tablespoon instant espresso powder

Place walnuts in food processor and pulse until chopped. Add raisins and cranberries and pulse until mixture is finely chopped. Add rice cakes; process until finely chopped. Add agave nectar, orange juice, vanilla, and cinnamon; process until mixture holds together. Transfer mixture to an 8-inch-square glass baking dish; cover with plastic wrap and press into a firm, even thickness. Remove plastic wrap.

Combine chocolate, milk, and espresso powder and place over a double boiler of simmering water. Cook, stirring constantly, until chocolate is melted and smooth. Spread chocolate evenly over rice cake mixture, cover, and refrigerate at least 1 hour before serving. Cut into 12 (3- x 2-inch) bars.

What's in it for you?	
Total fat	6 g
Saturated fat	2 g
Healthy fats	2.5 g
Fiber	2 g
Carbohydrates	13 g
Sugar	8 g
Protein	2 g
Sodium	10 mg
Calcium	9 mg
Magnesium	8 mg
Selenium	0.2 mcg
Potassium	132 mg

Lifestyle 180 Quinoa and Fruit Pudding

9 servings ❖ 130 calories per serving

1 cup organic quinoa

2 cups water

½ cup dried cherries

½ cup dried cranberries

½ cup unsweetened apple juice

2 bananas

1 teaspoon grated orange zest

1 teaspoon vanilla extract

½ teaspoon cinnamon

Rinse quinoa in cold water if saponin has been removed, if not rinse in hot water. Add rinsed quinoa to boiling water; reduce heat to low, and simmer for 7 minutes. Add dried cherries and cranberries and simmer until liquid is absorbed, about 5 to 7 minutes. While quinoa is cooking, combine remaining ingredients in food processor and puree until smooth. Remove quinoa from heat, combine pureed mixture with quinoa, and mix well. Place in serving bowls and refrigerate until ready to serve.

What's in it for you?	
Total fat	1 g
Saturated fat	0 g
Healthy fats	1 g
Fiber	4 g
Carbohydrates	28 g
Sugar	11 g
Protein	3 g
Sodium	0 mg
Calcium	16 mg
Magnesium	42 mg
Selenium	1.8 mcg
Potassium	197 mg

Simon's Popcorn

4 servings ❖ 61 calories per serving, 10 percent from fat

½ cup popcorn kernels

Flavored cooking spray (butter, olive oil, or garlic)

Garlic salt or cinnamon

Place popcorn in a 2½-quart microwave-safe container; cover and cook at high power 4 to 5 minutes, or until popcorn is popped but not scorched. If the microwave oven does not have a rotating turntable, use oven mitts to grasp and shake the covered container after 3 minutes of cooking. Immediately pour the popcorn onto a baking sheet and coat with cooking spray. To further flavor the popcorn, immediately sprinkle on your favorite seasoning blend such as garlic salt or cinnamon.

What's in it for you?

Total fat	0.8 g
Saturated fat	0.1 g
Healthy fats	0.7 g
Fiber	0.4 g
Carbohydrates	5 g
Sugar	0 g
Protein	1 g
Sodium	0 mg
Calcium	1 mg
Magnesium	0 mg
Selenium	1 mcg
Potassium	0 mg

101 FAQs

Since the first edition of this book, we've received more than 100,000 questions about weight loss (and waist loss). Here, we've chosen 101 of the most common to give you even more insight into ways that you can improve your health. They're grouped by subject matter (and some are combos of two or more questions) to make it easier for you to navigate to the questions you have—and the answers you want.

MAIN MEALS

Some Fats Make You Hungrier

Q: Let's face it, a salad is never going to satisfy my hunger like a good old slice of pizza. As long as I don't overeat, does it really make that much difference what I eat? *Lisa in Chicago*

A: Your logic says that if you eat a fatty bacon cheeseburger, you'll feel full and won't want to eat later. Nice try. Compared to healthy-fat meals with the same number of calories, meals high in saturated fat produce lower levels of leptin, the hormone that turns off appetite. And these saturated fats turn on your aging genes (see page 131). All fats, both saturated and unsaturated, have 9 calories per gram. Because they provide equal amounts of energy, you'd think all fats would satisfy your appetite the same way. But they don't. To get the highest leptin levels, eat healthful unsaturated fats. You'll find them in nuts, seeds, olives, fish, avocados, and vegetable oils.

Herbs for High-Powered Salad

Q: I love a salad for lunch, but I'm getting bored with lettuce, tomatoes, and cucumbers. What can I add to my salad to make it more interesting and better for me? *John, bored in Seattle*

A: You may be bored, but you're also smart. You could load your salad with such nasties that can quickly turn a healthy idea into a calorie-laden meal masquerading as salad (think salad dressings, cheese, croutons, and bacon). Here are our suggestions: Fresh herbs (sage, rosemary, marjoram, and thyme) add extra cell-protecting phenols to salads. In a recent study, these herbs added the most antioxidants to a salad. For spices, cumin soared up the salad chart, and second to cumin was fresh ginger. Wondering which vegetables pack the strongest polyphenol punch? Artichoke, beetroot, broccoli, garlic, a variety of leek, a type of radish, and spinach were top produce picks in a recent study. Adding onions also ups your antioxidant-polyphenol ante.

Bigger Breakfast, Smaller You

Q: You seem to indicate that loading up my plate could make me lose weight—if I do it at breakfast and if I'm smart about it. That seems just like diving in Lake Erie in January can make you a faster swimmer. Were you serious? *Don in Cleveland, Ohio*

A: OK, so you can't pile your plate higher than your inbox and hope to drop pounds. But when obese dieters ate a big 600-calorie breakfast of healthy protein and carbs (think scrambled egg whites, diced turkey, whole wheat toast, and a banana), they lost significantly more weight than dieters who ate only half that much. Why? It's possible that eating a large balanced meal in the morning with lots of fiber helps stymie carb cravings later in the day—especially if you're cutting them in an effort to slim down.

Let's Talk Soup

Q: I love a cup of soup for lunch because it is so easy to pack. Any recommendations on which soup might be the healthiest for me? *Jillian in Bethesda*

A: Soup for you? No problem. There are plenty of soups that pack too much fat, too much cream, and too much sodium, so you have to be careful. Our choice: tomato soup. It may protect your blood vessels from the damaging, out-of-control party that high blood pressure and inflammation want to start in your arteries. When a group of people ate about two cups of a tomato-based soup every day for two weeks, they had lower blood pressure, higher blood levels of vitamin C, and decreased markers of inflammation. Vitamin C, and possibly other compounds in the vegetables in the soup, may play a critical part in preventing the invitations from going out to the inflammation party in your arteries. People in the soup study were eating gazpacho, the cold soup made of tomato, pepper, and cucumber that's popular in Spain and other Mediterranean cuisines. But it's easy to make hot soup with tomatoes or incorporate these healthy fruits into other dishes. We recommend trying salsa-topped salmon: The fish oil–tomato combo makes a high-powered blood pressure reducer and inflammation stopper.

Make an Easy Meal Healthier—Fast!

Q: Soup is a great quick lunch at the office when I don't have time to get away from my desk. Is there a way to make it healthier? *Betty from Pine Bluff, Missouri*

A: When your schedule has less room in it than the Tokyo subway at rush hour, a bowl of canned soup is a good quick-and-easy meal option. But there's one thing that's not so easy about it: finding the veggies in it. Here's how to make it easy again: Soup up your soup with fennel. A spice, herb, and veggie all rolled into one, fennel complements many soups, from chicken noodle to tomato. And it's loaded with disease-stomping flavonoids. Look for this wholly edible root vegetable in the produce section: It looks like a bulb with feathered leaves and celerylike stalks. Just cut the bulb up, put it into a Baggie, and toss some chopped bits into your bowl before you nuke your soup.

Dairy Decisions

Q: I prefer yogurt with my granola in the morning, but my fiancé says I should be using milk instead. Tell me I am right. *No Soggy Cereal for Me*

A: We vote with you. Start your day with some yogurt (make it low fat, no sugar added). Later, have some more for a snack. Compared with their peers who never ate yogurt, people in a study who ate two or more servings daily had an almost 40 percent lower risk of bladder cancer. Cultured milk products like yogurt contain something that other dairy items lack: lactic acid bacteria. Just how the bacteria help stave off bladder cancer isn't clear, but the fact that they have an immune-boosting reputation is one possibility.

DRINKS

Get the Most from Your Morning Brew

Q: You've mentioned that coffee can help you live longer and be healthier. Can you get these benefits from instant coffee or only from brewed? *Anonymous*

A: Though brewed-coffee drinkers may turn up their noses at cups of the instant stuff, the caffeine and some of the healthy polyphenols (plant substances that help your body help itself) found in brewed coffee are preserved when it's made into instant. After all, instant starts its life as brewed coffee that's been either freeze- or spray-dried until the liquid is gone. While some of the polyphenols and the taste go too, that depends on which beans, what brewing process, and which drying method are used. But get this: the instant crowd is actually getting two-thirds more fiber than filtered-coffee drinkers are. A 12-ounce cup of instant contains about 3 grams of fiber, compared to about 1.8 grams in the same amount of brewed. Bonus: the fiber helps your body absorb those polyphenols.

Getting Creamed

Q: I like nondairy creamer or soy milk in my coffee and tea, but I've heard they wipe out the antioxidants in these drinks. Is that true? *Deanna in Lowell, Michigan*

A: The more you dump into your cup, the greater the chance of dumping fat onto your waist. So be careful about loading your drink with cream, sugar, syrup, and the like. But for your specific question, the research shows mixed results: In some cases, whiteners decrease the benefit of healthy compounds, while other studies show it makes no difference. Our take: You're far better off drinking tea than sugary sodas, especially if you drink tea and coffee without the sugar and with only skim milk. But here's a cool fact: You will get more healthy compounds to start with by—surprise—brewing a medium-roast coffee rather than a dark one, like French or Italian roast.

A Grape Solution

Q: I know a glass of red wine is healthy, but it isn't always appropriate to drink a glass a day (my boss is a stickler about drinking on the job). Is there another way to get some of the benefit without the wine? *Andy in San Diego*

A: Sorry to say, but you couldn't possibly drink enough wine to make it healthy because of the grapes alone. It's actually the alcohol that does the trick. But you can get a health boost if you have a lot of grape skins, because they contain chemicals called pterostilbene and resveratrol that work as a cleanup crew, mopping up nasty free radicals in your body so they're less likely to cause problems such as heart disease and cancer. And if you got the resveratrol of 180 bottles of wine, you'd turn on your sirtuin genes that also increase DAF-16 (sweet 16) (see page 131). And you'd slow aging that way too. Not to mention that they contain vitamin C and anthocyanins, which attack disease-fostering inflammation. But for now, it's the alcohol that is anti-aging. And instead of saucing up at your three-o'clock break, have your glass of wine as a great dessert; you can get the sweet taste, avoid traditional fatty finishers, and get the health benefits all in one shot.

Choose Cloudy Apple Juice, Clearly

Q: When I buy apple juice, I always look for ones that are clear because the cloudy ones look as if they have been on the shelf too long. Does it make a difference? *Dan in Fayetteville, New York*

A: Cloudy may not be ideal for summer vacation, but you can't beat it when it comes to apple juice. Depending on how much pectin is removed during processing, apple juice varieties are either completely translucent or a bit murky. Choose the cloudy stuff. It contains more disease-fighting polyphenols. Apples are full of cell-protecting phenols, antioxidant-like compounds that fend off aging and diseases such as Alzheimer's and cancer. When researchers compared see-through apple juice to the cloudy stuff, the muddy version was a clear winner: It had more phenols, and it mopped up more cell-damaging free radicals. Clear apple juice goes through extra processing that makes it translucent. And that process appears to zap the juice's phenolic content.

Time for a Tea Party

Q: I love joining my friends for afternoon tea at a local hotel. I am thinking about making tea a daily ritual for me. Is there a health benefit I can state when my husband teases me about lazing away the afternoon? *Anne in Philly*

A: Use this as antihubby fodder: Each daily cup of green or black tea helps beat down the risk of ovarian cancer. In a recent study, two or more cups per day helped cut the risk nearly in half. Within a group of women, those who drank green and black tea had lower rates of ovarian cancer than those who rarely or never did. And the more they drank, the further their disease risk plummeted. Powerful antioxidants called polyphenols may prevent cancer cell growth, hinder blood supply to the tumor, or encourage cancer cells to commit suicide. More studies are needed to confirm the results of the ovarian cancer study. In the meantime, tea boasts many other powerful health benefits, for both men and women.

FRUITS AND VEGETABLES

Bitter Fruit for Better Weight Loss

Q: My daughter told me she heard one of you on WSYR in Syracuse talking about grapefruit for weight loss—but not eating it, just smelling it. So she's been putting some grapefruit juice on her wrist every day. It's only been a week—it seems to be working. Why? *Janice in B-town*

A: Often the punch line of diet jokes, grapefruit does have some pretty startling benefits. In one twelve-week study, obese people who ate half a grapefruit before each of their three daily meals shed more pounds than their counterparts did. In the study, whole grapefruit also took a bite out of insulin resistance in folks with metabolic syndrome, a constellation of conditions that can raise the risk of developing several serious health problems, including diabetes. Although grapefruit juice and grapefruit capsules may also have pound-shedding potential, whole fruit was clearly the winner in the study, probably because the whole fruit has appetite-controlling fiber as well. The scent of grapefruit may help you too. Apply grapefruit scent to your wrist and smell before a meal; it may decrease your appetite, and it has worked in studies as well as for your daughter.

Black and Blue

Q: I love strawberries and raspberries but have heard that blueberries are a healthier choice. Is that true, and what about other black- or blue-colored berries? *Marie in Montpelier*

A: When it comes to rain clouds, dark isn't such a good thing. Not true when it comes to berries. The darker, the better (also true for real cocoa-based chocolate). Two lesser-known and darker berries, chokeberries and elderberries, are starting to get more attention because they're approaching superfood status (because of a nutrient they contain called anthocyanin). You can't eat them raw, but you should be seeing more of them in juices and other health-food products. That said, all berries are good. Eat them, enjoy them, and let them work their antioxidant or other form of black and blue and red magic.

The Good Stuff in Organics

Q: Organic food can be hard to find and more expensive than other produce in the store. Does it really make a difference what I buy? *Rachel in Rapid City, Iowa*

A: You probably buy organic to get less of the stuff that's bad for you, such as pesticides. But organic foods may have more of the good stuff too. More and more research is showing that fruits and veggies sustainably or organically grown have higher levels of disease-fighting phenols than traditional large-business-farmed produce. In a study, corn grown with little or no pesticides had almost 60 percent higher levels of phenols than conventionally grown corn. Strawberries were nearly 20 percent higher in phenols, and marionberries also had greater amounts. Researchers suspect that pesticide use somehow inhibits the formation of these powerful disease fighters.

Being Green

Q: My husband says that if former President George H. W. Bush doesn't eat broccoli, neither will he. I think he is making a mistake. Even George is probably making a mistake, but my hubby is whom I care about. What do you think? *Maxine in Mendocino*

A: We think it's great that you care about your hubby, even more than a former president. When it comes to the top ten list of vegetables people eat most, broccoli has a secure spot. When your blood sugar (glucose) is chronically high, the cells of your heart, eyes, kidneys, and nerves take a big hit. Hit after hit leads to permanent damage. But when researchers looked at what glucose did to blood vessel cells in a petri dish, they saw that sulforaphane reduced the damage—or oxidation—by as much as 73 percent. Broccoli and other cruciferous vegetables are the main sources of that sulforaphane. It also stimulates specific genes to turn on, one of which is a potent cancer fighter. Scientists have seen compounds in this vegetable stop ovarian, breast, and prostate cancer cells from spreading (in a lab and hopefully also in your body), cut the risk of laryngeal cancer, and inhibit other cancers. To get the most from broccoli, steam it to preserve its health-giving compounds and eat it with a little fat to allow your body to absorb them best.

Feel Good about Cranberries

Q: My family makes fun of me because I look forward to holiday meals just because I know there will be cranberry sauce. Give me some good news about cranberries so I can shut them up! *Cranberry-seeking Carrie in Rochester*

A: Hey, no need to wait until November to start salivating over your favorite in-mold fruit. Most of all, cranberries curb your risk of heart disease (cranberries were high on the list of best-for-your-heart foods in a review of 134 studies examining cardio-smart nutrition). Researchers suspect that an arsenal of polyphenolic compounds in the tart red fruit may help your ticker in several ways by decreasing inflammation, balancing blood fats, and cleaning out free radicals.

You Say Tomato

Q: I have eliminated added salt from my diet, but my blood pressure is still a bit too high. I don't want to take medication. What else can I do? *Tom in Denver*

A: Think Italian. In one study, people with hypertension who consumed tomato extract daily for eight weeks experienced a ten-point drop in systolic blood pressure and a four-point drop in diastolic pressure. Researchers credit the lycopene in tomato extract for the potential blood-pressure-lowering effects experienced by participants in a recent study, but it works whatever the mechanism. It wouldn't even be a difficult amount to add to your daily diet, only about 10 tablespoons of tomato sauce or 4 tablespoons of paste a week. Regardless of the blood pressure benefits, we already know that lycopene has anticancer and heart-protective effects, but if you're not a fan of tomatoes, you have other options. To get your lycopene fix, try watermelon, red grapefruit, and canned baked beans. In the meantime, remember that most of the salt we eat is in processed food and fast food, so be sure to know what you are getting by checking food labels and the websites of your favorite hangouts.

Brainpower Lunch

Q: People call me Popeye because I eat so much spinach. I say I will have the last laugh. I'm right, aren't I? *Strong man in Saint Pete*

A: And not because you have mountainlike biceps? Well, good for you either way. Filling up on that green can keep your brain so sharp you'll be the one who wins the million-dollar account, solves the global warming problem, and keeps doing the Saturday crossword puzzle in pen. Eating three or more servings of spinach and other leafy greens (such as kale and collard greens) slows mental decline due to aging by as much as 40 percent. Spelled out another way: Leafy greens can make your brain function more like the brain of someone who's five years younger! What makes these veggies so super for saving your smarts? Probably brain-friendly nutrients including carotenoids and flavonoids. Keep extra power in your spinach by not letting it linger in the fridge. If you store it longer than four days after you buy it, these carotenoids, flavenoids, and folate levels plummet, turning it into a wimpier green.

Produce Power

Q: How can I make the most of my fruits and vegetables? *Rita in Butte*

A: Buying produce and then not cooking it right is like paying for 172 cable channels including 18 ultimate premiums and using only 3 regular channels: It's a big waste. One way to get the most bang for your buck is to steam your veggies with spices you love. Boiling, sautéing, or roasting can rob some vegetables of vital nutrients. Steaming helps keep nutrients in and creates a nice tender-crisp texture. Add garlic, turmeric, onion, or basal. Steamy veggies with favorite flavors may also lower lousy LDL cholesterol more—at least when it comes to beets, okra, carrots, eggplant, green beans, asparagus, and cauliflower.

A Nice Wrinkle

Q: My mother still tells me that I should be eating prunes for breakfast. They aren't the most appealing fruit. Is Mom right on this one? *Anita in North Fork*

A: This is one wrinkle you want in your morning oatmeal: dried plums. They used to be known as prunes before they got a marketing team behind them, but by either name, adding them to your hot cereal may have huge advantages for your heart. Fiber-rich oatmeal protects your heart by helping you control your bad blood fats (not all fats in your blood are bad). Dried plums are no slouches in the fiber department either (delivering 1 gram per fruit), but what makes them such a great addition to your morning meal is that they're also chock-full of polyphenols. These are the compounds that have a reputation for stopping bad things from happening in your arteries, such as plaque ruptures that could lead to a heart attack or stroke.

SNACKS, SIDES, SAUCES

Nutty Times

Q: Should walnuts be eaten raw or cooked to get the maximum benefit? *Robert in Cleveland*

A: Love them as you love family members—unconditionally. That means you can have them any way you want (not including hidden in a gallon of ice cream). That said, the oils in walnuts are protected when they're fresh and raw. When walnuts are cooked at very high temperatures, the beneficial omega-3 oils seem to deteriorate. We like them roasted in a way that will also preserve the oils: Place walnut halves on a cooking sheet in a toaster oven for nine to twelve minutes at 275 degrees. Trust us on the flavor: You'll go nuts over it.

Snack Attack

Q: Any new snack ideas? *Jeanette in Portland, Oregon*

A: Ditch the chips and concentrate on getting balance into your minimeals by changing up colors, flavors, textures, and food groups. Some quick ideas: Stir whole grain cereal into plain nonfat yogurt and top with blueberries. Go British and eat sardines with mustard on 100 percent whole wheat crackers. Dip whole grain pretzels into low-fat cottage cheese.

Oil Changes

Q: I keep hearing about the benefits of olive oil—any new benefits to report?
May in Miami

A: Olive oil is making headlines again, and it has nothing to do with her relationship with Popeye. The unsaturated fat that's great for your heart is now getting attention for helping something a little lower down: your stomach. Research suggests that the polyphenols in olive oil may inhibit the bacterium that causes most stomach ulcers. To protect the polyphenols in your olive oil and get the most out of the stuff, store it in a dark bottle away from sunlight, and don't overheat it.

The Food That Makes You Healthier, Fast

Q: Everyone raves about the Mediterranean diet and olive oil. I don't cook with that much oil. Any other foods that have the same benefit? *Bernie in Boise*

A: We say "Mediterranean diet," you say olive oil (or "I'll take a Aegean vacation, please"). But there are other parts of the diet that are just as delicious, and they too are known to make your arteries more elastic and knock down your risk of cardiovascular disease. A new study of the Mediterranean diet gave people who already ate this way either a liter a week more of olive oil or about an ounce of mixed nuts per day. A year later, the olive oil eaters had a 6.7 percent reduced risk of metabolic syndrome, the cluster of health problems that can lead to heart disease, stroke, and diabetes. The nut eaters had more than double that reduction, reducing their risk by more than 13 percent. Plus, after just eight weeks on the Mediterranean diet—foods like roasted tomato basil soup, grilled tilapia with red lentils and kale, and other dishes filled with vegetables, whole grains, fruits, fish, and low-fat dairy products—your arteries start to become more elastic. After only three months, your risk of heart disease can drop by as much as 15 percent.

An Easy Way to Cut 220 Calories

Q: I barely eat during the day so I have room for my snack with the late-night TV shows and still I can't lose any weight. *In Love with Conan*

A: Removing 220 calories from your day could make a big difference to your waistline, right? So here's the simple way to make it happen: Set your DVR to record your favorite late-night shows. Then hit the hay. In a study, people who stayed up late—and got less sleep as a result—munched down 220 more daily calories than the hit-the-sack-early crowd.

VITAMINS, NUTRIENTS, ETC.

Vital Vitamin

Q: I spend time outside every day walking and puttering around the yard. Do I really need to take a vitamin D supplement? *Cody in Casper, Wyoming*

A: A D isn't great in school, but it is in your daily vitamin routine. If you're a health news buff, you know that getting enough vitamin D is important to your bones and just about every other body part. Adequate amounts not only reduce fracture risk and maintain muscle strength but also appear to—among other things—protect your heart, reduce diabetes risk, and lower the odds of developing certain cancers. We recommend getting 1,000 international units (IU) daily if you're under sixty years of age and 1,200 IU if you're over sixty. Just stay below 2,000 IU daily from food and supplements combined.

The Fats Your Body Loves

Q: What's the difference between DHA, ALA, and the other good fats? *Alan in Roswell*

A: We know that all the healthy fats sound more like acronyms for government agencies, but they're worth remembering. DHA is one of the omega-3 fats—the good fats that can protect your eyes, brain, and heart. Another important omega-3 fat is ALA (known as alpha-linolenic acid, if you want to get formal), found in chia, flax, and walnuts, which the body eventually (but in small quantities) converts to DHA. A third is EPA, found in fish oil (so is DHA). ALA is not a substitute for DHA. But we know ALA is healthy and that eating it is smart, especially when you choose foods containing ALA over those with omega-6 and saturated fats. That means:

- Snacking on walnuts instead of milk chocolate chips or other foods. Walnuts have about six times as much omega-3 as the next highest nut, and in one study, just twelve walnut halves a day decreased heart attack risk by 60 percent.
- Cooking only with canola oil, which contains ALA. Even better, use canola oil that's supplemented with DHA.
- Using chia instead of wheat as a grain.

Most people get far too little DHA, so we recommend getting 600 milligrams of DHA from supplements (we prefer the DHA from algae, but Mike has a conflict here—he chairs the scientific advisory board of a company that makes such stuff).

The Real Story

Q: Hey, you YOU docs have made me believe that high-fructose corn syrup was worse than the plague, but now there are all these commercials on TV telling me that it is fine. What's the real story? *Catherine in Bakersfield*

A: High-fructose corn syrup (HFCS)—once considered the "Frankenfood" fueling America's obesity epidemic—recently earned a presidential-style pardon. The American Medical Association concluded last June that this much-maligned sweetener was no worse than sugar. Recently, in *The American Journal of Clinical Nutrition*, a group of noted nutrition experts who've studied this processed sweet stuff agreed.

Even if you don't read medical journals or follow the headlines, you've probably seen the pro-HFCS commercials on TV—paid for by the Corn Refiners Association—featuring smiling moms reassuring one another that HFCS is perfectly safe and natural. (Of course, cyanide is also natural. Not that taking HFCS is the equivalent of ingesting cyanide, but don't think it has a clean bill of health.)

Hold that honey-mustard dipping sauce. Who said sugar was a great item to add to food? Further, almost all of the reports that found HFCS to be the same as sugar have been funded by groups that profit from sales of HFCS—including soda makers and their lobbyists. And we believe that the most important question remains whether big doses of fructose could trigger obesity in ways that go beyond all those excess calories.

Yes, we said fructose. But we don't mean the quantities found in fresh fruit, which come packaged with fiber and lots of nutrients. We're talking about the nutritionally empty megadoses added to soda, commercial sweets, and baked goods. We're also talking about all the little hits you're getting from foods that don't even seem sweet, such as ketchup and salad dressing. A growing stack of research suggests that getting too much fructose in your diet interferes with telling your brain that you're full and should stop eating. In a new University of Florida lab study, animals that ate a high-fat, high-calorie diet that was also high in fructose became leptin resistant and gained more weight than animals that ate a similar diet, minus the fructose. And fructose in large quantities overwhelms your liver's ability to process it without producing inflammation-producing compounds—see the science of the NASH on page 99.

Truth is, HFCS isn't the only source of excess fructose in the American diet. Table sugar has a similar makeup (roughly equal amounts of fructose and glucose). The reason HFCS comes under such fire is that the food industry's been pumping more and more of it into foods since the 1970s because it's cheap, mixes easily into beverages, and enhances flavor and shelf life. The result: we eat 1,000 times more HFCS now than when Richard Nixon was president—on average 63 pounds a year! That's over 230,000 calories worth. Per person! Per year!

The greatest cost differential in our global fight for jobs is health care costs: Health care costs are twice as expensive in America as in Europe since we have twice the chronic disease. Food choices, physical inactivity, tobacco, and stress cause 70 percent of those chronic diseases. So if all you care about is the potential for jobs in America, you'd ban tobacco and simple sugars like HFCS added to your foods.

The bottom line: Getting the obvious, and not so obvious, sweeteners out of your diet will save you hundreds of calories a day—and remove a substance that could be flipping metabolic switches without your permission. Here's how:

❖ Say no to soda and other sweetened drinks. The calories alone are enough reason to stop sipping liquid candy: A single eighteen-ounce soda, sweet iced tea, or fruit drink can pack 200 or more calories—courtesy of the fifteen teaspoons of sugarlike sweetener, usually HFCS, these beverages contain.

❖ If you're breaking a serious soda habit, transitioning to an artificially sweetened, 0-calorie version is a good stepping-stone on your way to healthier drinks: unsweetened iced tea, tea, black coffee, or skim milk. (Yes, coffee and tea are much healthier, according to much scientific data not sponsored by those who might profit from such.)

❖ Read labels to find hidden HFCS. Check the ingredients lists of all the processed foods you buy for HFCS (as well as other sweeteners you don't need, such as rice syrup). You'll find it in many breads, sweetened yogurts, and condiments. Buy only the brands without 'em, and certainly without them in the first five ingredients.

The B-All End-All

Q: What the heck is folate, and why do I need it in my diet? *Shanelle in Mansfield*

A: Like running with scissors, skimping on folate—an important B vitamin found in beans, greens, and fortified breads, breakfast cereal, and noodles—is an accident waiting to happen. Low levels can literally cause you to miscopy your DNA, raising your cancer risk by up to 40 percent. But more isn't better. New research shows that big doses of this B won't bulletproof your cells against cancer. In fact, there's emerging evidence that most of us should avoid high doses of this Jekyll-and-Hyde nutrient.

High-dose folic acid (the synthetic folate in supplements) did nothing to lower breast cancer risk in a new seven-year woman's health study. Nor did eight years of extra folic acid reduce colon cancer risk. In fact, it may even have raised the odds of developing advanced and multiple tumors, reports the University of North Carolina at Chapel Hill. And despite its early promise, this B vitamin hasn't been found to reduce the risk of heart disease either. So we advise 400 micrograms a day of folic acid from supplements and all the food folate you want.

When Sugar Is OK

Q: OK, guys, I'm finally purging the fridge, as you recommend. But while tossing things with more than 4 grams of sugar per serving, I noticed that my organic fat-free milk has 12 grams of sugar per serving and my nonfat plain yogurt has 6 grams of sugar per serving. Surely, they must be OK. What's the deal? *Penny, Pasadena, California*

A: And surely four pounds of bacon must be wonderful because it's natural too? The difference is between natural sugars, which are found in many foods, including dairy products, and added sugars, which are in chocolate chip cookies (and many times added to nonfat yogurts). The sugar in milk and plain yogurt is lactose (milk sugar), and your body is programmed to break it down and use it for energy (assuming you are not lactose intolerant). Added sugar is a different story, and you need to keep it down to 4 grams per serving (2 grams in snacks and sides).

But here's where it gets tricky: You can't tell the difference on an ingredients label. So trust your common sense. It's a sure bet that no one has added sugar to organic fat-free milk. The sugar is in the food itself. But chocolate milk? Yogurt swirled with syrupy fruit? Figure that most of the sugars on their labels were added (unless artificial sweeteners were used). How do you know? Read the ingredients part of the label; if there is a sugar, syrup, or food ending in an "-ose" in the first five ingredients, avoid it like the plague to avoid the plague of obesity, heart disease, and cancer—it is that important.

CONVENIENCE FOOD

What the 99-Cent Menu Costs You

Q: You guys often criticize fast food. But it's inexpensive and hits me when I need it; when I get off work, I can hit the drive-through and get two 99-centers quickly. Then I don't eat till dinnertime. *Don in Los Angeles*

A: When the people at the dry cleaner know your name, that's healthy community building. But when they know your order at the drive-through before you pull-up? Sign of a problem, son. The trouble with fast food (besides the fact that most of it is bad) is that it's not always obvious which items will turn you into an orca look-alike and which will leave you thinner than a guppy. Take, for instance, the fact that a Dunkin' Donuts reduced-fat blueberry muffin contains 400 calories and a glazed donut contains 230 (not that either of them is a good breakfast choice, of course). And would you know that two slices of a large Domino's pizza delivers 360 calories and a Southwest salad with crispy chicken at McDonald's brings you 430, without dressing?

It's true that these companies have made concerted efforts to add some healthier items to the menu. And New York City, the state of California, and the Cleveland Clinic are helping you make good choices by requiring chain restaurants to post their nutrition data.

But it's not that hard to make your own meals at home that taste far better than even the best options at the drive-through (and you won't spend ten minutes breathing the exhaust of the car in front of you). Example: Spread some tomato paste, stir-fried vegetables, olive relish, and sundried tomato bits on a prepared 100 percent whole wheat pizza crust. Top with herbs and a touch of shaved smoked mozzarella. Bake at 450 degrees for ten to fifteen minutes.

Who's Protecting Your Health?

Q: Is it possible to make every single edible item healthy? Nowadays even soda pop is fortified with vitamins. Should I buy products with additives in them to make them healthier? *Heather in Henderson, Nevada*

A: Think about it: Would cheese puffs laced with vitamins or ice cream pumped full of whole grains be great for you just because they added a good element? No. We're disturbed by this trend—soda "fortified" with essential vitamins and minerals, phooey. The U.S. Food and Drug Administration has started to crack down on these and other products recently—moves we applaud because this important agency has also taken a lot of heat for not being tough enough. In December of 2008, the FDA scolded Coca-Cola for nutrient claims on its new Diet Coke Plus, which contains a touch of magnesium, niacin, and zinc and some B vitamins. This soda's label violated the so-called Jelly Bean Rule, which says it's not appropriate to fortify snack foods and that 50 percent more than nothing is still very close to nothing. As in nothing good. That's not a huge flex of muscle by the FDA, but it was a bit of a warm-up for the new idea that the agency is not going to let iffy claims slip by.

Not sure of a product? Ask yourself these two questions when considering a product:

❖ Is this the best way to get the nutrients I need? A moderate-dose multivitamin cut in half and taken morning and night as well as supplements of vitamin D (1,000–1,200 IU per day), calcium plus magnesium (600 milligrams calcium plus 200 milligrams magnesium twice a day), and B12 (25 micrograms a day) are all the nutritional insurance most of us need to fill gaps in our diets. If you love the taste of a soft drink, go ahead and enjoy a low- or no-calorie version once in a while, but there's no need to drink pricey water to get nutrients you should be getting in other ways every day.

❖ Can I reach the same health goal by a safer route? Getting slender with a questionable substance—even if you do manage to slim down with it—may bring on far more problems than the extra weight did. Yes, cigarettes and cocaine are associated with weight loss (and early death and disability). Not worth the pain. Going the proven weight-loss route—a diet rich in fruits, vegetables, and fiber, plus regular exercise—might take a little longer, but the results also last longer and won't land you in the ER (unlike substances in supplements, which can interact with other medications you're taking).

Cook Fast, Drink Fast

Q: I love those great shopper club stores. I can get all my shopping done in one visit. Any foods that I shouldn't be buying in bulk and storing for future use? *Diane in Denver*

A: Shop there if you want. Produce? Buy all you can eat this week. Lean protein? Get that too. And see what the price is over there on the brown rice. But there are two things you probably shouldn't get at your next trip to the big-box store: green tea and olive oil. That doesn't mean you shouldn't have them. In fact, you should. But buying them in big quantities means they'll sit around your kitchen, and new research suggests that both these products lose big amounts of their disease-fighting plant compounds over six months, even when you don't crack the seal on them.

Green tea loses its catechins—free-radical-fighting compounds that fight inflammation and help you avoid the aging and energy drops that accompany chronic disease. So buy it in smaller quantities, brew it frequently, and squirt some lemon juice into the tea when you drink it; this increases your ability to absorb these valuable compounds. Similarly, hanging around on a shelf for three to six months messes with olive oil's ability to fight free radicals, the damaging compounds implicated in heart disease and some cancers.

HERBS, SPICES, ETC.

Lick the Salt Habit

Q: My friends try to hide the salt shaker from me, but I think all food benefits from a little salt. Surely the small amount I put on at a meal can't make that much difference. *Betty in Sarasota*

A: This is one instance when it's not good that a whole lot of shaking is going on. Is your blood pressure a little high? Taste your food before you salt it, because it seems that letting go of the shaker provides big benefits, not just for people with high blood pressure but also for people with prehypertension (that's above 120/80 but under 140/90). More than one-quarter in U.S. adults have prehypertension, a condition where the numbers are just a bit high but not high enough to be officially classified as hypertension. Still, research shows that even slightly elevated numbers boost the risk of heart troubles down the road. To solve the problem, limit your meals out, as restaurant meals are notoriously high in sodium. Also, make sure to read labels closely when you buy premade, prepackaged, or canned foods. Words to look for on ingredients lists include sodium chloride, monosodium glutamate, baking soda, baking powder, disodium phosphate, sodium nitrite, sodium propionate, and sodium sulfite. And put away the salt shaker. Instead, experiment with flavors such as black pepper, lemon pepper, garlic, curry, lime or lemon juice, and red wine vinegar.

Apple Vinegar a Day

Q: I'm taking apple cider vinegar as my diet to lose weight. Is this a good idea? *Marjorie in Bismarck, North Dakota*

A: The lore is that apple cider vinegar decreases appetite and speeds metabolism. But there is no data to substantiate these claims. On the other hand, a lot of people find that it does decrease their hunger. So if it works for you and is successful, great. If it doesn't work for you, there are other ways to decrease appetite. Try having 8 to 12 grams of fiber at breakfast and again at lunch; because those slow transit between the small intestine and the large intestine, your small intestine stays fuller longer and you have less hunger.

Battle of the Fats

Q: I love nuts and eat a handful or two every day. My wife says I should be upping my intake of olive oil instead. Please say that nuts are good for me. *Bob in Davenport*

A: Let's pretend for a moment that you have two options for improving your health: eat more nuts, or eat more olive oil. Which should you choose? Believe it or not, nuts could have a slight edge, especially if you're concerned about metabolic syndrome, a combination of health conditions that raises heart disease risk. Why the difference? Here's one theory: Olive oil is a fat extracted from olives, but nuts are a whole food with more good-for-you stuff in them, including fiber, protein, and minerals. Both olive oil and nuts can—and should—have a place in a healthful diet.

Rise with Red Pepper

Q: I recently visited some friends in the Southwest, and wow, do they like some hot food for breakfast! Why in the world would you want to put red pepper in your scrambled egg whites? *Jason in Omaha*

A: We think red pepper is hot—but not for the reasons you think. Red pepper, when eaten early in the day, decreases food intake later in the day. Try adding a little to your egg-white omelet in the morning. The capsaicin in red pepper may get the credit for decreasing appetite. The heat-giving ingredient appears to stop sensory information in the intestine from reaching the brain. It basically kills, or stuns, the message that you're hungry. Capsaicin may also give your metabolism a boost. For a breakfast that will really fire you up, add cayenne, hot red peppers, or jalapeño peppers to a frittata. These hotties all contain capsaicin.

The Hidden Healer in Your Pasta Sauce

Q: I like to grow my own herbs to add to pasta sauce. What herbs would you recommend for my cutting garden? *Jim in Brecksville, Ohio*

A: Oregano isn't just a way to add pizzazz to your pasta sauce. Use it to bring some zing to your salad dressing, chicken marinade, or vegetable sauté, and your cells may thank you too. This herb may have the power to prevent damaging inflammation in your body, and that prevents weight gain, as well as wrinkles, impotence, and cancer, to name only a few that might concern you. The essential oils in this herb contain a tongue-twisting substance called (E)-beta-caryophyllene—we just call it (E)-BCP for short. This compound binds to certain receptors in your cells in a way that means less inflammation. That's the effect it had in mouse studies, and it's likely that it has similar inflammation-fighting benefits in humans.

FEELING FAT

Break Your Sugar Addiction

Q: Help! Quitting smoking was nothing compared to quitting sugar! I am addicted and can't stop eating it. I want to eat a healthy diet but seem to be unable to because of the sugar. What can I do to combat this addiction?
Anonymous

A: We know that quitting an addiction can be tougher than hiking in Sahara-like conditions wearing Everest-type gear. Recent research found that rats get the same neurochemical kick from sugar as from morphine, cocaine, and nicotine. We think that this surge of pleasure is behind a sugar-bingeing addiction in humans too. The good part: the principles we teach smokers to help them prepare to quit will also help you kick your sugar habit. Here are seven ways to set yourself up for success:

1. Make a pact with yourself to cut sugar out of your life. Studies show that making a serious commitment to doing whatever it takes to break an addiction is one of the most important steps toward beating it.
2. Set a quit date at least a month from today. Give yourself time to mentally prepare for the quitting journey and clear your pantry, car, desk, and gym locker of sugar in all its forms, including food and drinks containing natural sweeteners such as honey or rice syrup and high-fructose corn syrup (that includes most ketchups, many sports drinks [we like sugar-free Verve], coffee creamer, and many processed foods).
3. Start walking thirty minutes a day. Exercise, like sugar, releases mood-enhancing hormones. Later, when sugar abstinence causes a dip in feel-good hormones, you can add a tension-relieving five-minute walk to this regimen.
4. Gradually cut back. Begin by cutting back on the sugar you add to tea and coffee. Then substitute something healthy, such as no-sugar-added yogurt and berries or unsweetened applesauce for two or three of the sweet foods you usually have.

5. Visualize a slimmer, healthier you going for a walk, sipping water, or practicing deep breathing when you're stressed. A little role playing helps you practice alternatives to eating under pressure.
6. Think of the three biggest reasons why you want to live a sugar-free life, write them on a card, and read them aloud several times a day.
7. Get a buddy and report to her all the sugar you ate each day. Make sure it is a buddy who supports your move.

With a month of practice behind you, you'll be ready to weather the cravings that come when you first abstain from sugar. In time, your brain chemistry will readjust and the cravings will stop. You will beat the addiction the food companies taunt you with.

Four Hidden Causes of Weight Gain

Q: Everyone told me it would get harder to lose weight as I got older, but I think I must be a medical mystery—I gain weight even if I eat only raw veggies. Help me! *Frustrated in Fresno*

A: You're doing everything right, yet your waist keeps expanding faster than a marshmallow in a microwave oven. The trouble might be your hormones:

1. **Thyroid levels.** Hypothyroidism slows down your metabolism like a tricycle slows down speed compaired to Lance Armstrong on a racing bike. You can't burn calories like you used to.
2. **PCOS, or polycystic ovarian syndrome.** This accounts for unexplained weight gain in 20 percent of women. It's insulin resistance caused by abnormal secretion of a hormone by your darned ovaries.
3. **Testosterone drops.** These can occur in older men and postmenopausal women faster than your libido if you gain belly fat, because belly fat converts testosterone to estrogen. Some say that's why fat single men hang out with guys and drink beer in bars—no libido and no aggressiveness even to try a line on a woman. But women with belly fat develop the problem too, as testosterone from their adrenals is a leading stimulator of libido.

And less testosterone means less muscle mass, which makes it harder to burn fat (leading to weight gain). The cure: resistance exercise. The sign your testosterone levels are dropping: if you have to shave less often than you used to.

4. **Growth hormone dips.** This can decrease as you age when you don't sleep at least ninety minutes at a time because you have to get up to pee, leading to weight gain. The best way to boost it naturally: get the right amount of sleep and exercise.

Low-fat Letdown

Q: I choose low-fat foods whenever possible (love those cookies), but I don't seem to be losing any weight or waist. What am I doing wrong? *Tania in Washington*

A: There are German-to-English dictionaries, English-to-Spanish dictionaries, even picture-to-word dictionaries. You know what else we need? Marketing-lingo-to-truth dictionaries. In the supermarket aisle, you can sometimes translate the words "low fat" into things like "high calories," "lots of sugar," and "not as healthy as you think." Foods labeled "low fat" may actually help you pack on the pounds. That's not only because people aren't good at estimating serving sizes of low-fat foods, so they eat up to 50 percent more calories than they would of the "full-fat" version, it's also because the lingo tricks you into thinking those products are good for you. But there are ways to protect your waistline. To boost the flavor factor, food makers often replace the fat in snack foods with extra sugar, flour, and other waist-busting ingredients. The result: low-fat foods with the same number of calories as the regular versions. Follow these three rules to help make low-fat foods work for your diet, not against it: First, check the calories. Stick with the low-fat version if it's lower in calories. But if it's not, the full-fat version may do a better job of satisfying you, as long as it contains mostly healthful unsaturated fats. Next, check the ingredients. Is white flour or sugar a main ingredient in the low-fat version? Opt for a low-fat product made with whole grains instead. And pass up anything that has more than 4 grams of sugar per serving (2 grams for snacks). Lastly, check the portions. Eating twice as much of the low-fat version doesn't do your waist any favors.

Feeling Fat Can Make You Sick

Q: Over the years I have put on the pounds, and I am sick about it. Literally sick, all the time. I need help! *Sara in Seattle*

A: It turns out that the higher percentage of weight you want to lose—even if you're not overweight in the first place—the more mentally and physically unhealthy days you have every month. Your BMI or actual weight doesn't have that much to do with it, researchers at Columbia University found. But the desire to lose weight does affect how healthy you are. How? It's likely that distorted ideas about what an ideal weight is lead to stress—and that stress precipitates bad-health days. And distorted ideas are common, especially in women. Only 41 percent of normal-weight people said they were happy with their weight (only 20 percent of overweight and 5 percent of obese people did). Try strength training. In one study, women felt more confident about their bodies after a twelve-week weight-training program.

Scale of Justice

Q: Are weight-control programs that require weekly weigh-ins more successful than those that don't? *Judy in Germantown, Tennessee*

A: That depends somewhat on your answer to our question: If you hop on the scale and see a bigger number than you expected, do you:

1. redouble your effort to eat less and exercise more?
2. drown your disappointment in a pint of dark chocolate ice cream?
3. find a buddy who encourages you successfully at the weigh-ins?

Though research has found that scale watchers are more likely to lose moderate amounts of weight and not regain it, frequent weigh-ins don't work for everyone. Besides, everybody's weight tends to fluctuate a pound or so from day to day. But if the number climbs even a little, some people get anxious or depressed or throw in the towel and reach for the ice cream. We recommend ditching the scale in favor of a tape measure. Tracking your waist size is a better way to monitor your belly fat, which poses the greatest risk to your health.

Cave to Cravings

Q: I often hear the siren sound of a doughnut calling my name, just begging to be eaten. You often say timing is key to eating, so if I'm going to cave in to its siren call, when? *Anne in Oakland, Michigan*

A: Wow, you must have really good hearing. Truth is, the later in the day you crumble, the more you'll probably eat to feel just as satisfied. Research shows that our capacity to feel satisfaction from food is stronger in the morning and grows progressively weaker throughout the day. In other words, thanks to the way your body's natural circadian rhythms work, you may have to really chow down (that means eat many cookies) at night to satisfy a craving, especially when compared to the number of cookies you need in the morning. That's great for Nabisco, not great for the button on your waistband, your risk of cancer, or your ability to stay young and enjoy sex.

Growl Now

Q: My stomach is always growling. How can I tame the beast? *Famished in Fort Wayne*

A: One of the best things you can do for your digestion and your weight is to slow down the speed at which your digestive system works. Why? Because it can mean feeling fuller longer—so you eat less. Here's how to take things nice and easy.

* ❖ **Eat often.** By never allowing yourself to get too hungry, you help turn off appetite-inducing hormones.
* ❖ **Have a healthy-fat appetizer.** Eating a little healthy fat before a meal, such as a handful of nuts, slows the rate at which your stomach empties, so you'll feel full faster from the meal.
* ❖ **Feast on fiber.** Fiber takes a long time to digest, which means your stomach empties more slowly and the time until your next meal won't seem so far away.

STRESS AND LIFESTYLE

Stocking Up

Q: I am ready to embrace a healthier lifestyle. I have emptied the fridge; now what should I put in it besides water and carrot sticks? *Ivy in Independence*

A: You'll find our complete list starting on page 277, but make sure to include fire-extinguisher munchies, good foods that will put out three-alarm starvation fires. Pick up ready-to-eat snacks for those times you're likely to reach for waist-killing chips or sweets. Our list includes almonds, peanuts, and walnuts; bags of prechopped fruits and veggies; dried fruit (apricots, cranberries); and edamame (soybeans—look for microwavable bags in the frozen food section). Plus, snacking on edamame will boost your bone health, and munching on a handful of nuts will promote your heart health.

Managing the Mayhem

Q: Every time I have passed a crisis (I almost have a car accident, one of my kids runs into the street after a ball, the boss gives me ten minutes to complete an urgent task), I get an adrenaline rush—my heart pounds, and I want to eat everything in sight. Why is that? *Susan in New Mexico*

A: When a stressful moment passes, you're immediately relieved that it's over (you can pry your fingers off the steering wheel now). But that doesn't let your ticker off the hook. There's a little thing called the aftereffects of stress that can have you raiding the cupboard and make your heart race faster than a Formula 1 driver. In one study, men and women were asked to complete a task that sent their heart rates climbing. Afterward, the men's appetites were unfazed, but the women looked to bland, fatty foods, such as cheese and plain popcorn, to ease their frustration. The moral of the story: stress reduction strategies aren't just an in-the-moment fix for an unpleasant situation. Think of healthy ways to unwind after a crisis has passed (see our tips for establishing emergency foods).

Feel-Good Foods

Q: Whenever I'm around my extended family, I feel I want to go crazy. Any foods that can help me? *Zelda in Rockville*

A: Need to chill out around patience-testing relatives or the bills? Nibble on some dark chocolate, or have a bowl of chicken soup. Both can boost serotonin, the feel-good chemical in your brain. Having healthy levels of serotonin may make you less likely to lash out under stress. So how can you get more even-keel serotonin into you? One option may be to eat tryptophan-containing foods such as chicken, chocolate, dairy products, tuna, eggs, and nuts. Your body needs tryptophan to produce serotonin. Notice that turkey isn't one—that's the turkey myth.

Breathe In

Q: The more stressed I get at work, the shallower my breathing, and then I feel exhausted, so I stress more about my productivity. Stop, I want to get off! *Stressed in Saginaw*

A: Want the chemical that will make your performance at the office bulletproof? You don't have to go to a well-connected ball player or do anything sketchy to get it. All you need to do is breathe. Inhaling deeply brings a chemical called nitric oxide from the back of your nose and your sinuses into your lungs. This short-lived gas dilates the air passages in your lungs and does the same to the blood vessels surrounding them so you can get more oxygen into your body. Nitric oxide also doubles as a neurotransmitter to help your brain function. Sounds like a no-brainer, but after age two, most of us never take a deep breath all day long (have you done it yet?). Take deep-belly breaths, using your diaphragm to pull your lungs down as you inhale. To exhale, suck your belly button toward your spine to push the diaphragm up and empty all the air from your lungs. Feel better?

Say No to One-night Hamburger Stands

Q: Every Monday a group of friends and I hit a burger joint for the Monday-night special; it's inexpensive but fried. A couple unhealthy meals won't really hurt me, will they? *Jennifer in Pasadena*

A: You think that just one trip through a bargain-basement grease center won't hurt, and it's true that one fast-food meal may not immediately go to your hips. The key is not to let the bad behavior turn into a habit. Still, even if one burger won't knock your dress size up, it will hit your blood pressure hard and fast. In one study of healthy young women, one group was given a fatty fast-food breakfast of two hash-brown patties, a sausage breakfast sandwich, and an egg breakfast sandwich. Another group had a low-fat breakfast of cereal, skim milk, fat-free yogurt, a fruit bar, and orange juice. Two hours later, the women performed a stressful task; the fast-food group didn't fare so well. Their blood pressure readings went extra haywire from the strain. This is especially bad, because hyper cardiovascular systems are associated with problems such as high blood pressure, arrhythmias, and sudden deaths. We're not sure one grease bomb is worth it.

Tuning Out Is Healthy

Q: I have to watch *American Idol, Lost,* and *The Office,* or I won't be able to join the water cooler conversation each day. Really, what's the harm? *Janice in Houston*

A: Hey, there's nothing wrong with enjoying Adam Lambert performing or Michael Scott goofing, but don't be fooled into thinking that couch time is all that beneficial. If you're finding yourself glued to the TV, at least hide the remote. Less time clutching your clicker could mean less risk of type 2 diabetes. More tube time may mean higher blood glucose levels, which could set the stage for type 2 diabetes, in which chronically high blood sugar levels can damage your eyes, heart, kidneys, and other organs. Our solution for absolutely addicted devotees: Do push-ups, lunges, sit-ups, and walking or yoga every (every!) commercial break for the entire length of the commercial. Nothing wrong with combining a little sweat with your laughs!

Good News for Late Exercise Bloomers

Q: I have never exercised (unless you consider moving from the couch to the fridge to be aerobic). Is it ever too late to make a lifestyle change? *Howard in San Antonio*

A: If we thought it was too late, we'd have packed up our message and sent it to the bottom of the ocean. It's never (ever) too late. If you want to make a change, you just have to start slowly and keep at it. Metabolic syndrome is not inevitable, even if you're currently spending more time on your butt than on your feet. What to do? Just start walking. Doing so today could slash your risk of the syndrome by as much as 24 percent within three years, even if you're over sixty years of age and carry a few extra pounds. One-quarter of adults have metabolic syndrome, and the number jumps to 40 percent after age sixty.

Party Foods

Q: My daughter is getting married in eight weeks, and there are a lot of parties planned in the weeks ahead. How can I fit into my outfit without passing up appetizers altogether? *Joan in Chicago*

A: This game is won not at the party but during the preparty. Eating a small amount of healthy unsaturated fat—think walnuts, avocado spread on whole wheat, apple slices dipped in a little peanut butter—twenty-five minutes before a meal triggers a chain reaction in your digestive system that slows the rate at which your stomach empties, which means you feel fuller faster. It also helps keep your blood sugar levels from spiking after your meal and makes it easier for your body to absorb fat-soluble nutrients, such as vitamins A, D, E, and K, as well as lycopene and lutein. It takes only about 70 calories of this fat to get the effect. That's about six walnut halves, ten almonds, one-fourth of a medium avocado, or half a tablespoon of real peanut butter (from peanuts alone). Once you're at the party, reach past the chips for the spicy almonds, olive tapenade, or walnuts. It's a great way to love evenings out—and also what you see in the mirror.

Reverse an Afternoon Slump

Q: I often do a face plant on my keyboard in the middle of the afternoon. No matter how I refer to it, an afternoon slump, power nap time, etc., rarely helps me get ahead. Do energy drinks or caffeine work? What can I do? *John in Albany, New York*

A: After you pry your forehead from the G key, consider this. Scientists call it the postprandial dip, the postlunch dip, or the secondary sleep gate. Our circadian rhythm means we're hardwired to have an energy dip between 1 p.m. and 4 p.m. (though no one knows why evolution thought that was a good idea). Taking a nap makes lots of sense but can be difficult to accomplish if you want to keep your job. Fortunately, you can at least compensate for it—and likely lessen it—with these strategies:

❖ **Make every meal count.** You can't just blame lunch for heavy afternoon eyelids—the postlunch dip can even hit people who skip that meal. Your energy level is affected by what you do or don't eat the whole day long—try to eat no foods with added sugars or syrups and no grain that is less than 100 percent whole—this keeps your blood sugar more constant and you more alert.

❖ **Try a little caffeine.** We said a *little*. It helps you sustain afternoon attention, but beware—it also might keep you from going to bed on time, creating an even worse dip tomorrow (morning).

❖ **Take a hike.** Or just walk to lunch the long way. People in one study felt less afternoon fatigue on days when they worked out during lunch. Regular activity is key; one workout on one drowsy day won't give you afternoon energy all month.

Thirty Minutes to a Faster, Better Brain

Q: At 5 p.m. I am still searching office coffee machines for that last cup of coffee to keep me going, but no one will start a new pot for me. What can I do to stay sharp all afternoon? *Mike from Buffalo, New York*

A: Zoned out in a meeting, and now your brain is stuck on "off" or "I'll do it tomorrow"? Skip the trip to the local java joint. You'll get your mind moving at warp speed if you walk, run, skate, jump rope, or just keep moving for thirty minutes. People who did a single, half-hour bout of light exercise were able to think more quickly and experienced less frustration when they returned to work. (Bonus if you do this, too: You'll be at least $2 richer and not have coffee breath, although we like coffee too.)

What to Eat While Watching TV

Q: I know you recommend not eating after 8 p.m. and definitely no mindless snacking in front of the TV, but some nights I just gotta have a little something—throw me a bone! *Baffled in Biloxi*

A: We'll throw you a bone, but it's not going to be a T-bone. Love snacking your way through football on Monday nights . . . *American Idol* on Wednesdays . . . and *Grey's Anatomy* on Thursdays? You won't end up being a *Biggest Loser* contestant if you put aside the potato chips, cheese curls, and other fatty fare and snack on this: airpopped popcorn. You can eat up to six cups of certain low-fat—or no-fat—microwave brands (or make your own—see Simon's Popcorn on page 390) for about the same number of calories you'd get from just seven or eight chips. So that reduces your risk of health-threatening obesity right there (no fat—just put the kernels inside a Pyrex covered dish in the microwave and enjoy the noise, then spray with canola-based spray, put on your favorite spice or salt, and voilà). Of course, you'll undo all the good of perfectly popped popcorn if you drown it in butter and salt à la those movie-theater tubs.

Comfort without the Food Coma

Q: When I'm stressed out, nothing makes me feel better than some chocolate-covered pretzels, but thirty minutes later I feel terrible again. I crave foods that give me comfort. What are some better choices? *Candy in Carson City*

A: The trouble with turning to chocolate-covered pretzels or a bowl of ice cream for a pick-me-up is that it becomes a let-you-down and harms you long term. Fortunately, there are better ways to enjoy food and help it keep you healthier. Reach for the following:

❖ **Fortified cereal.** Healthy 100 percent whole grain, no-saturated-fat-added cereal (we're not talking Cap'n Crunch here!) gives you a boatload of energy-boosting B vitamins, which work to curb tension, moodiness, irritability, and depression.

❖ **Foods made with saffron.** Small studies have found that saffron, a trademark of many yellow-hued Indian, Moroccan, and Asian dishes, can ease symptoms of depression with virtually no risk of side effects. Although this spice isn't cheap (no surprise: it takes 75,000 flowers to produce a pound of the stuff!), a little bit goes a long way. Use it instead of salt to kick up the taste of chicken, pork, and veggies.

❖ **A little bit of last night's salmon.** People with low blood levels of EPA and DHA, compounds found in fatty fish, are more likely to show symptoms of mild to moderate depression. So have some sardines on a cracker or finish off the salmon from last night's dinner.

The Health Benefits of Being Cheap

Q: Times are tough, and I can barely pay the bills. I want my family to be healthy, but they also need to be full. Any suggestions? *Miserable in Missoula*

A: Whether you call it cheap, frugal, penny-pinching, or prudent, we call saving money smart, especially when it involves eating one of the cheapest sources of protein, fiber, and flavor available. Humble, tasty beans have an impressive portfolio of benefits. Here's what you'll cash in on when you cook with them:

❖ **A healthier heart.** Beans reduce your levels of C-reactive protein (CRP), a likely indicator of heart disease risk. How? Probably due to their fiber. Black beans have 7 grams of fiber per half-cup serving, which gets you well on your way to the 25 grams a day recommended for optimal health. Remember to add Beano so you do not clear out every elevator you get into. Beano does not in any way eradicate the benefits of beans.

❖ **Lower blood pressure.** Get your protein from plants, and your blood pressure may be lower than if you get protein from animal sources. The amino acids (building blocks of protein) in vegetables might help keep blood pressure low, and the magnesium and other nutrients in them may help keep arteries relaxed. Some beans even contain more protein per serving than lean meat. Example: kidney beans have 16 grams of protein per cup; 3 ounces of turkey contains 12 grams.

❖ **A smaller waist.** Bean eaters weigh as much as 6.6 pounds less than non-bean-imbibing folks do. Makes sense when you consider that beans are not only full of satisfying fiber and protein but low in calorie-laden fat.

Personal Energy Crisis

Q: I recently went back to school (nursing school) and find that with the change in schedule and stress of studying—plus taking care of my family and living on a farm—I'm tired all the time and feel bad about myself. Last summer, I was walking about two to four miles most days of the week, and now I can't fit it in. Can you give me some advice on how to fit exercise into my busy life? *Gail, Prairie Farm, Wisconsin*

A: Before trying to do more, you need to think about doing less. True, exercise is energizing and good long walks help your mood, but it's not a cure-all for lack of sleep and having too much to do. You're in an energy crisis, so instead of squeezing exercise into an already crowded schedule, swap it for something else on your to-do list. Is there a chore you can delegate? Can you postpone some tasks or accept "good enough" instead of perfection? If you don't feel better soon, ask your doctor to help you do some detective work, starting with some blood tests to rule out health issues such as hormonal imbalances, anemia, or a low-grade infection. You shouldn't ignore fatigue for long—you don't have to live with it or the bad feelings that hitchhike with it.

Off to a Good Start

Q: Every morning, I have great motivation to diet. But when I get home from work, my resolve goes out the window, and all I want to do is eat, even though I'm not skipping meals. How can I handle this? *Jorge, Chicago, Illinois*

A: The first thing to do (after having a breakfast with eggs and 100 percent whole grains) is stop blaming yourself. It makes perfect sense that your motivation would slip at the end of the day. Here's why: When you wake up well rested, you're not particularly stressed or emotional. You're busily doing your get-out-the-door routine, and tuning out the desire to hang out in the kitchen and eat comfort food at 7 a.m. is a no-brainer. Now look what happens when you come home from work: You're stressed, maybe you're even a little emotional (you're nearing fifty, it's that time of month, or your spouse is going to the Cavs with his buddies again), and you're staring into the pantry, wondering what to make for dinner. Try these three strategies to head off the habits and hormones undermining your motivation:

- ❖ **Don't let yourself get hungry.** When your stomach and intestines are empty, they release ghrelin, which sends an I-want-to-eat message to your brain. Carrots and apples join walnuts as terrific antistress foods because they have a tinge of sweetness to satisfy a craving and give you something to crunch when you feel frustrated.
- ❖ **Cook on the weekend.** Planning meals and shopping ahead cut your chances of impulse buys, foraging in the fridge, or giving up entirely and calling Domino's. Even better: prepare and freeze entrees so you have your own healthy version of fast food. The less time you're in the kitchen, the less time you're in the path of temptation. Think one-dish meals, like hearty soups, bean casseroles, and pasta, that you can zap and serve.
- ❖ **Be accountable.** One way to reprogram yourself is by writing down everything you eat. (Yes, even the three M&M's you swiped.) To make a food diary more fun, try one of the calorie-counting applications for your PDA and keep an ongoing tally.

Tune In

Q: I can't seem to tear my kids away from the TV to eat dinner. And when I do, all they will eat is hot dogs and chicken nuggets. They will eat when they are hungry enough, right? *Harriet in Houston*

A: Are SpongeBob SquarePants and Dora the Explorer sitting at your dinner table sabotaging your child's eating habits? Too much TV is associated with poor eating choices and amounts in kids, and there's no doubt about that. A recent survey of more than a thousand parents found it to be true. The survey also revealed that eating meals together as a family tends to increase consumption of fruits and veggies. So flip off the set and switch your clan's focus to what's on the plate and who's around the table. (See page 495 for more info on getting kids to eat right.) This is true for parents too!

Avoiding Restaurant Catastrophes

Q: You gave some tips on eating out. Please give me more. *Paul in Saint Louis*

A: Manage your meals at the most dangerous points: the first and last ten minutes.

The First Ten Minutes

❖ **Dip in olive oil.** If the restaurant brings you whole grain bread, dip it in olive oil. People who opt for this over butter eat less bread. Better: ask for veggies instead of bread.

❖ **Request the bottles.** Order oil and vinegar on the side. Relying on the kitchen or the waitstaff to dress your salad for you—even with oil and vinegar—can deliver as many as 450 extra calories!

The Last Ten Minutes

❖ **Share.** Get one dessert for every four or five people at your table, and have just a few bites. Not four or five desserts, split in half. Get one, share with one or two other people, and freeze the other half for a special occasion at home.

- ❖ **Savor your wine.** Ending a meal with a glass of wine lets you avoid the cloying postsweets aftertaste—and helps you avoid calorie bombs too.
- ❖ **End with a salad.** Make the salad the last thing you eat.

Easy Ways to Increase Your Energy—Fast

Q: It doesn't matter what I do—eat right and exercise—I'm still tired all the time. Is there something wrong with me? *Dead tired in Denver*

A: Some ill-advised folks might say that the greatest nutritional discovery of the last decade has been the Baconator (a whopping 830 calories—we don't think so). The real nutritional hero: ribose. This special sugar is made in your body; it doesn't come from food, but you can get it in a supplement. What it does is help build the energy factories of your body. Of all the things you can do to combat the effects of knee-dragging fatigue, taking a daily ribose supplement is the one that seems to really turbocharge some people with fibromyalgia and chronic fatigue syndrome, diseases associated with low energy. The only side effect is that some people feel too much energy. The data isn't good enough to recommend ribose for everyone. But if you want to give it a try, start with 500 milligrams three times a day for a week or so until you get used to the taste (or find a smoothie, coffee, or tea to put it in). Then go to 5 grams three times a day for three weeks to get a sense of the effect. After that, you can scale back to 5 grams twice a day. Prefer to go with an energizer that's more proven? Go green—tea, that is. Although green tea has one-third the caffeine of black tea, it's been shown to yield the same level of energy and attentiveness. And your heart and arteries get something out of it as well: four times more health-protecting polyphenols than black tea.

Middle Man

Q: It seems as if the dry cleaner shrunk another pair of my pants, or could it be that the three-cappuccinos a day habit is catching up with me? A little extra around the middle doesn't hurt, does it? *Mohammed in West Bloomfield*

A: Whether you call it a muffin top, spare tire, or beer gut, that extra belly fat nudges your blood pressure higher, even if you're young, have a healthy overall weight, and currently have a low blood pressure reading. When belly fat inside your kidney capsule (didn't know the kidney was shrink-wrapped, did you?) presses on your kidneys, the bean-shaped organs feel smothered, and they panic. In response, they flood your bloodstream with hormones that raise your blood pressure. Think of abdominal obesity as your early-warning system for high blood pressure. A thick middle and pants that feel too tight signal that this health risk may not be far behind. The key formula to remember is that your waist size should be less than half your height, no matter what your age or sex.

EXERCISE

Your Easiest Workout Ever

Q: Exercise studios blare upbeat music during exercise classes. Would it help me to have a sound track for my daily run? *Janice in Northampton, Massachusetts*

A: Do you lose that loving feeling for your workout about halfway through? Take along your iPod, and don't be surprised when you go longer and stronger than you've ever gone before. In one study, men who worked out to tunes found themselves going 11 percent longer without feeling they were exerting themselves more. Why? Music may simply be an effective distraction from your "Don't know how much farther I can go" or "There are other things I should be doing right now" thoughts. Or it may boost your mood enough to take your mind off that jelly feeling in your legs. Or it may cause a brain change that actually makes the physical activity more automatic and less requiring of thoughts of sweat. It doesn't matter if you get more from Mozart than Metallica, or vice versa. What may matter more than the type of music is that the beat matches or is just slightly faster than the rhythm of what you're doing. (And keep it low: Though you may be going for weight loss, you don't need hearing loss along with it.)

At a Loss

Q: I've lost fifty-five pounds by following *YOU on a Diet* but ran into a problem you warned about if I try to advance my workout too fast: I have foot pain. Thumbing through an in-flight catalogue, I noticed an ad for a nighttime splint for plantar fasciitis. I've recently experienced serious heel pain when I get out of bed in the morning, and I wonder if this product will help. I can't walk, and I know that is a basic of waist loss. *Anonymous*

A: It might, but there's a cheaper and more comfortable way to ease the pain than plunking down $50 or more for a castlike device to wear while you sleep. The pain you're feeling in the morning—as though you're being stabbed in the heel with a burning spear—happens when there's inflammation in the tough, fibrous fascia that connects your heel bone to the base of your toes. That tissue absorbs shock when your foot hits the ground. When your arch isn't properly supported, especially if you spend a lot of time on your feet, the fascia picks up the slack, sometimes damaging itself in the process. As you've probably noticed, once you've managed to walk around a bit in the morning and have stretched that fibrous band, the pain usually eases. Splints like the one you saw advertised are designed to do something similar; keep the fascia from contracting while you sleep. They're effective for some people but not others, and there's no way to know until long after your credit card has been charged.

So try this instead: Before you get out of bed, sit up, bend forward, and touch your toes (or get as close as you can). Keep your foot flexed toward your knee to lengthen the tight fascia. Stretch your Achilles tendon throughout the day (put the ball of your foot on a step, hold the railing, and let your heel hang down). Still hurting? Try icing your heel for twenty minutes three times a day, and take a nonsteroidal anti-inflammatory drug such as ibuprofen. Give your feet a rest from the treadmill or the tennis court until the inflammation resolves.

Can Workouts Make You Wealthy?

Q: I love to walk, but I have trouble convincing my slave driver of a boss that a workout break for me would help the company's bottom line. Any ammunition I can use to win this argument? *Alicia in Asheville*

A: The best way to keep your job might be to leave your desk. That's right: The less time you spend sitting on your bottom, the better it might be for your—and your company's—bottom line. In a study of entrepreneurs, people who worked out regularly also had companies that performed well. In fact, those who ran regularly were better at meeting their personal goals and their companies had better sales than those owned by nonrunners. (The researchers didn't ask about walkers.) People who stuck to a strength-training regimen were also better at meeting their personal goals than people who didn't lift weights—but their businesses weren't doing off-the-charts better. Researchers suspect that the boost in confidence and energy that people get from regular exercise may spill over into their careers, giving them an edge. Ultimately, taking time to work out may actually help you get more done during the workday. The best time to work out? Whenever you'll do it. But we recommend setting your alarm thirty to sixty minutes earlier than usual and getting moving first thing.

Short and Intense: A New Way to Get Fit

Q: I believe that if an activity is good for you, it will be even better if you do it faster. Why walk a twenty-minute mile when you can run it in ten? But everything I have read says that the benefits are the same. Say it isn't so. *Michelle in Hyde Park*

A: If you'd rather race for thirty seconds than trudge for an hour, seems you might have your wish and get something for it too. Short, intense bouts of exercise may boost muscle fitness as effectively as longer sessions do. But you won't burn as many calories, and you should check with your doctor first. In one study, men who worked out really hard on a stationary bike for just a few minutes each week, in thirty-second intervals four to six times a day, every other day, experienced muscle fitness gains on a par with those experienced by the guys who cycled at a moderate pace for 90 to 120 minutes daily. But for longevity and weight loss, we recommend a mix of exercises—from strength training to cardio workouts to walking.

Foods That Stop the Ouch

Q: I just finished a great workout, and I know that I'm going to pay for it tomorrow. And I'm starving. What should I eat to fill me up and help me feel great for the next workout? *Meredith in San Diego*

A: What's the best thing to grab after a major workout? A shower and water, yes. And right after that? One of these foods.

❖ **Cereal.** A carb-rich snack can help you overcome fatigue by restoring glycogen, the all-important stuff your muscles use for energy.

❖ **Curry.** Curcumin, a substance found in the Indian spice turmeric, may help quell the muscle inflammation that you know as next-day stiffness and soreness.

❖ **Coffee.** When there's inflammation in your muscles after exercise, your body releases adenosine, a substance that can cause you pain one or two days later. Caffeine is thought to help mute adenosine, which may reduce your ouch factor. A small new study suggests it may also reduce the perception of muscle pain even while you're exercising.

The Itch to Exercise

Q: Why do I get a crazy itch around my tummy and thighs when I jog? *Anonymous*

A: Your workout clothes are possibly to blame for your "itchy pants syndrome." We don't know whether the synthetic material stimulates a reaction in sensitive people or if there's some finishing chemical on the fabric behind it, but wearing 100 percent cotton gear—washing it before you put it on for the first time—helps many, including pro baseball players, stop scratching. If exercise still makes you itch, you may be triggering an allergy you didn't know you had. As you heat up, your body may react to a food that normally doesn't bother you. (Sometimes a similar reaction occurs if you warm yourself in a sauna or hot tub. Allergists report exercise-induced reactions to seafood, celery, wheat, and cheese.) You might also be reacting to aspirin or nonsteroidal anti-inflammatories (NSAIDs) if you took those beforehand.

Crunch Time

Q: Will crunches get rid of my belly fat? *Theodoros, Addis Ababa, Ethiopia*

A: Not by themselves. Combine ab work with other resistance exercises, aerobic exercise, and calorie restriction, though, and you'll lose the muffin top and maybe even have a six-pack to show off. Traditional crunches strengthen and tone the muscles that connect your rib cage to your pelvis, helping you stand tall and look more slender. But to lose the roll, you've got to empty those fat storage depots that sit on top of the muscles, and that's what diet, muscle building, and aerobic exercise do. Raising your heart rate helps reduce the unhealthy, deep fat that lies beneath your abs—another storage depot that crunches don't touch.

Curb Your Appetite with This Combo

Q: I am so hungry after my workouts that I think I would lose more weight if I stopped working out. What can I do? *Nancy in Newton*

A: Ever emerge from your workout hungrier than a lion on a bug-only diet? Well, changing what you do in the gym may have the power to make you eat less. The magic formula? Doing both cardio and strength training. When men in one small study did both for sixteen weeks, they consumed significantly fewer calories than the men who did either aerobics (sixty minutes) or weight training alone or who did no exercise at all. And people doing the combo weren't in the gym longer—in addition to weights, they did only twenty-two minutes of cardio. It's possible that the cardio/strength pairing has a favorable effect on blood levels of fats, glucose, amino acids, and satiety hormones, adding up to powerful hunger control.

Of course, there's physical appetite, which this combo seemed to squelch, and there's emotional appetite. The latter means using the "I deserve it" theory to binge on more calories after exercise than they burned. And the gym probably can't help you with that. What can: Being aware of how your emotions can steer your desire to eat. Help squelch emotional eating by aiming to keep your feel-good hormones level by getting the right amount of sleep, by eating a healthy balance of foods, and by working hard to create a more authentic and happier you in your life and relationships. And sleep.

DISEASES AND CONDITIONS

Too High

Q: What causes high triglycerides? What can I do to lower them? *Anonymous*

A: Triglycerides have a bad rep, but these fatty molecules serve a useful purpose: storing energy until you need it. However, like wine, real chocolate, and exercise, too much can do you in. Levels above 100 mg/dl of triglycerides in your blood can thicken the walls of your arteries and increase your risk of heart attack and stroke. Bringing down your triglycerides to healthy levels calls for some serious waist management. That's because belly fat is a key player in raising your triglyceride levels (not to mention your cholesterol count and pants size). Avoiding simple sugars and syrups is also a key to unlocking the secret to triglyceride reduction.

Large Liver

Q: My doctor told me I have a severely fatty liver, but I don't have cirrhosis. Since I started taking the diet drug Alli, I have lost ninety pounds. I now eat a low-fat diet, exercise regularly, rarely drink alcohol, and take milk thistle every day. Is there anything else I can do? *Patty, White Haven, Pennsylvania*

A: You're already doing the most important thing: losing waist. Obesity is notorious for causing too much fat, especially triglycerides, to be stored in your liver. Simple sugar causes it too. So anything with a sugar added to it (usually sugar—they usually end in "-ose"—or a syrup in the first five ingredients) should go too. Ironically, however, rapid weight loss can also cause liver trouble. So if you have more to lose, take it slowly. But you can stay on the Alli; it may help alleviate fatty liver. Your waist loss and workout regimen are smart, and milk thistle's powerful polyphenols could help protect your liver against inflammation. Consider adding a multivitamin (half in a.m., half in p.m.; buy a pill splitter). Finally, skip the booze entirely, at least till your doc tells you your liver has returned to normal. Your liver has to filter everything you consume, from walnuts and jelly beans to the fries you swiped from your friend's plate. It doesn't need the stress of filtering out any more toxins than it has to.

This Is Only a Warning

Q: I eat right and get regular exercise, and I feel great. If I were at risk for disease, I would have some warning signs, right? *Bob from B&N*

A: And you thought your 401(k) statement was scary. How about the fact that more than half of all heart attacks strike people who seem perfectly healthy—no high LDL cholesterol, no high blood pressure? Don't cue up the menacing music yet: There are other known factors, and you can control them relatively easily. Heart attack risks are also a risk for stroke, impotence, kidney failure, and even wrinkling. A major cause (not the only one) of all of these is arterial aging, and though arterial aging is typical, it is neither normal nor necessary.

One reason a heart attack, stroke, or impotence happens to seemingly healthy people like you is that there's a stalker in their arteries: inflammation. If you're in good shape otherwise but have this villain, and you have been treated for many low-grade infections like prostatitis, vaginitis, periodontitis, or sinusitis, then taking a statin drug such as Crestor in a low dose could slash your risk of a horror-story heart attack by 50 percent. Does this mean you need a statin, even if your cholesterol level's not high? Maybe. But the drugs-or-not debate obscures the more important issue: Don't wait until you need a drug to get serious about inflammation.

Meds You Don't Need

Q: I understand that regular blood pressure checks are important, but my numbers are all over the map. How can I find out what my real blood pressure really is? *Gary in Green Bay*

A: It's one thing to guess how much pressure your tires have, another how much your arteries have. High blood pressure is often called the silent killer, because you don't "ride funny" when your pressure is wrong. The only way to know is to have your blood pressure taken. Or when you have a stroke (too late then). So learn your blood pressure numbers today, even if only with one of the inexpensive home automatic devices (and we think anyone with possible high blood pressure should have one). Little things such as talking or having a full bladder (and it doesn't require talking with a full bladder) can throw your readings off. The leading cause of inaccurate measurements? Operator error, even at the doctor's office. Make your next reading right on with these rules:

1. Sit quietly for three to five minutes before you're measured.
2. Make sure the cuff fits.
3. Have your BP measured at least twice, and use the average.
4. Sit comfortably in a chair.
5. Avoid caffeine, cigarettes, and alcohol for at least thirty minutes before you measure. They can cause a temporary increase in pressure (or lower it, in the case of alcohol)—just as they can in life.
6. Always measure at the same time of day.

Against the Acid

Q: I have GERD and take Nexium for it. I was wondering if reducing the amount of acid in my stomach would slow down the digestion of food. *Tracie in Boise, Idaho*

A: Not likely. Proton-pump inhibitors (PPIs) such as Nexium and Prilosec reduce the amount of acid in your stomach, which tames your pain from GERD. But there is still plenty left to help digest your food. In fact, even when you take those drugs, the stomach goes about its normal business, reducing stomach acid during sleep and fluctuating naturally throughout the day. Also, keep in mind that digestion isn't confined to the stomach; your mouth (and the glands that produce saliva) and your intestines (and the bacteria inside them) do a lot of the work too. But keep in mind that PPIs can make it harder for your body to absorb calcium, and they don't allow you to absorb B12 from food very well, so you may need to take a supplement.

The Secret of Feeling Rested

Q: My husband snores all night, and I'm the one who ends up sleep deprived. How can I get him to stop so I can get the beauty sleep I so desperately need? *Teresa in Duluth*

A: Want to wake up feeling rested and more energetic than a ten-year-old in the Guitar Hero play-offs? Hide the Oreos. From your spouse. It might nix your bedmate's sleep apnea and some of the snoring that goes with it. In one study, when a group of overweight people with mild sleep apnea—meaning they stopped breathing for more than ten seconds at a time while sleeping—went on a very-low-calorie diet, their apnea and lives improved (they lost weight too).

It's no big surprise that weight loss helps limit sleep apnea. After all, part of the problem is that there's obstruction of the free flow of air through the passages in the back of the mouth. When fat accumulates there, this blockage becomes even more likely. But the study did suggest that if you catch sleep apnea in its early stages and intervene with weight loss, you may be able to cure it or at least prevent it from getting worse. Sleep apnea isn't just an inconvenience: When you stop breathing, your body wakes up (hey, breathe, will ya?!) and prevents you from getting the rejuvenating benefits of sleep. And that means a higher risk of high blood pressure, obesity, memory loss, and stroke. People in this study lost weight with a restrictive 600 to 800 daily calories. They might have been easier to be with during the night, but probably not during the day. We recommend losing both the weight and the apnea by dropping only one to two pounds a week.

Five Foods Your Heart Loves

Q: I am sure all those foods in fancy New York specialty shops are healthy, but I live in small-town America. The local food market in my town doesn't stock anything more exotic than kiwifruit. What choices do I have? *John in Clay Center, Kansas*

A: You don't have to eat raw fish or hard-to-find vegetables (unless you want to) to keep your heart healthy. Simply stock up on these ubiquitous—and delicious—foods:

- **Red Delicious apples.** These are particularly rich in compounds called phenolics that do something magical to your bad cholesterol. They make the blood fats more stable, so they're less likely to oxidize, stick to the walls of your arteries, and cause a dangerous blockage.
- **Sesame seeds.** Women who took a little more than 3 tablespoons of sesame seed powder daily for five days reduced their total and bad (LDL) cholesterol. They also had higher levels of heart-protective vitamin E and lower blood levels of substances linked to cell damage.
- **Walnuts.** Studies have found that an ounce of these nuts a day decreases the incidence of heart disease by a whopping 60 percent. All nuts are good for you, but walnuts are best, since they're highest in omega-3 fatty acids, which reduce triglycerides, stabilize your heartbeat, make platelets less sticky, and may knock down blood pressure.
- **Salmon and trout.** Fatty fish like these are high in heart-protecting omega-3 fatty acids (and low in mercury and PCBs). Feast on them three times a week.

Should I Stop Eating Soy?

Q: I'm wondering if it's dangerous for me to eat a lot of soy-based foods, since I'm at higher-than-average risk for breast cancer (my grandmother died of the disease and my sister was recently diagnosed with it). I'm also a vegetarian and like to get my protein from soy. *Jeanie in Seattle*

A: Considering that protein-packed soybeans also contain a hefty helping of compounds that act like weak estrogens in your body, you might cut back on soy to balance your meatless meals. An occasional tofu scramble or skim soy creamer in your coffee is unlikely to be harmful, but moderation is key. The reason to curtail the soy is that some of the estrogen compounds in soy may stimulate some types of breast cancer cells, and since you're at higher-than-average risk of breast cancer, you don't want to increase the possibility of any abnormal cell growth. Your best choice is to eat cruciferous veggies such as broccoli, which stimulate a gene to produce a protein that decreases the risk of breast cancer. Discourage your sister from eating large amounts of soy, and teach her the joys of broccoli, cabbage, cauliflower, and Brussels sprouts. Meeting your daily recommended 46 grams of protein (men need 56 grams) without relying on soy is about as hard as speeding in a Ferrari if you eat a varied diet that includes eggs (6 grams per egg), low-fat dairy products (8 grams per cup of nonfat milk), nuts (about 5 grams per ounce), and beans (12 to 18 grams per cup, depending on the variety). Eating them along with brown rice (5 grams per cup), whole grains, and a mix of vegetables will keep your body well stocked with protein. And since you have two relatives with breast cancer, you might get genetic counseling and testing to see if you are at risk and should consider some other options.

Ask about Aspirin

Q: I've been doing a low-carb diet, and I'd like to take a regular low dose of aspirin for its heart-health benefits, but I have gout and have read that aspirin could make my gout worse. Is that true, and if so, what foods should I be eating? *Anonymous*

A: It's true that aspirin can aggravate gout—it may increase the uric acid levels in your blood. Deposits of tiny, needlelike crystals of uric acid in the joints are what cause your painful problem to begin with. But there are plenty of other things you can do for your heart that are just as good as or better than taking aspirin, and once you get the uric acid levels down to normal, you can take 162 milligrams of aspirin a day (if your doc agrees) with half a glass of water before and after. In particular, the omega-3s in fish oil and algae (DHA) reduce inflammation, and the EPA helps prevent artery-blocking clots, part of what aspirin does. And while aspirin can cut your risk of heart attack by 44 percent, studies have shown that eating oily fish even once a week or taking DHA daily can cut your risk by 50 percent or more. So grab the salmon or trout (they are the only fish sold in America that consistently contain omega-3s). Don't like fish? Pop 2 grams of fish oil daily, or take the active ingredient, 600 milligrams of DHA, from a vegetarian source, algae. By the way, it is high doses of things that increase uric acid levels—red wine, tomatoes, and red meat—that make gout worse.

A Note about Bloat

Q: My lower abdomen is always bloated, making me look as if I'm about three months pregnant. No matter what I eat, I blow up like a balloon. I exercise every day, work out my abs regularly, and drink plenty of water, but nothing seems to help. I'm often constipated and have stomachaches too. *Anonymous*

A: Any discomfort that sticks around is your body's way of putting you on alert, and it sounds as though you have three loud and clear messages: bloating, bowel problems, and pain. Whatever is causing your trouble could be as easy to fix as changing your diet, as challenging as tracking down a food allergy, or as life-threatening as cancer. So, before you do another thing today, pick up the phone and make an appointment with your gynecologist. No doubt you'll need some diagnostic tests, maybe including a transvaginal ultrasound (if the doctor doesn't suggest one, ask for it) and a test for gluten allergy. The bloating and abdominal pain you describe are classic warning signs not only of a gluten allergy (see "Go G-Free" on page 100) but also of an ovarian tumor, and it's not unusual for women to have constipation as well. Other red flags are pelvic pain, feeling full quickly when you eat, and urinating often. Back pain, feeling tired, or painful intercourse may signal a tumor too. We don't say that to scare you but to urge you to act quickly. Ovarian cancer used to be considered a silent disease, but in the last few years, researchers have discovered that 90 percent of women diagnosed with it had early symptoms of disease. The key to early detection, when cancer is most treatable, is paying attention to your body. You know it better than anyone else, and if anything unusual persists for more than a few weeks, see a doctor.

Flu Fighters

Q: I know that avoiding obesity can help the immune system, but are there foods that can also help fight the flu? *Jasper in Louisville*

A: The flu virus loves it when you stay up late doing the work of three people in your office who got downsized. It loves when a road trip, the red-eye, or a supertough workout wipes you out physically. When your body is under unremitting stress, the flu virus, like a jewel thief around a distracted salesperson, seizes its moment to slip by your body's defenses. Fortunately, there are a few delicious things that the virus doesn't love: Apples. Broccoli. Tea. Red onions. These are rich sources of a flavonoid called quercetin. The normal dip in immunity that comes with physical fatigue is pretty much canceled out by this flavonoid. Also, get a flu shot every year, and wash your hands. Washing is one of the most powerful things you can do to protect yourself from viruses (not to mention bacteria and fungi). And take a probiotic and vitamin D if you aren't already. Finally, you should also avoid sugar, which decreases your immune response.

Is Watermelon the Next Viagra?

Q: I know that losing weight can help erectile dysfunction, but I read an article claiming that eating watermelon is as good for erectile dysfunction as taking medications is. Have you heard this, and is it true? *Anonymous*

A: If it were true, watermelon would be a lot harder to find than it is. When it comes to treating the 30 million men suffering from erectile dysfunction (ED), watermelon and prescription drugs aren't equal—yet. However, watermelon is loaded with a nutrient called citrulline that helps produce nitric oxide, a powerful blood vessel dilator that's critical to healthy blood flow. Viagra and other ED drugs work on a similar principle: They temporarily let much more blood flow into the penis. But in watermelon's case, evidence that more citrulline means better sexual functioning hasn't yet been found (and may never be). Still, it can't hurt to help keep blood flowing to all the right places by eating watermelon and other foods high in citrulline: almonds, cocoa, dark chocolate, chickpeas, peanuts, salmon, soy, and walnuts.

Pill Power

Q: If I'm prescribed pills that say, "Take on an empty stomach," and I have already eaten a meal, how long do I need to wait before taking them? *Anonymous*

A: After a normal meal, your stomach is generally empty enough for you to take a medication in about two to three hours. Note the phrase "normal meal." It's no surprise that it takes longer for your stomach to empty if you've overeaten (which happens only occasionally, we hope!). After a heavy meal, wait four hours before taking your meds.

Number Management

Q: I am very deficient in vitamin D and also have high cholesterol. I am afraid to eat certain foods for fear that they will raise my cholesterol. What can I do to manage these problems? *Janice in Billings, Montana*

A: Your cholesterol number needs to be broken down into LDL and HDL measurements. If your cholesterol comes from high HDL, you have a trump card and don't have a problem. (Play that ace, and go to Las Vegas.) On the other hand, if it reflects high LDL, we would advise you to radically decrease sugars, syrups, and saturated fat (that's four-legged fat plus palm and coconut oil) in your diet. You may need to take niacin with aspirin one hour beforehand, a statin drug, or omega-3s to decrease your LDL (see your doc about this). As for vitamin D, low levels increase arterial disease, cancer, and bone weakening, so get that up now. The best way we know to get more vitamin D is to take it as a supplement. We both do so every day: 1,000 IU of D3.

Spice Up Your Knees

Q: My knees crack more than a squirrel in a walnut tree. Do you have an alternative to surgery? *Crickety in Clarksburg*

A: Hey, nice one (couldn't have said it better ourselves). One new contender for soothing Rice Krispies knees: ginger. When people with stiff, sore, osteoarthritic knees took a ginger extract for six weeks, they felt significantly better than their placebo-dosed pals. For other classic treatments and prevention strategies, see *YOU: The Owner's Manual*, New and Expanded Edition, pages 123 to 131 and 467 to 468.

Sugar Coating

Q: I have diabetes, and eating only one fruit a day keeps my blood sugar in check (I eat three to five servings of vegetables too). You suggest eating four servings. Isn't that dangerous? *Anonymous*

A: No; the key is tailoring your fruit plate to your body's response to it. Fruit is tricky—ripe, dried, or cooked fruit might send your blood sugar soaring, while raw fruit might be fine. Having fruit first thing in the morning raises one person's glucose but doesn't make waves in another. Eat the fruit twenty-five minutes after a few walnuts—that way four fruits a day are fine. The trick is monitoring your blood glucose to see that it doesn't raise your blood sugar level too high.

Armor against E. coli

Q: Why is it that some people seem so naturally resistant to bacteria like *E. coli* while others fall victim every time they eat a turkey sandwich that has been out of the fridge for an hour? *Chris in Scranton*

A: Fiber is fab. You already eat it to stay regular and to feel fuller longer. Now there's another reason: gut protection. Research shows that fiber-rich foods help derail illness-causing bacteria that may otherwise have you running for the bathroom. In a lab study, researchers exposed a variety of foods to several strains of *E. coli* and salmonella. The results? The bacteria adhered to fibrous foods such as pumpkin, artichoke, and flax—a good thing, because if the bacteria latches onto intestinal tissues instead, it might reduce some gut-churning consequences.

Eat This, Flex Better

Q: My family has a history of heart disease. I want to do everything I can to keep my waist, heart, and arteries healthy. What are some foods that would keep me out of the hospital? *Fred in Fort Wayne*

A: When it comes to making your arteries as flexible and open as your mind, there's a food you can rely on: grapes. The evidence: just three hours after eating the equivalent of one and a quarter cups of grapes, people had better blood flow through their arteries than did people who drank a sugar solution. The blood-flow benefits were even better after three weeks of daily grape eating. At only 75 calories in a cup and a quarter, the habit is easy on your waist too. We've known about the cardiovascular effects of fermented grapes (as in wine) for years. And this shows you can get at least some of the healthy cardiovascular benefits without the risk of slurring your words or telling blonde jokes to the wrong hostess.

How Weight Loss Helps Your Colon

Q: I just got a colonoscopy, and some benign polyps were removed. How can I make my next procedure polyp free?

A: Cutting a few pounds not only will help you toward your ideal weight but also may cut down on colon growths. Add 162 milligrams a day of aspirin with a glass of water, 600 milligrams of calcium twice a day, and 1,000 IU a day of vitamin D, and stay away from those five aging foods.

Better Blood Sugar

Q: My blood sugar level is creeping up, and I want to get it back to a normal level before it becomes a problem. What should I be eating?

A: We know that hearts love a Mediterranean-style diet. But here's big news: so does your blood sugar. Yep. Mediterranean fare—rich in olive oil, vegetables, fruit, nuts, cereals, legumes, and fish—may reduce your risk of developing diabetes. And not just a little.

The Blood-Pressure-Friendly Breakfast

Q: I need to bring my waist measurement and blood pressure down. Any suggestions for a way to start the day off on the right foot? *Concerned in Connecticut*

A: Here's a great morning meal for better blood pressure: Grind up some flax-seeds and sprinkle them on your whole grain cereal. That's right. Whole grains are good for lowering blood pressure, and flaxseeds may help bring it down a bit as well. Give those omega-3s another round of applause.

Teatime

Q: I've heard that chamomile tea can help lower my cholesterol. Is there any truth to that? *Becky in Colorado Springs*

A: Chamomile tea is good for many things, including helping you relax and maybe even boosting your immune system, but it won't help get your cholesterol levels where they need to be. The better bet is to limit saturated fat, eliminate trans fats, and eat healthy fats, not to mention increasing your fiber intake and making sure you walk thirty minutes a day.

GETTING OLDER

Slowing Down

Q: A year ago, as I was going through menopause, I quit smoking. Now I have no metabolism! I'm eating the same as always and I exercise on an elliptical trainer thirty minutes a day, but I've gained thirty pounds. I'm on high blood pressure medication and take Synthroid to counter a sluggish thyroid. *Eileen in Angola, New York*

A: Quitting smoking shouldn't be the cause: We've found that people who go through our quit-smoking program—which involves walking thirty minutes a day and weight lifting ten minutes three times a week—are an average of two pounds heavier six months after quitting. The difference between them and you could be the strength training. So get yourself some weights, check out some exercises (we have plenty online) and the workout in this book (page 233), and start lifting yourself today.

Aging Taste Buds

Q: I have noticed over the past couple years that food doesn't taste as good as it used to. I've started to eat more fish as I've hit age fifty-eight. Is this why? *Monica in New England*

A: Don't blame the tuna; your tongue's the culprit. If those pretzels don't seem as salty as they used to and the sweet-and-sour pork isn't so sweet or sour, it's likely because you're losing taste buds as you age. The average person is born with about 10,000 taste buds, but only 5,000 may be left by retirement years. People regenerate new taste buds every three to ten days, but the buds renew at a slower rate as you get older. Plus, it could be that you're losing your sense of smell too. Researchers say that three-quarters of how we taste food comes from how we smell it, and your ability to smell—like your sight, your hearing, and your ability to leap over cars—can diminish with age too.

SKIN CARE AND APPEARANCE

Green Tea for Great Skin

Q: Every day I hear something new about how green tea beefs up metabolism. Are there other benefits as well? *Michelle in New Jersey*

A: You're right. You won't just find green tea in convenience store fridges; you'll also find it at the cosmetics counter—in cleansers, moisturizers, and sunscreen. Studies suggest that the polyphenols in green tea (if the tea is consumed, not applied) may help revive aging skin cells and even aid in the healing of wounds. For a green tea face refresher, soak a cotton ball in green tea (cooled to room temperature, smarty pants) and swab it over your face. Place cucumber slices over your eyes, and lie down for fifteen minutes. Voilà—an instant skin pick-me-up. (One caveat: Before applying green tea to your face, test your skin's sensitivity to it. Dab a small amount behind your ear and wait twenty-four hours to make sure your skin doesn't react.)

The Fruit That Fights Wrinkles

Q: I've lost weight, and I'm starting to notice more wrinkles (because of the loss of fat, I'm told). Is there a best food for preventing wrinkles? *Dorrine in Houston*

A: Go ahead, feed your face (that may be the only time we ever say those words). Eating the right stuff makes you look younger, and one fruit in particular leads the charge: papaya. What makes it so perfect is that it's brimming with vitamin C. And getting lots of that vitamin may mean more youthful skin. A recent study in women over age forty found that women who consumed that vitamin had fewer wrinkles and less thinning and dryness of their skin. Of course, you can put it on your face at night (that's when you won't oxidize it—see our book *YOU: Being Beautiful*) to really achieve youth-giving levels in your skin. Vitamin C is essential for making collagen, the protein fibers that give skin its strength and resiliency. C also disarms free radicals that would otherwise chip away and weaken those fibers.

Sweets That Save Your Teeth

Q: I am trying to get added sugar out of my diet, but if I don't eat something sweet soon, I'm going to book a trip to the Hershey factory. There must be something that's both sweet and good for me. *Mary Jo in Talladega*

A: When it comes to sweets, not all of them will help your dentist buy a third home in Cabo. Sweet, delicious dates may leave holes in his schedule, not your teeth. That's right, these candies from nature have one up on chocolate Kisses and Gobstoppers: They contain a substance that may help strengthen tooth enamel and guard against plaque. Dates are rich in the element fluorine, a relative of fluoride, the enamel-friendly compound that can actually help reverse early tooth decay. Raisins may also save you from extra trips to the dentist. Phytochemicals in these fruits appear to inhibit the growth of certain types of bacteria that mess with your mouth and help prevent them from sticking to your teeth.

Skin Savers

Q: I'm starting to lose weight, but I know appearance also has to do with how your skin looks. When the fat is gone, what can I do about acne and awful-looking skin (not including expensive creams and treatments)? *Debbie in Duluth*

A: Beautiful skin doesn't start in a jar or at the dermatologist's office. It starts with what you eat. We've always said that what's on your plate can influence what pops up on your nose the night before a big presentation. And preliminary research agrees. It found that people on a low-glycemic-index diet—meaning they ate vegetables, lean poultry and fish, and only 100 percent whole grains rather than refined and sugary foods that spike blood sugar—saw their acne improve. And more than 90 percent of people taking acne treatments decreased the dose or the amount of treatments they were using while on this diet. That's no surprise to us. One other culprit in breakout-prone skin is inadequate intake of omega-3 fatty acids. When you trade sugar (and meat) for avocados, walnuts, and salmon or trout, you boost those valuable fats—and help control acne.

Appendices

This Is Your Fat on Drugs

The Medical Jump Start to Waist Management

Diet Myths

❖ Using weight-control drugs is a sign of failure.

❖ OTC weight-loss drugs are harmless.

❖ Caffeine makes you hungry.

In sports, drugs are viewed as cheating. In school, drugs are viewed as a quick ticket to suspension. In music, drugs may be viewed as another member of the band. But in weight-loss circles, drugs have the reputation for being extreme or even being the dirty way to lose weight. Used the right way, under the right supervision, however, pharmaceuticals that influence weight can help change your brain chemistry to help you reach your goals.

Myth Buster

Why? Because they're kick starts for times when you may reach a plateau after you've started to succeed with diet and exercise with the YOU Plan. They're what can help you get over the hump.

Myth Buster

YOU-reka! Weight-control drugs—in the form of doctor-supervised drugs, not OTC weight-loss fads—help you regulate your brain chemicals, so you think less about "dieting" if you need help to break plateaus.

It's like a coach helping an athlete through a slump. Whatever their use, you do need to know that they're not miracle weight-loss methods, at least not at this point. They won't microwave fat from your belly in thirty seconds. But they can help you achieve about a 5 percent to 10 percent weight loss while you're taking them. That's significant, especially when you're stalling. But the only way to maintain the change is to simultaneously incorporate and supplement with the lifestyle and behavioral changes that we discuss in your overall waist management plan. Here are some hard numbers for the average person: Lifestyle change alone will usually get you 7 percent loss of your total weight without major difficulty. Drugs alone will get you the same benefit, on average. But if you combine efforts, you can double the benefits to 14 percent.

Because these drugs have side effects, prescrip-

A Good Side to Bad Drugs?

It could be a $20 billion market (yes, with a *B*), so pharmaceutical companies are searching for drugs to help control appetite. Some of the searches have their biochemical roots in the mechanisms of illegal drugs. One of the newer classes of weight-loss drugs—cannabinoid blockers, one of which is called rimonabant—didn't pass muster in the United States due to side effects. But more of this class and others will come along. This class is used to prevent cannabinoid receptors from making you hungry. Those receptors in your brain are the ones that are activated when someone smokes marijuana (cannabis is the scientific name for

marijuana) and goes on to devour the top two shelves in the pantry (hence the marijuana munchies). How do they make you hungry? By blocking CCK and leptin, which encourages hedonistic eating. Drugs that block cannabinoid receptors are suspected to work because those blockers help reduce cravings. The cannabinoid receptors are also found in your liver, muscle, and belly fat and they affect how your body uses and stores food. Blocking these receptors results in less fat in the blood (triglycerides), less risk of diabetes, and more of the healthy HDL cholesterol, dude. Unfortunately, some bad side effects appeared. Stay tuned.

tion weight-loss medications should be used only by patients whose complications from obesity are more serious than the possible side effects. They're not to be used for cosmetic weight loss. They're approved for people with a body mass index of 30 or above (see Figure A.1 on page 455), or 27 or above with obesity-related conditions such as high blood pressure or diabetes. For many people, though, obesity causes an altered body image that also has medical consequences. We are comfortable prescribing them for women with a waist greater than 36 inches or men with a waist greater than 39, or for people who have diabetes, depression, sleep apnea, arthritis, high blood pressure, low self-esteem, or significant arterial disease. But the one prerequisite is that the patient has earnestly attempted changes in eating and activity. None of these drugs has been shown to sustain effectiveness once it is stopped, but the weight losses obtained while the drugs are taken have an added effect: In our and our colleagues' experience, they've helped patients gain confidence, get off the plateau, and lose the sense of guilt and shame associated with obesity.

Here's how these kick starts work: They help control the balance of chemical reactions in your brain, so that your appetite is never in a monsterlike free-for-all for food. (The downside is that you may revert to old habits when you come off them.)

Generally, drugs that influence weight are classified by the mechanism through which they work. Many, like the ones listed below, work by controlling pathways in the brain (specifically through the brain chemicals that we discussed in Part 3), while others, which we'll explain later in this appendix, have an effect on the digestive process.

YOU WHO Barbie

It turns out that your waist divided by your height is as valuable as the BMI in predicting the risks of obesity to your health. Your waist height odds (WHO) should be less than 50 percent, but keep in mind that Barbie is 25 percent and Ken is 36 percent. The average for men is 58 percent and for women is 54 percent. But average is not healthy. Go for less than 50.

Tale of the Scale

This body mass index (BMI) table lets you easily see what category you fall into. Just find your weight across the bottom and your height in the left column to see where the lines cross. The most common way governments and doctors keep track of our fat is through tables like this BMI table.

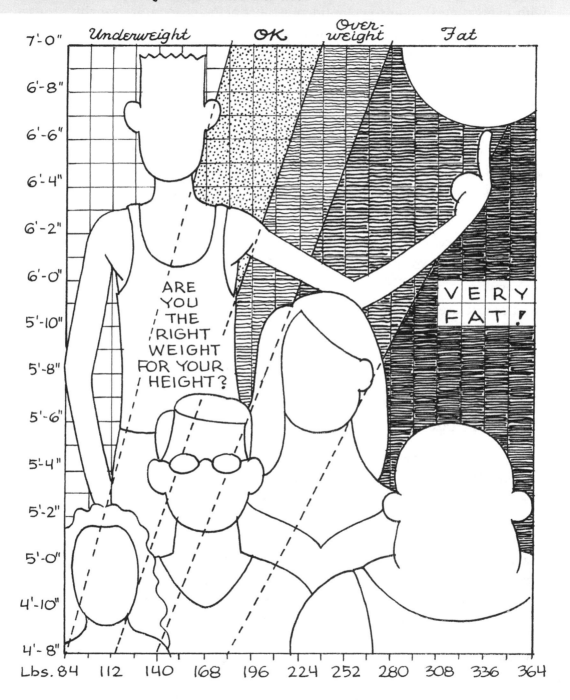

Drugs That Influence Norepinephrine: Some antidepressants work to control eating by easing anxiety, so that you don't experience the mood shifts associated with overeating. While some antidepressants actually increase weight, at least one—called bupropion (Wellbutrin)—has been shown to be effective for weight loss by influencing levels of norepinephrine (the fight-or-flight neurochemical), as well as increasing the pleasure-seeking dopamine. It creates a synthetic saber-toothed tiger: The norepinephrine increase that suppresses hunger causes your heart rate to increase and your blood pressure to increase, also speeding your metabolism. One study showed that people who took Wellbutrin maintained a seven- to twenty-pound weight loss for a year. (The downside is that the study was done with a dose of Wellbutrin that is associated with an increased risk of seizures—300 to 400 milligrams.) Wellbutrin is often used in conjunction with a class of drugs called SSRIs (selective serotonin reuptake inhibitors) to reverse the weight gain and sexual side effects (decreased libido and delayed orgasm) that are sometimes associated with some SSRIs like Zoloft. (Some SSRIs like Celexa and Lexapro are shown to decrease appetite by increasing CCK and oxytocin.)

Caffeine and nicotine also work as appetite suppressants the same way—by

Drug Thugs

You think you're doing something right: You're overweight, which causes high blood pressure, so you go on medication to bring your BP down. Or maybe you're depressed about being overweight, and you take an antidepressant to help deal with self-esteem issues. The irony of it all? Many of the drugs used to treat those issues have been shown to make you *gain* weight. Beta-blockers, one of the drugs most commonly used for hypertension, for instance, have been shown to cause weight gain and decrease metabolic rate by 10 percent. Several classes of antidepressants have also been shown to increase body weight, as has insulin (used to help control diabetes, which can be caused by obesity). The lesson: Don't automatically assume that medications—even ones designed to help a specific problem—will help your weight-loss efforts. We recommend that you ask your doctor about weight side effects of drugs and try addressing weight issues with nutrition and activity levels first, before starting a prescription regimen that may leave you with an increase in the very thing you're trying to decrease.

Get the Message? Neurons communicate with each other by sending and catching chemical signals. Serotonin, for instance, makes you feel good when your synapses are catching it. When there aren't enough for your neurons to catch, that's when you feel depressed. Drugs that stimulate the feel-good aspect may help promote weight loss.

increasing norepinephrine, suppressing appetite, and speeding metabolism (and heart rate). These drugs can be an effective part of a waist management plan (just not in the form of actual cigarettes). The herb ephedra, which is found in many "miracle" weight-loss solutions, has the same mechanism of action but can cause heart attacks. Just because something is natural doesn't mean it's good for you; tornadoes and bubonic plague are natural too.

Drugs That Influence Serotonin: The drug sibutramine (Meridia) has been shown to suppress appetite by acting like the feel-good brain chemical serotonin, so you don't experience the dramatic increases and decreases in brain chemicals that lead to hedonistic eating. Most folks can lose roughly 7 percent of their weight but not much more with this drug alone. By the way, the popular weight-loss drug phen-fen had the same physiological action too, but it was taken off the market because of its link to pulmonary hypertension (that's high blood pressure in arteries that supply the lungs). An interesting side note: Increasing serotonin has been shown to reduce carbohydrate intake, so it becomes a physiological chicken-egg discussion: Do comfort foods work to help curb depression? Or do we eat because we're depressed?

Drugs That Influence Dopamine: Currently, no weight-loss drugs work by changing your reward-seeking dopamine levels, but dopamine may hold

The Future of Gut Drugs

One of the most promising drug therapies involves the injection of CCK or things that have a chemical structure similar to the Crucial Craving–Killer peptide. (Remember, CCK causes your stomach to hold on to food for a long time and sends messages to the brain through the vagus nerve to say you're full.) The body produces specific enzymes in the small intestine to degrade CCK, but new developments show that you can stop that action. Ingesting or inhaling CCK that can access the bloodstream may help increase satiety levels.

the key to why you crave the foods that make you feel good. Sugar's been shown to increase dopamine levels—and that spins you into a cycle of addiction. You eat sugar, which makes you feel cloud-high. When that feeling diminishes, you crave sugar to feel good, and so on. Of course, another radical direction is to address the psychological pain directly instead of using food as an emotional bandage.

Drugs That Influence GABA: Drugs that affect gamma-aminobutyric acid (GABA) levels are used for anesthesia and antiseizure medications, because GABA acts to slow you down, calm you down, and put you to sleep. We don't recommend a lifetime of general anesthesia for weight control, but two anti-seizure medications—topiramate (Topamax) and zonisamide (Zonegran)—have been shown to promote weight loss. They work because the drugs calm the nerve activity in your brain that signals you to eat (plus, you can't very well snort down a dozen glazed doughnuts when you're snoozing head-over-chest on the recliner). Topiramate, in fact, is a drug of choice for some weight-loss docs, but its class of drugs does have potential side effects; these drugs can make you feel disoriented, as if you're in a zombielike state.

Drugs That Influence Your Gut: While a number of weight-loss drugs can help change the circuitry in your brain to help you control your weight, other drugs influence the functions of your gut. The drug orlistat (also known as Xenical) and its over-the-counter smaller size (Alli) work by inhibiting the digestion of fat—specifically by blocking the enzyme lipase, which is responsible for breaking down dietary fats to prepare them for bile and absorption. When fat isn't broken down, the body can't absorb it, so you'll take in fewer calories. Orlistat seems to be safer than other weight-loss drugs and effective at helping you lose about 10 percent of your body weight. And it also seems to help with cholesterol, because it inhibits the absorption of fat. One disadvantage of orlistat and Alli is that you absorb less of the fat-soluble vitamins A, D, and E from your food, so you need to take a multivitamin at night. Another side effect is that you experience a toilet trifecta: more frequent stools, more gas, and caca that's oilier than a mechanic's garage. Luckily, you can counteract the effects with natural fiber in the form of psyllium husks, which seem to reduce the symptoms by bulking up your stools. You can also reduce the side effects by having a little fat (and less fat, in total) with each meal instead of all of your daily fat at dinner alone. Too much fat, and you'll know it with a full-time appointment with your bathroom if you want to avoid soiling your undergarments. There is a question of rare liver injuries with this medication.

The drug works by not allowing your body to absorb fat, effectively teaching people what foods have fat. It's like a candle for many patients—it teaches them how close you can get to the fire without getting burned. Just because a package says the food is cholesterol-free (or the like) doesn't mean it's free of fat. (You'll know by the fact that fat will go right through you.) Many docs say this drug is useful as it teaches you which foods have hidden bad fats in them so you avoid the aging that hidden saturated and trans fats cause in addition to losing weight. Many specialists find orlistat a very useful addition to a successfully started waist-loss program that has stalled. Other gut-related drugs are also worth exploring.

❖ Because the drug glucophage (Metformin) increases insulin sensitivity, and seems to decrease DAF-2 (see page 130), it seems to reduce inflammation in the liver, so the hormonal cross talk that is so important to prevent metabolic syndrome or polycystic ovary disease is preserved. Sugar levels return to normal as insulin is able to perform its role in pushing these tasty molecules into cells for consumption (blocking the production of new sugars that are made every half hour as energy stores are used up). Side effects include gas and nausea, not a bad combo to force less calorie intake. If you become dehydrated, this drug can cause severe problems—so it is not for those who like to exercise for two hours or more at a time.

❖ Acarbose (Precose) works in a similar way to the drug orlistat, but on sugars. While orlistat inhibits the absorption of fat, acarbose inhibits an enzyme in the metabolism of carbohydrates—meaning that it blocks carbohydrates from breaking down in the gut and being absorbed by your body. (The side effect is that sugars can cause diarrhea and also can be fermented, resulting in more gas.) Think of this as a subtle reminder to eat the right foods.

YOU TIPS!

Drugs: Just Say Maybe. Any of the drugs we discussed earlier in this appendix are practical jump starts to use when you've reached a plateau or need help getting over a hump. So when you start your diet, schedule an appointment with your doc when you're likely to hit the hump—about day thirty. If you fit the BMI or waist profile from earlier in the appendix, we suggest you and your doc think about Wellbutrin. The drug is thought to work by helping emotional eaters decrease cravings. The reason why it works: It helps us not think and obsess over food. It can program our bodies to get back into our natural position—that is, not substituting a six-pack of Hershey bars for a spouse who doesn't listen, a boss who doesn't understand, or a child who feels like rolling soup cans down aisle four. Very soon, more and more new classes of drugs will be developed to help curb cravings and appetites, and they're worth exploring with your doctor. But these are short-term boosters to help you along your path.

Try a Waist Management Cocktail. When many people quit smoking, one of the first things they'll do is complain about the weight they've gained after quitting. There's something to that. While cigarettes are bullets to your lungs, they do seem to help people control weight—possibly, in part, through the destruction of taste buds. But they also seem to help by increasing metabolic rate

Myth Buster by up to 10 percent as well as helping to reduce appetite.

Well, the chances of our offering up cigarettes as a waist-control method are roughly the same as the eight-track tape making a comeback. We don't want to rule out nicotine as one of those early-program jump starts you can use to jump over a hurdle to increase your metabolism and reduce your appetite. Studies have shown that nicotine—in the form of patches and gum, *not* in the form of cigarettes—when combined with a modest dose of caffeine (as in two cups of coffee) can help reduce weight for those who use it. It's not a long-term solution but one that can help you adjust and automate. We've prescribed a 7-milligram nicotine patch to help some over a hurdle, combined with two cups of coffee (average cups, not the high-test espresso type—it would be only two-thirds of one of those babies). Of course, we ensure that the patient doesn't have side effects triggered by the caffeine, such as migraine headaches, GERD, increased heartbeats, or anxiety. Caffeine will raise your metabolic rate just a tad to burn more calories. Combine the two if your weight-loss program stalls. They can act as that crutch to help you over the hump. This is one tip, like all others in this appendix, that you should share with your doctor, to play it safe. Plus, you need a prescription.

Skinny Skin Skin

When Plastic Surgery Is an Option

Diet Myths

- ❖ If done well, plastic surgery pretty much guarantees bodily happiness.

- ❖ Liposuction can help you lose a lot of fat fast.

- ❖ Some procedures can eliminate cellulite.

One of the reasons many of us want to lose weight is to look better, but sometimes—even after losing weight—that doesn't happen. That's because all that fat you were carrying around has stretched your skin to the size of a hot-air balloon and made it droopier than a basset hound's ears. But unlike some side effects, there are ways around this one. If you've gone through the rebooting process and then experience the effects of saggy, stretchy skin, you might be considering adding another player to your waist management team: the plastic surgeon.

Like a relief pitcher in baseball, a plastic surgeon can come in to complete your new image by sculpting, shaping, and rebuilding your body. Before we start, let's make two things clear: Plastic surgery isn't about perfection, and it has its risks. In reality, plastic surgery can very well be about trading in one deformity (saggy skin) for another (scars that can run longer than the Amazon), but for some people the trade-off is worth it.

We know the knock: Only egocentric people use plastic surgery in a quest for exterior perfection. (Say that to someone who's lost a lot of weight and has stomach skin hanging down to the knees.) But you don't have to be desperately seeking saline implants to benefit from plastic surgery. For many who undergo plastic surgery after weight loss or as a supplement to weight loss, some procedures can improve health as much as they improve appearance. That hanging skin can trap sweat, leading to rashes and yeast infections. Skin removal can cure that problem. Of course, plastic surgery isn't for everybody, and it's not something we endorse if the idea makes you squirm. Having plastic surgery doesn't turn you into a Barbie, doesn't make you vainer than a mirror-hogging gymgoer, and doesn't make you

FACTOID

Anyone who claims he can remove fat cells without surgery is more fraudulent than a credit card thief. Ads for "mesotherapy" appear in the yellow pages, on telephone poles, and in your inbox—but stay away. They purport to do it by injecting a cocktail of drugs into your skin over the course of ten to twenty sessions. The drugs in these treatments haven't been shown to be effective, and some states have even tried to ban this procedure. Some chemicals such as sulfuric acid—might actually work, but we'd prefer you save such chemicals for clogged sinks. See YOU Tips for a new process.

a cheat. If you're comfortable with it, you can view it as the polish on the washed car, the foam on the tall cappuccino, the kiss after the first date. It helps make your weight loss feel complete—so you can be comfortable with your newly reprogrammed body.

Stretching the Truth

Anyone who's gained or lost weight knows what it can do to your skin: Pack on too much fat, and you'll create stretch marks that look like a family of earthworms. Lose a lot of fat, and your skin will pour off your body like vats of pancake batter. Of course, we all know that skin is elastic and has a rubber band's ability to expand and snap back; one look at a woman who gives birth and regains a flat tummy a few months later is evidence of that. So the question for those of us who lose a lot of weight is this: Why doesn't our skin snap back to normal after our weight does?

Think of your skin as one of those large Hefty plastic garbage bags. When it comes out of the box, it's folded up nice and tight. Fill it up with trash, and it expands, stretches, and bulges. Durable yet flexible, most bags can withstand the typical dumping of cans, papers, turkey carcasses, anything you throw into it. Your skin works the same way—it's durable, it stretches, and it can withstand most of the junk you toss into it. But what happens when you put on too much weight? When you fill your human Hefty bag with pies, nachos, and turkey carcasses? It'll keep stretching and stretching and stretching, but the leather of the skin, the strong collagen layer, can't grow too fast. So if you pile too much linguine Alfredo into your thighs, the undersurface of the skin will

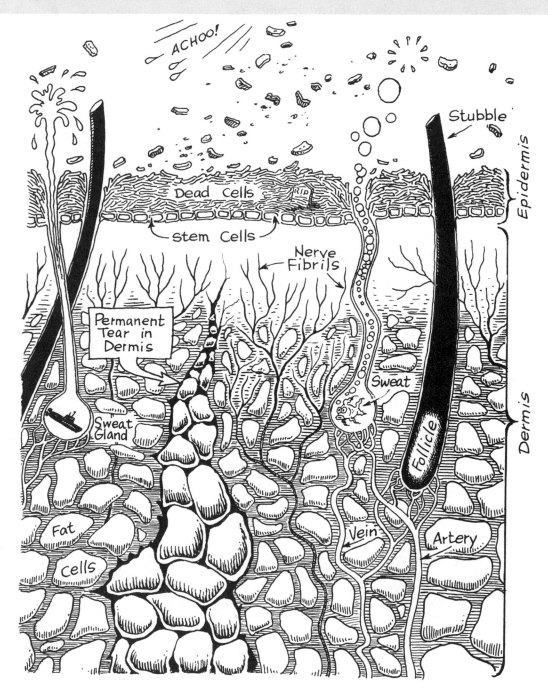

actually tear (see Figure B.1). It will tear at the level of the dermis—that's the lower level of your skin, which makes new cells, not the outer level of skin called the epidermis, though the stretch marks associated with weight gain do appear on the outer level. Your body sees those stretch marks as an assault, and nasty inflammation results. That's why they look red for a few months. As the inflammation subsides, the redness goes away. It's predictable enough for skin creams to be able to claim they cure stretch marks. They can't, they don't, but that doesn't stop the false claims.

The same way the bag becomes stretched to the point of tearing, your skin does too—and at that point it's too late for it to snap back in place. So even if you take the trash out of the bag (by losing fat), you won't be able to restore the bag to its original state (of nice, tight skin). So it's very likely that you'll keep the skin of your 250-pound body, even if you now weigh 150.

The Plastic Possibilities

Whether you've lost a lot of weight or a little, you can fine-tune your skin with some small-scale procedures. These are the most common and—as long as you use them for the right purpose—reasonable solutions for specific problems.

FACTOID

It's about as easy to remove cellulite as it is to remove a suspect-looking mole with a plastic spoon. It can't be done. About 90 percent of women have some of the cottage-cheese-looking fat in their thighs or butts, and that's natural. Human skin is tethered to the underlying muscle by connective strands of collagen, which prevents excessive motion. Dogs lack these; that's why their skin can move so easily. No creams (which mostly use caffeine as the active ingredient), medicine, lasers, or massage will work to remove cellulite marks. One technique vigorously marketed out of France is called Endermologie. It may temporarily reduce the appearance of cellulite. But the result is only temporary and not worth the big bucks (or even little ones), in our opinion.

Myth Buster

Tummy Tucks: Given the number of plastic surgery shows on TV these days, flat stomachs are everywhere. Tummy tucks aren't for people with massive weight loss but primarily for people who develop a football-size pouch under their belly button (they're done mostly for women who develop a pouch after childbirth).

> ## FACTOID
>
> You'll find nearly 700,000 websites for that ever-elusive stretch mark cure. Whether they can be prevented is a hotly debated topic, but once the dermis tears apart and stretch marks are born, there's nothing you can do. A lot of people recommend lotions with alpha-tocopherol (vitamin E) or retinoids (vitamin A) in them. No research has shown that these vitamins or any other cream will make stretch marks fade. Once the layer underneath the skin is ripped, in theory you can only prevent it from getting worse. If you wait long enough, all stretch marks look better. While stretch marks are red, avoid the sun or use sunscreen to prevent the red marks from turning brown. Some of our medical friends do swear from patient and personal experience that applying aloe and/or vitamin E will reduce the size and improve the look of stretch marks. Things that make stretch marks worse: getting fatter and lack of exercise. Steroids and sun damage also weaken the skin's collagen. By the way, one thing that does facilitate skin healing (though not the total disappearance of stretch marks) is walking. In one study, identical wounds healed in twenty-nine days for walkers and thirty-nine days for nonwalkers.

Here's how they work: The excess skin is lifted from the pubic area right up to the ribs, and the skin up to the belly button is then removed. During pregnancy or with weight gain, the rectus abdominis muscles (the six-pack muscles) drift to the sides of the body. Unless you're very lucky, they don't return to the middle even by the time your kid is in high school. So your belly will pouch forward, your buttocks will shift backward, and you'll get a little lower back pain. That's where your plastic surgeon will sew the muscles together with stitches that will outlast your body. Because the rectus is attached to the external obliques (the muscles on the sides of your torso), the tightening will improve the overall tone of all your abdominal muscles, potentially decreasing back pain and improving your posture and lower-body strength.

Some of the newest procedures in plastic surgery are big-time body-contouring procedures such as body lifts, thigh lifts, and arm lifts. Not for the faint of heart, these procedures remove huge pieces of skin and stitch the body back together like a piece of clothing. With a monthlong recovery period and complication rates that approach 25 percent, these procedures are reserved for

people who have lost huge amounts of weight and are miserable with all the extra skin.

Face- and Neck-Lifts: Once you've lost all that weight, your grape might look like a raisin and your plum might look like a prune. Wrinkles that were hidden by all your fat might now be visible from across the room. Plastic surgeons stay up at night thinking of new ways to stretch, fill, Botox, and laser those wrinkles. The genetic reality is that some people have more chins than Elvis has platinum records. If, thanks to your ancestors, you store fat in your neck even when the rest of your body is as sleek as a jaguar, you can have the walrus rings removed from your neck. To tighten the skin on your face, the surgeon will make cuts that run from the sideburn area to the top of the ear, continuing in front and then to the back side of the ear. There seem to be as many names for these new face-lifts as there are plastic surgeons, but the common thread is that today's face-lifts use "short scar" techniques. One more cut is made under the chin to fix the two neck bands. Then the surgeon can remove excess fat from your neck and jowls with liposuction (see below), pull your facial skin up and back, trim off the excess, and stitch it back to the line where the cut was initially made. The new face-lifts are "ponytail friendly," showing almost no scars even without makeup.

Liposuction: Straws may suck the cola out of cups, and vacuums may suck the crumbs out of carpet fibers, but when it comes to the fat removal process, liposuction sucks big time. A fairly safe procedure (with three to five days of recovery time), liposuction has a place in a waist management plan. **YOU-reka!** But know this: Liposuction is no better as a weight-loss technique than a leg amputation. Liposuction is a sculpting technique; it'll help remove fat from problem areas, but it won't help you lose a significant number of pounds. Most plastic surgeons feel that suction of more than five liters (ten pounds) is dangerous. If you can grab a fatty area within one hand and think you'd be happy if it were gone, you might be a good candidate for liposuction. Or if you are dis-

Myth Buster

proportioned (a size 4 upper body and size 10 lower body), liposuction might match the parts better.

Liposuction has little effect on weight because fat is light. Remember that loving barb, "fat floats." A liter of fat weighs about two pounds (and the lipo max is five liters of fat removed). The ideal patient is about 10 percent above the ideal body weight, with isolated fat in one area (and that one area is often genetically driven; in other words, all the members of a family have excess fat in the same place). People who undergo massive weight loss can still use liposuction, but it should be in combination with other procedures to get their bodies into the proportions they want.

Here's how it works: Get ready for a little embarrassment, since your surgeon will draw on your absolutely naked body and paint you from head to toe with the bug killer betadine. You'll then climb onto the sterile operating table, and the next thing you'll see is the recovery room ceiling. About ten minutes before the actual sucking procedure, but while you're anesthesized, you're pumped full of fluid in the area of focus. The fluid contains saline (a salt solution) and epinephrine (to control bleeding by making the arteries in the fat constrict or spasm). Though some surgeons add lidocaine to the mixture (to numb the pain), we think that's unnecessary and even dangerous. If you're having the procedure done with general anesthesia, you'll get different amounts of these drugs, which is important, because too much lidocaine causes many of the most serious complications associated with liposuction. When the fluid is pumped in, you'll swell

FACTOID

You'll need to ask your insurance company whether your procedure is included in your plan—that is, whether and what percentage will be covered. Since many plastic surgeries are health-related and help fix and prevent serious health problems (rather than being purely cosmetic), they may be covered by insurance (for instance, breast reduction for treatment of back pain). If you are initially denied, though, you can fight; be persistent. One survey showed that patients who appealed denied insurance claims were successful in getting paid in about half the cases, although it does seem to be more and more difficult. One thing that particularly helps: enlisting your doctor's help. Have him or her write a letter explaining why you need the procedure; submit lab results of your blood work that support the procedure; find information on trends for your particular surgery. The plastic surgeon may be able to help your doctor write the letter. Finally, try to get your case in front of the insurer's medical director; a doctor will usually look at your situation sympathetically and support good patient care.

up like the Michelin Man because you'll be given an amount of fluid equal to the amount of fat that's going to be sucked out (about one liter of fluid in for one liter of fat removed, depending upon the technique being used).

Then doctors suck out the fluid and fat in several ways. In the first procedure, they take a tube of straw-shaped metal, shove it under the skin, and push it to where it needs to go. They shove it in and out, in and out, cutting little tunnels of fat that are then removed. In the second procedure, they use ultrasound energy to break up the fat. In the newest variation, they pop the fat cells with lasers before they are suctioned out. Though the newer procedures may not be better than the older ones and may actually have higher complication rates, all are acceptable procedures in the right hands and allow for precise contouring. The key phrase? "The right hands." See "Do Your Own Checkup" on the following page to find a plastic surgeon.

FACTOID

It's best to keep a new surgical incision moist with a gentle moisturizer; it will heal faster. Once the wound is healed, sunscreen is the only thing proven to help scars. UV light will permanently color red scars brown. Our general rule: You shouldn't put any medicine or anything else on your skin that you wouldn't put into your eye. But get this: One study showed that covering a scar with porous paper (such as paper tape) for six months reduced the likelihood of an ugly scar—probably because the tape helped keep the healing scar moist.

FACTOID

Smoking worsens the tears made in your dermis by interfering with microscopic healing processes and depleting the short-lived gas nitric oxide that preserves the elasticity of your skin. That's why smokers get wrinkles around their lips (plus the inflammation in arteries that cigarettes cause).

YOU TIPS!

Maintain Your Holding Pattern. Before you have any kind of plastic surgery for your skin, your doctor should insist upon a healthy nutritional status (that is, maintaining a diet with healthful ingredients), primarily so you can heal properly after surgery. You will also have a much better outcome if you actually train for surgery as you would for a road race, by exercising. You will need to be sedentary after surgery, so being strong beforehand will make you bounce back better. Your doctor will also use diet and exercise to assess your ability to stay at your current weight level. The doctor will want to know if your weight's been stable over the last six to twelve months. If you've been fluctuating either up or down, there's no point in having the surgery. If you're prone to gaining weight again, you'll simply stretch the skin out again and defeat the purpose of the surgery. And if you're still losing weight, the surgery may be a bigger waste of money than a psychic hotline, because you run the risk of sagging again after the surgery.

Take a Reality Check. It all sounds more blissful than an oceanside piña colada: no more fat; no more loose skin; ah, the ideal body. But many people have a tough time adjusting to life in the plastic era. Why? There are psychological reasons: Weight gain occurs slowly—and most times, with the exception of some surgical procedures, weight loss happens slowly as well. You have time to adjust psychologically to your new body, whether it's getting bigger or smaller. But when you have plastic surgery (especially with skin removal), the changes are fast, drastic, and, in some cases, emotionally heart-stopping. It took ten years to get fat and mentally adjust to your sense of "you," but when somebody whacks off twenty pounds of excess fat and skin and stitches you up like Grandma's needlepoint pillow, it takes a whole different mind-set to deal with the effects. Yes, losing weight and losing excess skin are what you've always wanted, but you need to be prepared for the scars, for the body adjustments, for the attention you'll be given. While some people bask in the compliments they receive on their new bodies, others are embarrassed or shamed by positive feedback, because it reminds them of how noticeably overweight they once were. And the new scars may give you new reasons not to go to the beach. Sometimes it's a good idea to discuss possible cosmetic surgery with a psychiatrist or psychologist to be sure you're mentally ready for the knife. Lots of obese people never look in the mirror, so your new body may take some getting used to. There are also physical reasons that people are disappointed after plastic surgery. It's not like blowing your nose. Some of these surgeries are quite invasive, and there are drains, swelling, some pain, immobilization, and other discomforts that come with them. Some patients expect to look twenty-five years old when they're done. That just isn't realistic. The best you can hope for is a fitter, well-rested, ten-years-younger you.

Do Your Own Checkup. With some skin-altering procedures, it seems as if everybody and his mother's gardener thinks he can do them. But for any of these procedures, you need a surgeon certified by the American Board of Plastic Surgery. Liposuction docs should perform more than fifty procedures a year, and those doing surgeries for massive skin reduction should be doing a minimum of one and hopefully more a month. Remember that even if your surgery is performed in an office or surgicenter, your surgeon should have hospital privileges to perform that procedure. That gives you another assurance that the doctor has had oversight. Both the board-certified plastic surgeon and the facility must be equipped to handle complications (remember, in liposuction procedures, the fat is stabbed, and one potential risk is the stabbing of vital things and things that bleed a lot residing under or in the fat).

It doesn't matter whether you sign up to have surgery done in a hospital or an in-office doctor's OR; there's only one way to determine if the facility meets standards of high quality for service and cleanliness. That is, it needs to be accredited or state-licensed. Reliable accrediting organizations include the country's health care do-gooder group called the Joint Commission and the American Association for Accreditation of Ambulatory Surgical Facilities (AAAASF). You can search for facilities at www.jointcommission.org. or www.aaaasf.org. These organizations give you the reassurance you need when someone's about to slice a few bricks' worth of skin off your belly. Just because the corner guy is offering the "latest" or "newest" or "most cutting-edge" procedure doesn't mean you should be first in line. The plastic surgery field is full of fraud, and you don't want to be a lab rat in someone else's experiment. Make sure the tool, technique, or procedure has scientific backing. Check out the surgeon's website and learn about his or her credentials. If the surgeon has published scientific papers in journals about a particular procedure, that's a hint that he has some experience in it. In a consultation, ask to see photos of other patients. You might even be able to talk to some of that surgeon's prior patients. Some plastic surgeons specialize in extreme-weight-loss patients and can show pictures with disappearing bat wings and shots with and without skin aprons. But remember that no one shows off images of complications or poor results, so ask to see at least a dozen pictures. It also helps if the surgeon is a member of a plastic surgical society such as the American Society of Plastic Surgeons (ASPS), the American Society for Aesthetic Plastic Surgery, the International Society of Aesthetic Plastic Surgery (ISAPS), or the American Association of Plastic Surgeons (AAPS)—which means having to keep up

FACTOID

When you try a new recipe, the proof is in the taste test. When you have plastic surgery, the proof is in the before-and-after photos. Computers can modify anything, so computer-generated images or models of your potential results (morphing) shouldn't be enough to convince you of the benefits of being "cut." They can be used as a method of communication between you and your doc, but insist on seeing before-and-after photos of other patients as well. Anyone in the field will admit that if a plastic surgeon's office burns, the first things to be saved would be the before-and-after images, so anyone of the quality you deserve will have a dozen samples of folks similar to you.

with the latest and greatest. And remember, just because the corner plastic surgeon buys a quarter-million-dollar device doesn't mean he or she is a great plastic surgeon.

Now Stop. We've all seen pictures of them; they're people who treat cosmetic operations like massages. The more they have, the better they feel. The truth is that these people have more plastic than an in-debt college student. Yes, it's tempting to have additional procedures, but plastic surgery can be as addictive as any drug. The sign that you're in a constant quest for—*watch our fingers making quotation marks in the air*—"perfection" is that you're planning your next surgery as soon as you're finished with the one before it. So, yes, find your trouble spots and decide what will make you happy. Then pick an end point where you want your body to be and deal with the reality of what you're going to look like when you get there. Look in the mirror, tell yourself what changes would give you satisfaction, and then stop. If you can't stop—if you're constantly considering lipoing this or tucking that—then it's not your skin you need checked, it's your head. Bottom line: Before deciding on a procedure, you have to accept the fact that you're not seeking perfection; you're seeking improvements in your body and your happiness.

Make a Sound Decision. The next big thing in plastic surgery is noninvasive fat removal. As one of the "holy grails" in plastic surgery, the Ultrashape device promises the removal of fat without making any incisions and, in fact, without surgery. Sound has energy—that's how loud, high-pitched voices can actually break glass. But the challenge has been to focus just the right pitch of sound to bust apart your fat cells. The future is just about here. Without an incision, without anesthesia, and without pain, the Ultrashape device focuses unhearable sound energy into a tiny space aimed just under your skin. And voilà—that pizza is history! (Well, not really, since the fat is actually released into the bloodstream and picked up by other fat cells somewhere else in the body, or excreted via kidneys or deposited into your arteries.)

The Ultrashape device is now available around the world and very soon will be approved in the United States. This computer-driven marvel can destroy as much as 6 ounces of fat around the belly in a little over an hour. It's certainly not a replacement for the pounds of fat that liposuction can remove, but then again, it's without surgery. And after three or four sessions, a lot can be removed. Future devices may remove even more fat. The big question facing you and the FDA if you want this is where does that fat go? Will it make heart disease and memory loss worse as it creates inflammation in the short term, or make both the outside and the inside of your body look better? It is approved in Europe, so this is one time where those continentals may test the safety for us in North America. You'll have to keep listening to see if these sound waves make good vibes inside and out.

The Extreme Team

What to Do If Your Weight Is Out of Control

Diet Myths

❖ Weight-loss surgery is the easy way out.

❖ If you have gastric bypass surgery, you never have to worry about dieting again.

❖ Once you have the surgery and recover from it, the hard part is over.

For basketball players, desperation is the full-court shot at the buzzer. For accountants, desperation is 11:59 p.m. on April 15. For parents of an antsy kindergartner, it's a malfunctioning SpongeBob DVD. But for people struggling with weight issues, desperation is the feeling that comes when you've morphed from being overweight to going overboard. But here's the difference between most desperate situations and this one: While basketball players rarely make full-length heaves and 1040s can't be completed in sixty seconds, people with extreme weight situations do have a life raft that can change desperation to salvation: weight-loss surgery.

Most people view weight-loss surgery the way they view steroids in sports—that it's cheating, it's unnatural, it's an unfair advantage, it's cutting corners. But there are plenty of people—way too many, in fact—who have coffin-enticing obesity in the form of a body mass index of 35 or higher, with consequences like diabetes and high blood pressure. And for this segment of the population, especially if they have repeatedly tried and failed at a diet and exercise regime, weight-loss surgery may be an effective solution.

Myth Buster Some people simply can't lose weight like everyone else and often beat themselves up about being undisciplined or out of control. Many are very disciplined, successful, and in control in other aspects of their lives but are just wired differently in the weight department. Finally, there's a real alternative for people who are incapable of succeeding without help: weight-loss surgery.

In nearly every other medical situation in our lives, we experience a symptom, we try to treat it ourselves, and then we seek professional help if we can't. We need to start thinking about obesity as if it's any other health problem that prompts you to see a doctor—be it a bullet wound, a lump in your breast, or cholesterol numbers that need commas.

The truth is that many people have tried every over-the-counter antiobesity option; they have a library of diet books, a garage full of exercise equipment, and neurons full of frustration. But no matter what they try to do to lose weight, they either can't take it off or can't keep it off. For these people, the answer isn't always the over-the-counter way, because a life of obesity requires more than a commitment to a three-day all-juice fast or some ab machine that claims to banish your belly using electrodes. Heavy-duty bodies require heavy-duty help.

And that's OK. If you—or someone you love—falls into this category, then you have a serious condition that should make you feel you'd do whatever you could to try to reverse it. Technically, it's defined as 100 pounds above the ideal weight for men and 80 pounds above the ideal weight for women, or men with 48-inch waists or larger and women with 41-inch waists or larger.

Think for a second: If you had prostate or breast cancer (which both have about the same risk of death per year for people over fifty as does a waist size of 38 for women and 45 for men with risks like high blood pressure, sleep apnea, diabetes, and cholesterol problems), you'd take action. You'd talk to doctors, you'd schedule surgery or radiation therapy to remove the tumor, and you'd make lifestyle changes that would help lower the chance that you'd ever contract the disease again. You wouldn't pop a cough drop, then throw up your hands in defeat if menthol weren't the magic tumor killer. You'd get professional—even drastic—help. You would even let someone cut you open if the therapy was effective.

It's a mistake to think you're a weakling or a fool if you consider the operation option. Morbid obesity (morbid!) is as concrete a health problem as a sprained ankle, a heart problem, or cancer. In fact, at least 5 percent of morbidly obese people have a specific genetic problem that renders their brains unable to receive the leptin signals that they're full. So no matter what the cause of your weight problem, there's no shame in seeking one of the most effective cures for obesity that modern medicine has developed. Weight-loss surgery works. And it works more effectively—and faster—than any traditional dieting method for people with morbid obesity. Surgery can reduce your excess weight by half, whereas weight-loss drugs get you only 5 percent to 7 percent while you're on them, and lifestyle changes buy you *on average* another 7 percent of total weight if you're on your best behavior.

The success of weight-loss surgery is defined first and foremost by changing the expression of genes that promote type 2 diabetes, hypertension, and arthritis. As you start to lose weight and waist, whether by diet and exercise alone or combined with surgery, you lose the diabetes, hypertension, and arthritis. Your genes don't change, but they turn off—in fact, within six weeks after surgery, 60 percent of patients might lose their type 2 diabetes, and 75 percent do so within six months. The other way of defining success is the loss of excess weight—that is, not how much total weight you lose, but rather the difference between your current weight and your ideal weight. (For women, the ideal weight is 105 pounds for five feet of height, and 5 pounds for every inch after. For men, it's 106 pounds at five feet and 6 pounds for every inch taller. Those are for medium-framed people. Some adjustments are made if you're larger or smaller framed.)

Surgical options aren't for people who are just a little overweight. They're not for people worried about losing their runway-model job or their clothes not fitting. They're for people whose health is at extreme risk, who are four fries away from putting the grave-digger on speed-dial, because the effects of excess fat increase your risk of developing such day ruiners as coronary artery disease, hypertension, sleep apnea, infertility, chronic back pain, hernias, infections, gallstones, and depression.

Still, these options are the foundations for tomorrow's cutting-edge (and cutting-weight) procedures—the operations that may help people who don't have extreme weight problems. Of course, we still want you to adopt lifestyle changes, like regular walking and pushing away the corn dogs (to be successful with surgery, you have to adopt more lifestyle changes than ever). But you should also know there is help that can save you and improve your quality of life if you are completely out of control.

Alternative Routes: Have You Got the Guts?

If you were driving along and came upon an urgent flashing sign that warned you of a twenty-mile backup a few miles ahead, you'd peel off at the next exit, hop onto back roads, stop at gas stations, and find your way around the mess. You'd do anything to avoid staying stuck in the same spot for hours. You wouldn't want to feel like you were going nowhere. And you'd probably take your chances that the country roads would turn out to be more effective than the parking lot of a freeway.

Well, if you're in an extreme waist situation, you're in the parking lot. You're stuck. You've stalled. You might even be running out of gas. And you haven't found that magic car-carrying helicopter that can take you from the desperation of feeling like a refrigerator to the healthy, happy feeling that doesn't always revolve around the refrigerator. But some nice alternative routes can get you out of this disastrous jam of yo-yo dieting and morbid obesity. Even better, they're the foundations for future waist management procedures that can change the way we all live.

Most important, these solutions are real options with life-changing results. Consider these statistics:

1. A twenty-five-year-old obese man (with a waist size of 40 inches or greater) has a 22 percent reduction in his longevity (that is, he will lose twelve years of his life).
2. A twenty-pound weight loss corresponds to a 53 percent reduction in obesity-related deaths—and most of these procedures are designed to help people lose five times that much weight.
3. Weight-loss surgery reduces diabetes-related deaths by 80 percent—and some procedures can even *cure* diabetes in over 90 percent of the cases. They do not change your genes; the early weight loss turns the diabetes genes off.

What's most amazing is that changes in your risk factors like hypertension and cholesterol, but especially diabetes, start before the significant weight loss even starts in the first few days after surgery. (We know, it sounds like a tabloid headline: "Drop Your Cholesterol in Half! By 3 p.m.!") Your body, the smart little devil that it is, senses that the trend of weight and waist gain or loss is more important than your actual body weight or waist size; for these risk factors, it's not necessarily your waist size or how much you weigh that influences the risks, but which direction your body is heading in. Again and again, patients are off their insulin and hypertension drugs by one month or less after surgery. And they get rid of their C-PAP machines, sleep apnea, and daytime sleepiness. After surgery, your body starts behaving the way a normal body might behave, regulating the ghrelin and leptin cycle and other ways that your gastrointestinal tract may signal satiety and appetite. One patient told her surgeon that she was sure that he had operated on her brain, not her stomach, because the voice that continually told her she was hungry was turned off for the very first time. Weight-loss surgery may also work by decreasing markers of inflammation in your blood (like C-reactive protein) almost immediately. No matter the mechanisms, the effect is clear—and fast.

So, if obesity has forced one foot in the grave (and ten fingers in the pie), there's no reason to ignore surgery like a two-toothed hitchhiker. It isn't magic and won't create permanent success without lifestyle changes, but it will absolutely make a huge change in almost everyone who does it. Our understanding of how the stomach works has allowed us to develop procedures that manipulate the physiology of the stomach and the digestion process, to help people better control their weight and to take away hunger. While a bunch of different surgical procedures exists, they all fall into two categories. They're either restrictive— meaning the procedures limit the room in your stomach and thus the amount of food you can eat. (This is sort of like saying you can't cram any more people into a phone booth; there's only so much it can hold.) Or they're malabsorptive— meaning that they change your body so you can't absorb all the excess calories. Nearly all of them can now be done through a thin, flexible scope, or laparoscopically, without cutting your muscle wall. Some procedures combine the best of both tactics. Below, we'll outline how they work. For more logistics and specifics about weight-loss surgery options and preparation, see www.realage.com.

But let's be clear: These are major surgeries that, like skydiving and bumper cars, have as many risks as they have rewards. Most of all, you

Myth Buster have to know going in that you have to commit to preparing for the procedures and changing your postoperative lifestyle with an appropriate diet and behaviors. Do that, and they'll turn out to be effective procedures that aren't just about improving your looks or sparing your desk chair—they're all about improving your health. Dramatically.

And you also have to be prepared to define what success is. Success isn't defined by how happy you are or how thin you are. It's defined by continuous weight loss of 50 percent of your excess weight and the reversal of side effects of the formerly big waist. In those terms, surgeries, along with you making changes in food choices and physical activity, have a success rate of more than 90 percent at one year, with an average over five years be- **Myth Buster** tween 55 percent and 70 percent.

You also need to understand that two of these procedures are permanent and irreversible, and you will need to commit to certain routines (like taking a multivitamin and B12 daily; drinking lots of water; taking it easy on alcohol, caffeine, sodas, and acidic foods; and not drinking during meals and doing physical activity regularly) to stay healthy for the rest of your life. You also need to know that every patient reacts a little differently, so while some patients breeze through, others have a lot of adjusting to do to regain their vitality.

Gastric Banding: Restrictive

In this procedure, the surgeon places a belt-like band around the stomach—up high on the stomach. When the belt is tightened, it constricts the stomach to form an hourglass shape (see Figure C.1)—leaving a very small pouch at the top of the stomach for food to get stored as it enters from the esophagus. The band creates a

one-lane road that needs to accommodate dozens of lanes of traffic, a bottleneck that slows the movement of food through your GI system, so there's no way you can physically get more traffic into the bottom half of your stomach. When your food has to travel through that belt-tightened hourglass to the intestine, it means that you stay full for a long time, and you literally can eat only a small meal (this also forces you to eat slowly and chew thoroughly).

The big-band effect is that it simply limits your food intake so you can't eat (and store) excess calories. Doctors can also tighten or loosen (adjust) the band depending on how much you're able to get down, so this is a procedure that has some flexibility to it. (Think of it as when Popeye squeezes Bluto's neck. When he squeezes, Bluto's head gets bigger. When the band gets tightened, it creates more of a bulge in the stomach and a tighter hole in the middle of the hourglass.) Some say these adjustments take less than three months but are necessary two to four times a year to take away your hunger. That's the key: No desire to eat, no waist gain. The pluses: Like an intramural-team T-shirt, it's reversible, and it has the lowest risk of all surgical options. The downside is that because your stomach shrinks, you have to cut food down to the size of the nail on your pinkie, which means you may be more likely to eat junkier foods than bulky foods such as spinach.

Duodenal Switch: Malabsorptive

Take a driving trip of any distance, and you know the difference between Route 1 and Alternate Route 1. Route 1 may take you right through the city's downtown so you can stop at the shops, see the houses on the historical register, and putter through the thirty-five traffic lights within a half-mile drag. Fine, in some cases. But if you're just trying to get to the other side of town, then you'll take Alternate 1—the loop that goes around the town, avoids the lights, and gets you from the post office to the pet salon without having to worm along in traffic that's slower than a sedated slug. A malabsorptive procedure is Alternate Route 1: It

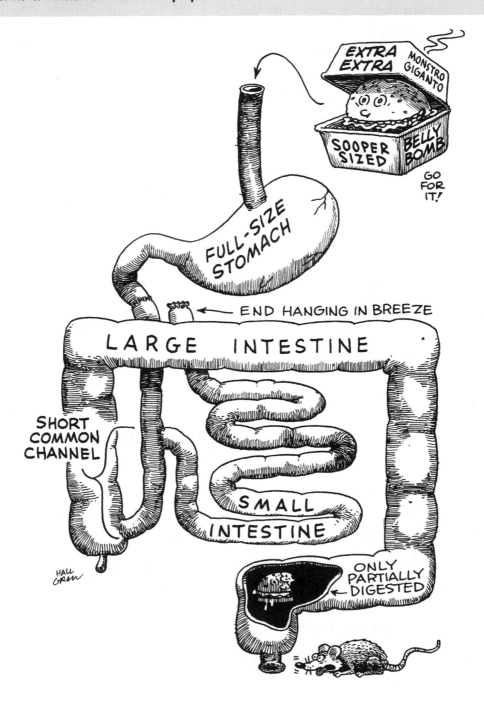

cuts out the gastrointestinal main street so that food can go tollbooth to exit ramp without having to stop at fat-storing traffic lights along the way.

In the duodenal switch (see Figure C.2), the intestines are cut and reattached, to quicken the time it takes food to go through the system so that not all the nutrients can get fully absorbed. (It cuts out about 80 percent of the distance food travels in the intestines, from 600 centimeters to 100 centimeters—from more than nineteen feet to about three feet.) The switch allows the intestines to separate the flow of food from the flow of digestive juices like bile, and that's what helps you avoid absorbing all of the calories. Farther down the intestinal line, the two paths get reconnected where the food and fat juices get mixed together like a margarita before you launch it into your municipal sewer system. During the time the two paths are separated, less fat will be absorbed into the bloodstream and eventually stored on your belly. It's a simple physiological statement: If you can't absorb excess calories, you can't store them.

In a way, restrictive procedures like banding and the sleeve (see Factoid box) are a little bit like having a smaller gas tank. If you cut the size of your fuel tank to one-tenth its original size, your car simply won't be able to hold as much gas. But malabsorptive procedures are like having a leak in your tank. With a leak, your engine wouldn't even be able to get the gas, no matter how much you put in there. In malabsorptive procedures, your body doesn't get the excess calories to store as fat—and in a way it leaks them out of your body (out your back alley).

The switch is typically the most effective procedure and allows people to eat normal-size portions. But you'll probably need to take supplements for the rest of your life (see www.realage.com for specifics), because your body won't digest the nutrients you do eat. Plus, the draconian nature of this operation leads to the highest complications rates of any bariatric procedure.

FACTOID

A new procedure called gastric sleeve surgery is designed to help extremely obese patients who aren't ready for invasive procedures such as gastric bypass. In the procedure, the doctor removes about 60 percent of the stomach (to form the shape of a tube or sleeve). It's performed laparoscopically and helps the patient lose weight until he or she is ready for bypass or duodenal switch surgery, if it is later needed.

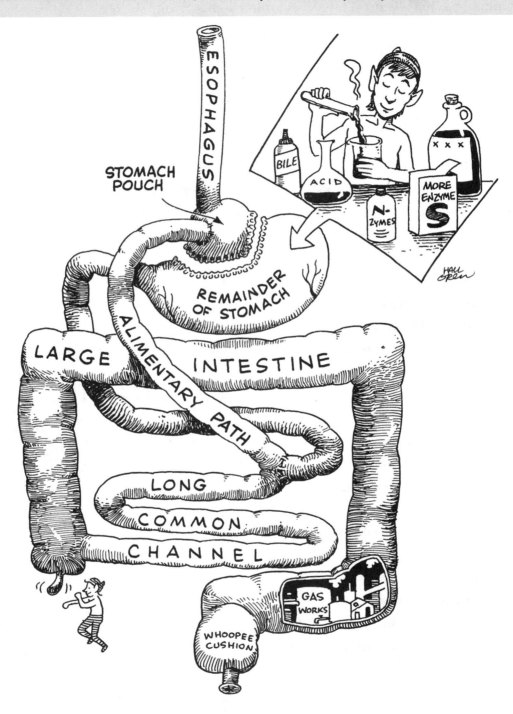

Gastric Bypass: Restrictive and Malabsorptive

Like a good doubles team, a healthy marriage, or oatmeal topped with fruit, gastric bypass has the strength of two parts molded into one. Traditional bypass surgery combines the best of both restrictive and malabsorptive methods—and that makes it the right answer for lots of people who desire surgery. In gastric bypass, surgeons staple off a little pouch of the stomach (about the size of an egg) to accept the food you eat (see Figure C.3). That's the restrictive element, since you can't eat too much food at once without getting sick. The remainder of the stomach drains into the first section of the small intestine, but no food passes into this section of the intestine, so no absorption can take place. To allow some absorption, a downstream limb of the intestine is sewn to the top of the stomach. So the food goes into the little stomach pouch and then passes into the midpoint of the small intestine, where it continues along the normal pathway for 200 centimeters (about six feet) before it hits the large intestine. In the end, about one-third of the small intestine is bypassed, but not as much as with a duodenal switch. That's the malabsorptive element. In addition to keeping you from absorbing large amounts of excess calories because key components of food digestion are cut out of the process, there is a change in hormonal response to foods that leads to satiety.

How did surgeons ever figure out this crazy idea for losing weight? They latched onto the fundamental ideas for this procedure when removing stomachs in people with ulcer disease (before antacids, H2 blockers, or proton-pump inhibitors). Surgeons went in there like special-ops forces and just took out what was causing the problem. But they found that patients developed symptoms and couldn't eat when food bypassed the stomach and got dumped right into the intestines; in that scenario, nutrients entered the bloodstream too quickly, as they got mainlined directly into the sensitive absorptive areas of our bowels. This ailment earned the title dumping syndrome, and suffering patients would feel nauseated, clammy, and sweaty. That all sounds about as appealing as a piping hot cup of Budweiser—unless you're trying to change your size from a redwood to a twig. The surgeons found that those patients who were not experiencing diges-

The Future of Weight Loss?

We know what you're thinking: Why can't they just make a pill that allows you to burn fat and maintain a healthy weight no matter what you eat? Future innovations may not be that simple, but they might be just as effective. One such procedure is called deep brain stimulation. It sounds like something out of an Orwellian book, and it sort of is. In this procedure, electrodes are implanted in the brain to change the way it functions (like the way a pacemaker changes a heart). It's currently done with Parkinson's patients and is being experimented with in other areas, but in the future, doctors could be using it to help control obesity. How? The electrodes would be used to target the satiety center, the hypothalamus, creating a kind of biological "off switch." Of course, with brain surgery comes complications, and it would be used not for people looking to lose a few inches but for those with morbid obesity with high health risks.

tion problems were eating smaller portions—and eating healthy foods, since high sugar content really got the dumping syndrome cooking. So that made researchers believe they could curb appetites surgically by bypassing the stomach during the digestion process.

Forcing food to skip some of your small bowel will fix your metabolic problem almost immediately by triggering chemical changes that reverse high blood sugar and hypertension. While weight reduction is fast (about four to seven pounds a week at first), the procedure also has a higher complication rate than the more popular gastric banding.

The Gastric Liner: Artificial Intelligence

Surgeons are so inventive. Instead of an operation to bypass the absorption of nutrients and calories in your small intestines., why not just place a plastic barrier against that area in your intestine, preventing food from reaching the absorption surface? The one now being tried is about 60 centimeters (about two feet long) once deployed. It's inserted through your mouth, and like its mother, causes malabsorption. It's been used in about 250 patients to date (as opposed to over 100,000 a year for established procedures like the gastric band). But its results are promising: About 40 percent excess weight lost and reversal of type 2 diabetes in a large percentage.

Gastric Pacing: The Procedure of the Future for All of Us?

Throughout the day, we receive lots of signals that make us want to eat: come-hither burger commercials, coupons for $2.99 buffet specials, unopened bags of sugar wafers flirting with us every time we pass the pantry. But the future of waist-control surgical procedures could come in the form of a message-delivery system that sends signals that help keep us full or feeling full. This system was developed just like bypass procedures—by surgeons working on ulcer disease. They found that when they cut the vagus nerve, the brain no longer stimulated the stomach to make acid, and intestinal contractions slowed down. In effect, disrupting the vagus nerve sent a message that put the intestines to sleep, and the doctors realized that if you could control the message, then you could control the feelings of satiety.

To do that, scientists developed a gastric pacemaker that can be placed on the stomach near the vagus nerve. That pacemaker sends signals to the brain that you're always full by mimicking the actions of CCK (remember, Crucial Craving Killer). So that means it will take a lot less to get you full—and you won't eat as many calories because the pacemaker will send the signal that it feels like Thanksgiving dinner even if you've had only carrot sticks. Clinical trials are now being done, and the really exciting part about gastric pacemakers is that they could become the option for those in the middleman's zone—those with a large enough waist to be frustrated by dietary stalling but not wide enough to risk gastric banding or bypass surgery. Even better, the pacemaker could be adjusted for voltage to adjust the signals depending on your needs. How well does it work? We don't know yet, but the early reports are that it doesn't work as well as restrictive procedures; however, it's less invasive because no organs are being manipulated, and eventually it could even be placed endoscopically, with no cuts at all. And most likely, its descendants will serve as the basis for hybrids and new technologies that will be developed for people with any kind of waist issues.

YOU TIPS!

Interrogate Yourself. We have nothing against using crutches when we break an ankle, tear a knee ligament, or need to trip a purse-snatcher, so there's no reason not to consider weight-loss surgeries if you qualify for them. They're effective, they're fast, and they have the potential to turn a blimp of a body into a dragster. But they don't come without risks and potential complications, and they necessitate long-term behavioral changes.

Weight-loss surgery will do more than give you the confidence to reintroduce tank tops into your wardrobe. It can also save your life. Still, you have to know that it's not for everyone—and it can be challenging. So when you investigate options, be aware of the ways to lower your risks and increase your odds of success. Your first order of business is asking yourself these two questions:

Are You a Candidate?

You're eligible for surgery if you fit one of these three categories:

- ❖ If you're 100 pounds or more over your ideal weight.
- ❖ If you have a BMI over 40.
- ❖ If you have a BMI over 35 with hypertension, diabetes, arthritis, sleep apnea, serious lipid abnormalities, or altered body image.

For any of these procedures, you need to be willing to make the life changes—exercise and diet—that will make these procedures work. Without them, these procedures won't be successful. After an initial "bounce" downward, you could be back at marathon munching before you know it. You will also need to be realistic about the potential side effects, like hair loss, dumping, diarrhea, and vomiting.

Whom Do I Trust to Switch My Duodenum or Band My Stomach or Bypass My Gastric?

You wouldn't want an orthodontist removing a tumor, an orthopedic surgeon doing a heart transplant, or a urologist doing a nose job. So the same rules apply here: Find a specialist. Ideally, you'll use a facility and team that will do the procedure laparoscopically, as opposed to open. Laparoscopy means that the surgeons will make small incisions and do the procedure through tubes (it'll appear as if they're working with chopsticks). Laparoscopic surgery means you'll heal faster with less pain, but sometimes the surgeon has to resort to the old-fashioned way.

You'll want to find a hospital that does at least 150 procedures a year (yes, 150—no exceptions)—such hospitals have much lower complication rates than those that don't. Whoever your surgeon is, be sure there's an entire team of support both pre-op (to minimize complications) and post-op (to give you the best chance for success), including a nutritionist and psychiatrist. You can eat your way through—and thus destroy—any of these procedures. A support team can help you prevent post-op pudding backfires and give you resources to call upon as you're adjusting to your new eating habits—and new body. You should choose a hospital certified by the American Society for Bariatric Surgery (ASBS) (www.asbs.org).

Waist Management Under Age 18

Getting Your Kids to Eat Right

Diet Myths

❖ Kids can easily outgrow early baby fat.

❖ Kids will naturally eat the right foods because their bodies crave it.

❖ You can't change what a child likes and doesn't like.

Of all the superpowers we'd like to have (and we can think of quite a few), we wish there was one that would allow us to magically change some popular sayings and slogans: "Like a kid in a candy store," "Trix are for kids," and "Have a Coke and a smile."

Our versions may not be all that catchy, but they sure would be a lot better for the long-term health of our children: "Like a kid in a produce aisle," "Sugary cereals are for garbage disposals," and "Have a pop, an insulin shot, and pair of size-53 pants."

While you may be struggling with your own weight issues, childhood obesity has become a capital-*H* huge problem that we absolutely need to address head-on. In fact, it's the single most prominent chronic disease in childhood—and the problem, like the collective waistband of our country's kids, is getting bigger every day. In this appendix, we'd like to address the delicate balance of getting kids to eat foods that give them energy, satisfaction, and nutrition, even when faced with obstacles such as the relentless marketing messages that simmer in their minds every single day.

The truth is that although adults have a lot of biological underpinnings they can blame their obesity on (thyroid issues, for one), children very rarely have a genetic or medical condition (other than genes that make saturated fat, sugar, and salt addictive) that contributes to obesity. The main cause of childhood obesity, while certainly multilayered, is really simple: bad eating **Myth Buster** habits. That's not to dismiss, of course, the fact that kids get some of their bad habits even in utero—that is, some habits are coded into a child's genome because of how a mother may have eaten energy-sapping stuff with saturated fat, straight sugar, and salt during pregnancy. Kids do have the ability to change those codes through a process called epigenetics (which we discuss in detail in *YOU: Having a Baby*).

Yup, that's right. You, as a parent, really have the ability to control your children's metabolic destiny by establishing the right eating habits that they will carry with them through childhood, adolescence, and **Myth Buster** adulthood. The trick, as any parent knows, is that children can be as hard to move into action as a 300-year-old tree trunk. What we want to do is give you some of the strategies that will help you help your children make smart, nutritious, healthy choices throughout their lives. The big battle cannot happen at home after they get their little hands on the packaged goods. The big decisions have to be made in the supermarket aisle as you select foods that create only acceptable eating options at home.

First, however, we want to make sure you understand the seriousness of this issue. Just consider these stats and ramifications:

❖ There was a 54 percent increase in obesity in children under the age of thirteen from the 1980s to the 1990s. Currently, 20 percent of children between six and nineteen are obese.

❖ Your chances of being obese as an adult are dramatically increased if you are obese as a child. For example, there's a 41 percent chance of being an obese adult if you're obese at age seven, a 75 percent chance if you're obese at twelve, and a 90 percent chance if you're obese as an adolescent.

❖ The medical consequences of childhood obesity are staggering. There's a huge increase in the risk of developing hypertension, type 2 diabetes, coronary artery disease, joint problems, stroke, and cancer as well as many other conditions. That's probably not the life you want for your kids.

❖ The psychological consequences can be just as damaging, albeit in other ways. Overweight kids have a harder time interacting with peers, they're less often chosen as preferred playmates, they have lower self-esteem, and they have to deal with negative stereotypes and discrimination all throughout life. (We tend to think that kids who suffer through these troubles would gladly trade in their sugary cereals for smoother relations with their peers. Take that, Trix!)

We could spend a lot of time playing the blame game, because, frankly, there's a heck of a lot of blame to go around. We could blame the aforementioned marketing and our easier access to junk foods. We could blame the increased time kids spend watching TV and decreased time playing outside. We could blame the limited physical activity that kids get in school. We could blame the busy lives of parents, who don't have the time to cook healthful foods. We could blame the poor quality of school lunches. We could blame the lack of safe streets, which keeps kids playing indoors instead of playing outside. We could blame cookies. We could blame candy. We could blame grilled cheese or mac and cheese or Cheez Doodles.

But you know what? We don't want to play that game (actually we just did, didn't we?). We want you to roll the dice and move forward. Follow the *YOU: On a Diet* strategies below to get your kid going in the right direction. If you allow your own waist to get out of control, there's a very good chance that you will send your child directly to the jail of omental obesity. Unfortunately, if you can't find a way to turn the situation around, it may very well be a life sentence.

YOU TIPS!

Throughout this book, you'll find our specific food recommendations; the same principles hold true for kids. The good foods will rock your body; the bad foods will rot your body. With kids, though, it's not always about knowledge; it's about a parent instilling good habits, making healthy living fun and engaging, and teaching them the fundamentals that will become second nature. And you'll make them more emotionally involved with their bodies—a good thing, as they will value themselves more. Here, we present some of the ways you can combat this weighty issue.

Eat Together. In this era of soccer games, dance recitals, Mom working late, sister's having a Pluto project, and brother's putting together a PowerPoint, it's easy to fall into the trap: Eat quick, eat in front of the TV, eat junk. Big mistake. Of all the things you can do to influence the health of your child, perhaps the most important is to make family dinner a priority. Research shows that having family dinner more than twice a week can positively influence a child's waist, eating behavior, and overall psychological development.

Play Red Light, Green Light. Kids love this game on the playground, but you can also play it in the kitchen to teach young kids about healthy foods. For young kids, make a short list of green-light "yes" foods (such as vegetables, fruit, nonfried fish), red-light "no" foods (such as soda), and yellow-light "treat" foods (the 100 percent whole grain, 100 percent omega-3 chia muffin or Lifestyle 180 Bar after dinner). It makes it fun for kids and teaches them principles that will last. Other cool games that work well with some kids:

- ❖ Find the best cereal in the store (based on what you learn from labels; see below).
- ❖ Have a kids cooking day (pick one healthy meal that your kids could assist with).
- ❖ Toss out the junk at a friend's house (with said friend's approval).

Create a Mantra. Kids can be motivated to change their behavior if you introduce a fun system that gets their little imaginative and competitive minds churning. One we love: The "5 to 0 Go!" system developed by the Cleveland Clinic. Basically, you come up with a daily checklist of 5 things you need to eat or do every day, 4 things, 3 things, and so on. Throughout the day, you track what they've done to meet the goals, and you can even make it a daily competition between siblings. Here's an example:

- ❖ 5 veggies/fruits
- ❖ 4 servings of nonfat dairy (for calcium and vitamin D3)
- ❖ 3 compliments (create a positive environment)
- ❖ 2 or fewer hours of screen time
- ❖ 1 hour or more of play/exercise

❖ 0 sweetened beverages, other than nonfat milk (children under age two [some say all children] need full-fat milk)

Start Early. A basic biological fact: Kids will not crave foods they're not familiar with. So as soon as you are pregnant, or if we've already missed that date, as soon as your kids start eating solid foods, really concentrate on the YOU strategies—no added sugar or syrups, less than 4 grams of saturated fat per meal, no trans fat, and only 100 percent whole grain foods. If your kids don't taste high-sugar foods such as candy, cereals, and soda, they won't grow to like them (and won't "please-Mama" for them all day long). We also recommend that you teach your kids to start reading labels (but please, don't make it an obsession; some think that obsessing too much can instill eating-disorder behavior in children). See the figure below for the big things to consider when looking at labels.

Myth Buster

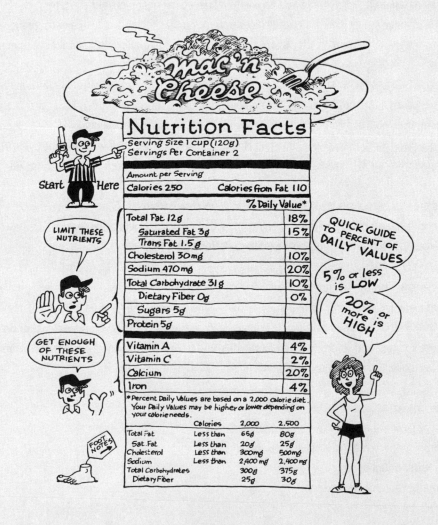

Don't Go Too Far in the Other Direction. We've seen it happen: Parents have success on a low-fat diet, so they decide that the kids need to follow it too. Not a great strategy. Kids need healthy fat for brain development. So though you don't need to calculate every single meal, a good ballpark figure is for kids to have about 20 percent to 25 percent of a day's calories in protein (important for muscle building), 15 to 30 percent in healthy fat, and 50 to 60 percent in healthy carbs. Another note about nutrients: Teens should consume about 1,500 milligrams of calcium, children 800 milligrams, and toddlers 500 to 600 milligrams daily. Since 60 percent of bone mass is accumulated during puberty, you want to make sure kids get enough for building a strong skeletal foundation.

Don't Talk About It. Some research shows that the majority of teasing about a child's weight doesn't happen in school, the neighborhood, the locker room, the mall, or even via cyber means. It happens at home. And that's what directly influences a child's self-esteem. Instead of criticizing (and teasing, of course), it's more effective to talk less and do more, by making your home environment more conducive to healthy eating and physical activity. Do not use body dissatisfaction as a motivator for change; instead, you'll be more effective using some of the game-playing methods detailed above. Also, don't use the word "diet" at home for parents or for kids; it tends to backfire when kids believe they're "on" some kind of temporary solution to weight issues.

Make Some House Rules. Part of establishing a healthy routine is establishing guidelines, principles, and traditions that will make healthy living automatic. Some easy ones that you can instill (and enforce):

❖ Set a limit for daily TV and video games, and take them out of the kids' bedrooms.
❖ Don't eat in front of the TV or computer (it leads to mindless eating, not to mention the fact that your metabolic rate decreases as you watch TV, making it a double downer).
❖ Make at least one family activity a week something that involves physical activity (a hike or bowling night instead of a movie and popcorn).
❖ Pack healthy lunches, rather than relying on less healthy in-school options.

How to Handle Teens. Since teens and tweens spend more time texting than talking, U r going 2 have 2 come up with some different solutions. They're not going to take too kindly to supermarket games, especially because they don't like to listen to adults anyway, so the task is a little more delicate. To be most effective, you want to give them strategies that will allow them to make choices rather than follow orders. Some strategies that you can try for an older child who's battling weight issues:

❖ It can be more effective to tell your teens why good foods are good, rather than what those good foods are. The rest of the book will give you those answers and aha moments.

❖ Make one night a week your child's cooking night. He can choose what to make—as long as it fits the nutritional guidelines. Thinking about what is healthful will get him considering nutritional facts but still give him freedom to create and experiment. Provide some ideas: Maybe a whole wheat pizza (with low-fat cheese and lots of veggies). Or even start out with salsa or guacamole.

❖ If your teen is an outdoor type, start a garden and grow some vegetables. Lots of kids like the idea of seeing food as it comes up from the ground.

❖ Hike, hike, hike. Long walks through nature are about adventure and exploration (and, as a side effect, calorie burning). Look up local trails, and let your kid pick the path for the day.

❖ Bike, bike, bike. More and more communities have bike paths, and cycling is another great family activity.

❖ Establish a reward system. If your teen reaches his or her goal (maybe a waist size, a dress size, or whatever other goal she sets up), reward it with something special: a pedicure, the newest sneakers, a fun outing with her friends.

Focus on Mental Resilience More than Weight Loss. Kids are often embarrassed to speak directly about their developing bodies. To avoid the awkward discussion, start the conversation by teaching kids how to become tough enough mentally to deal with the world they're growing up in. Teach them that the best way to hone their mental resilience is to control what they put into their bodies, since they are making this decision unilaterally. The conversation can evolve into a weight-loss tool if appropriate. For more great ideas, check out www.healthcorps.org to see how kids teach other kids about staying fit.

Play, Play, Play. Buy some balls, go outside, run, run, run. We've gotten so far away from the days when kids would play for hours outside, and we need to get some of that back. There are many creative ways you can get your kids moving without having them feel as though they're doing a workout. Routine walks create physical time for parents and kids and are also good one-on-one time. For those of you who want a little more structured routines for the kids, try this kid-friendly workout that will get their bodies moving—and their minds engaged.

YOU Workout for Kids

1: CRISSCROSS

Builds heart strength, helps improve coordination

With feet shoulder width apart and your hands on your waist, jump your feet into a crisscross position. Go back and forth, switching your feet from back to front. Do for thirty seconds. For a more advanced exercise, reach your arms out at shoulder height, palms up, and imagine you are holding glasses of water on your palms. As you crisscross, try not to move your hands, so that you don't spill the water.

a.   b.   c.   d. advanced

2: GROUND TO SKY

Improves balance and strengthens every muscle

While balancing on one foot, reach down and touch the ground with both hands. Then reach up toward the sky while simultaneously swinging one foot up in front of you, ideally bringing your knee into line with your hip. Do ten times each leg.

a.   b.

3: HAMSTRING HANG

Stretches hamstrings and back

With your feet wider than shoulder width apart and your toes pointed forward, slowly drop your hands toward the ground between your feet. Hold for ten seconds. Walk your hands to your left foot and hold for ten seconds, then to your right foot and hold for ten seconds. Move back to the center for ten seconds. Really relax your neck and think hanging down instead of reaching down. Take deep breaths the entire time.

4: ARMCOPTER

Stretches shoulders and gets the blood flowing in the arms

With your feet together circle your arms five times. Try to clap your hands in front of your face. Your goal is to make circles as big as feels comfortable. Relax your shoulders, and resist bobbing your neck; keep your head upright. Do twice.

5: AIR ANGELS

Strengthens entire back

Lie face down on your stomach. Close your eyes and reach your arms above your head, your palms facing down. With your feet together, lift your legs off the ground and keep them there. Keeping your arms straight, reach your hands back toward your hips. Go back and forth twenty-five times, making an angel. For a more advanced exercise, move your legs as well. The higher you lift your knees and armpits, the harder it is.

a.

b.

advanced

6: TRICEPS PUSH-UPS

Works triceps and chest

While on your stomach, bring your hands underneath your shoulders, palms down and fingers spread. Kick your heels up so your legs are at right angles, and cross your ankles. Keeping a straight line between the top of your head and your knees, do twenty push-ups. Keep your elbows flush against your sides so that they rub against your shirt. Keep your abs tight. For a more advanced exercise, balance on your toes rather than on your knees.

a.

b.

advanced

7: DONKEY KICKS

Strengthens quadriceps and shoulders

While on all fours with your shoulders over your hands and your hips over your knees, lift your knees one inch off the ground. Now bounce and lift your feet one inch off the ground. Do twenty-five times. Try to float your feet off the ground, and make as little noise as possible. Do twenty-five times. For a more advanced exercise, try to kick your feet up behind you like a donkey while maintaining a soft landing.

8: QUAD BEND

Stretches quads and knees

Kneel and position your feet and knees a little wider apart than your hips. Maintain a straight line with the outsides of your lower legs and point your toes directly behind you with the soles of your feet facing up. Drop your tailbone between your heels; lower yourself only as far as feels comfortable for your knees, or else drop all the way down and lie down on your back. Hold for thirty seconds. Scan your body and take deep breaths, releasing any tension.

9: ZIGZAG

Strengthens the entire core

Lie on your back with your legs bent and your feet flat on the ground. Interweave your fingers behind your head. Open your elbows to the side so you cannot see them. Lift your head off the ground and hold it there; maintain a relaxed neck. Lift your feet an inch off the ground and zigzag them out until they are almost straight. Go only as far out as you can keeping your lower back flat on the ground. Then zigzag them back toward your tailbone. Do twenty zigzags.

a.

b.

side to side

10: BACK BEND

Stretches abs and chest

Kneel and place your palms on your back with your fingers pointing down. Looking up toward the ceiling, bring your elbows toward each other. To increase the stretch, gently press your hips forward. Take five deep chest breaths.

11: BREAK DANCING

Strengthens entire body; great for agility

Get into the "up" push-up position. Walk your feet around clockwise toward the outside of your left hand. When you get to your left hand, lift it off the ground and put it back on the exact same spot. Keep walking your feet around in front of you until you get to your right hand. When you do, lift it off the ground and put it on the exact same spot. Do five clockwise circles, then switch and do five counterclockwise. Focus on always having your middle finger pointed up and your elbows barely bent. For a more advanced exercise, do it faster.

a.

Crab Walk

Lift Arm

b.

walk walk walk

c.

Keep on Crabbin'

walk under your hand

d.

12: ONE-FOOT HOP

Improves balance: strengthens legs; improves cardio
With your hands on your waist and balancing on one foot with your standing leg slightly bent, hop around in circles five times. Switch directions and do five more. Do twice. For a more advanced exercise, do a shoulder press on every hop. Resist looking down; look straight ahead.

Hop!

Rotate

13: INVISIBLE CHAIR

advanced

Stretches hips and lower back and improves balance
Standing in place, lift your right ankle up on top of your left quad. With your hands on your waist, slowly lower your tailbone until you get a stretch in your hip. (For a more advanced exercise, straighten your arms above your head, palms facing, and bring your thumbs back as you squat lower.) Hold for twenty seconds and switch sides. Take long, deep breaths throughout the stretch.

Acknowledgments

Ted, Ted, Ted, Ted. We cannot say his name enough. Ted Spiker brought the multiple complex pieces together in an accessible and humorous fashion that is edgy but never condescending. Gary Hallgren continues to amaze us with his wit and raw artistic talent. He takes challenging concepts and contorts them into engaging cartoons packed with critically important content. View his illustrations with great care to observe every nuance. Craig Wynett is a seer and had the vision to bring us together. He always busts through the clutter with the big ideas that change the way we (and you) should think. These massive ideas are woven through the text and constitute many of our YOU-reka moments. The Lifestyle 180 team of master chef Jim Perco, nutritionist Kristin Kirkpatrick, and director Dr. Beth Ricanti created sixty new Lifestyle 180 recipes that fit YOU guidelines, that taste terrific (some didn't and got trashed), and that Mike can cook in thirty minutes start to finish. Linda Kahn's great editorial advice and attention to detail and data made this edition better. Dr. Ellen Rome's brilliant intellect and dedicated desire to contribute information that would benefit the younger readership made her a crucial ally. She was crucial to the appendix on obesity control under age eighteen. Jeff Roizen's remarkable ability to gather raw data and interpret the sometimes disparate results helped us teach America about the hard science of obesity research. We thank Joel Harper for his tireless efforts to make the YOU Workout the perfect tool for us to get procrastinators to exercise. Dr. Keith Roach's clinical insights kept our aim on target. While the hours of conference calls, research, and writing were sometimes exhausting, this powerful team always pulled in the same direction to resolve content and style conflicts. Steve Phillips helped us with his very sophisticated understanding of emotional eating. Finally, our agent Candice Fuhrman's superb insights and honest commentary allowed this book to grow into the manuscript America deserves. Arthur Perry is the plastic surgeon supreme who guided our appendix on removing excess skin. And the shrinking John Ellis made important suggestions to this edition.

We also want to thank the group at Free Press (Simon & Schuster) who so enthusiastically supported this material and dedicated themselves to bringing our ideas to the world. Thanks especially to our insightful editor, Dominick Anfuso, and his assistant, Leah Miller. We appreciate the courageous leadership of Martha Levin, and the tireless support of Jill Siegel, Carisa Hays, Linda Dingler, and Suzanne Donahue.

We are indebted to our wonderful collaborators at RealAge.com, including Charlie Silver, Dr. Keith Roach, Meredith Wade, and especially Val Weaver for coming on strong at the end (and for the two *Vegetarian Times* recipes), and the former Discovery Health team, including Eileen O'Neil, Donald Thoms, John Grassie, and, of course, Billy Campbell. The patients depicted in the wonderful shows on Discovery Health and the PBS special *YOU: On a Diet* were real and are still inspirational: Jodi now weighs less than anytime since grade school; sixty pounds into her weight-loss journey, she tried again to become pregnant and subsequently had a beautiful daughter. Jillian went from a size 18++ to 6. Howard lost weight steadily until meeting his ideal. We've received more than 80,000 thank-you notes since first publication—all along the lines of "I've tried many others, and this one worked, and I'm not yo-yoing anymore. Thank you for the inspiration." We get more than 800 questions a week—keep them coming. From this, more than 100,000 questions and answers, and we've chosen 101 of the most common to include in this edition. Thank you—they help us learn too.

In a book of this scope based in science, no one human commands all the needed knowledge, so we sought advice from many world experts who selflessly shared their insights in the true academic tradition. We list them all here without details of their contributions in order to save space for the actual book, but we deeply appreciate their dedication to their specialties and willingness to sacrifice their time in helping craft the most scientifically accurate book on obesity possible. We thank Dr. Linda Bartoshuk, Dr. Mark Bessler, John Campodonico, Jason Conviser, Kathy Chambers, Irwin Davis, Ruth Davis, Dr. Lisa Deosimo, Mark Eldaief, Dr. Kevin Fickenscher, Michael Gershon, Donoyan Green, Tracy Hafens, Dr. Byron Hoogwerf, Dr. William Inabnet, Gail Jolly, Evan Johnson, Paul Katz, Judith Korner, Ivan Kronenfeld, Dr. Jon Lapook, Karen Levin, Dr. Ben Lewis, Chris Malcom, Dr. Beth Mintzer, Dr. Michael O'Donnell, Susan Petre, Dr. S. Sethu Reddy, Dr. Paul Rosenberg, Sean Shilinsky, Nancy Unobskey, Sidney Unobskey, Meredith Uran-Skuro, Dr. Bernard Walsh, Jim Wharton, and Dr. Jim Zins. This book became a number one bestseller in six countries and sold more than 8 million copies because of the tireless work of so many. Thank you.

—Michael F. Roizen and Mehmet C. Oz

Mike's Acknowledgments

Most diets and diet books fail you because you regain more than you lost—and that is an epic tragedy of wasted effort. I need to thank the many special people who helped us make this book one that leads to your ideal waist size. So I am grateful to the many other people who did much more than discard the emails when we asked them (sometimes desperately) to help us explain what hadn't been known even five years ago about hunger and satiety. John La Puma, a doc-tor who doubled as a chef at Rick Bayless's Chicago restaurants, taught me more than I now know about food and cooking. And Donna Szymanski had the patience to correct me and make the recipes more times than can be counted on all fingers and toes.

I need to thank the twenty or so fourth-year medical students each year who took the ten-day, ten-hour-a-day course that Dan Zakri and I taught—you taught me more than I taught you. I'd like to also thank the numerous tasters who visited our home to participate in the yearlong quest for perfect recipes that were great-tasting, were easy to make, and contained only foods that made you healthier. And the Wattels of Lettuce Entertain You indulged and encouraged even when their own patrons shunned the food with hearts next to them in the late 1990s ("times will change"). Our family was fully engaged—with Jeff as our MD, PhD, research assistant and Jennifer and Nancy as critical tasters and reviewers; joined at times by the "enlarged family" of the Unobskeys and Campodonicos, and Dr. Axel Goetz, Ruth Klein, and Irwin Davis. Ruth especially made the diet chapter easier to follow and helped create the shopping lists. I also need to thank Tracy Hafen, who taught me a magnificent amount about exercise; Sukie Miller and Anita Shreve, for saying the early chapters were just what she wanted to read; the many gerontologists and internists who read sections of the book for accuracy; others on the RealAge team who validated and verified the content, and contributed their expertise to the book; and Shivani Chadha and Kate Poneta, the research associates who worked tirelessly to analyze the nutrients of all the recipes we tested.

I also want to acknowledge the passion and tough love from the staff of the former Center for Partnership Medicine at Northwestern Memorial Hospital in Chicago, especially Dr. Dan Dermann, Drew Palumbo, and Dean Harrison. And my partners who allowed me the time to complete the work: Dr. Aaron Gerber and Mike Kessel.

My administrative assistant, Beth Grubb, made this work possible: She made sure the weekends (and most nights) were free of CAVs games to work on YOU, YOU-Turns, and YOU-reka Moments. I could not have done this were The Institute of Anesthesiology, which includes Critical Care Medicine and Pain Management at the Cleveland Clinic and its staff not the best in the world. But it is and they are. Add to that the now wonderful and innovative staff and associated at the Cleveland Clinic Wellness Institute, including Jim Perko and Kristin Kirkpatrick, who worked tirelessly on the Lifestyle 180 recipes, and their medical director Dr. Beth Ricanati. It's no accident that the Cleveland Clinic has been ranked by *U.S. News & World Report* number one for fifteen years in a row in cardiac care: Toby Cosgrove, Joe Hahn, Martin Harris, Joe Patrichek, and Paul Madsen are the best at their positions and insist on innovation and simple excellence—they understand the need to prevent illness and promote wellness. And to the Wellness Institute and staff, especially Quintene Graham, who hunted down so many studies, and Nabil Gabriel, who provided so much support. And thanks to all the outstanding colleagues at the clinic who answered our many questions. And my prior and current other associates: Anne-Marie Ruthrauff, Michelle Lewis, and Candy Lawrence, each deserve special thanks, as do some of our original RealAge partners: Martin Rom and Charlie Silver; and Diane Reverand, who told me not to worry about offending medical colleagues—as long as the science was solid, they would understand we were trying to motivate YOU to understand that you can control your genes and jean size.

Nancy and our children, Jeffrey and Jennifer: I want to thank you for more than your critical reviews and scientific expertise. Your encouragement and patience, constant love and support really are saint-like. Thanks, Saint Nancy.

I hope and believe this book will help YOU to take control of your waist. That would be the best reward any physician could want.

—Michael F. Roizen

Mehmet's Acknowledgments

I thank my colleagues in Cardiothoracic Surgery for supporting the belief that surgeons can heal with our pens as well as with the cold steel of a scalpel edge. They freed me to write and brainstorm, especially Dr. Eric Rose, Dr. Craig Smith, Dr. Yoshifuma Naka, Dr. Mike Argenziano, Dr. Henry Spotnitz, Dr. Allan Stewart, Dr. Barry Esrig, and the other superb surgeons on our team. The physician assistants, especially Laura Baer, and the nurses in the OR, ICU, and floor cared so meticulously for my patients that in my free time I could turn my mind totally to this book without the need to "pick up the pieces" from my clinical work. My clinical office manager, Lidia Nieves, has a razor-sharp mind (and memory) that prevented any patient's care from being compromised. My administrative coordinator, Michelle Washburn, not only made sure that all the tasks surrounding the book were done on time, but also read countless drafts of the text and provided incredibly insightful commentary. Finally, our divisional administrator, Diane Amato, shared her precious intellect with me without concern for her time and provided critically important edits and broad opinions about the direction of our work. We would have had an inferior book without their advice and support.

Thanks to all my colleagues in other specialties who provided quality control by offering thoughtful feedback on our writing. We list them in our joint acknowledgment by name, but their tireless responses to my sometimes tedious questions will always be appreciated. Thanks to the wonderfully talented (and busy) public affairs group at New York–Presbyterian, including Bryan Dotson, Alicia Park, and Myrna Manners, who have taught me to communicate complex messages in an accessible fashion. Thank you, Ivan Kronenfeld for all your guidance.

My parents, Mustafa and Suna Oz, taught me to work hard for my life goals and never let go, even when success appears a fading hope. My parents-in-law, Gerald and Emily Jane Lemole, shared their strong value system and desire to look for the more profound answers in seeking truth. Thanks to my wife and coauthor, Lisa, who all our friends unanimously agree is the "brains" of the family. It is fun to marry and work with one's soul mate. Our siblings—Seval, Nazlim, Laura, Emily, Michael, Samantha, and Christopher—selflessly offered honest commentary on our work. Our four children—Daphne, who inherited the bug and has written her first bestseller; Arabella; Zoe; and Oliver—bring joy to our lives with their every breath. Thanks for sacrificing numerous weekends in the name of "Waist Management."

—Mehmet C. Oz

Index

impact of, 98–101
and impact of fat on health, 108, 110
impact on health of, 114
and inflammation, 76, 81, 97, 98, 100, 101
and perfect storm, 200
and psychology of dieting, 167, 168, 177, 178
response to, 98–101
and stimulation for eating high calorie food, 20, 24
strategies for reduction of, 418
types of, 89–90
YOU-reka about, 90
stretch marks, 466, 467, 468
stroke
    and children's eating habits, 497
    FAQs about, 401, 402, 434, 435, 436, 437
    and impact of fat on health, 108, 117, 121, 126, 133
Stuffed Whole Wheat Pizza (recipe), 271, 276, 331–32
subcutaneous fat, 110, 112
substitution, 178, 204, 207, 258
Suck in Belly (exercise), 12, 161, 194, 227, 232, 242, 243, 419
sucrose, 57
sugar
    addiction to, 413–14
    and appetite, 52, 53
    and children's eating habits, 496, 500
    and digestive system, 55, 62, 63, 64, 65, 67–68, 71
    and elimination diets, 104
    and emotions, 187, 191, 193
    Factoid about, 89
    FAQs about, 404, 405, 407, 413–14, 415, 422, 428, 434, 441, 442, 443–44, 447, 448
    and fast foods, 283
    and "fat free" products, 94
    and history of human diets, 29, 31
    and hormones, 142–43
    and impact of fat on health, 120, 121, 122, 123, 124, 126, 129, 135
    and inflammation, 79, 80, 104–5
    and labels, 269, 281
    and muscle, 154
    and perfect storm, 200, 206
    and psychology of dieting, 168, 169
    and ready-made meals, 287
    and Rule of 5, 53, 270
    in sports drinks, 151
    and stress, 92
    and weight-loss drugs, 459, 461

and weight-loss surgery, 490
and whole grains, 282
and YOU Diet, 258, 263, 264–65
and YOU strategies, 225–26, 227
See also artificial sweeteners; blood sugar; glucose; sweeteners; specific recipe
sulforaphane, 398
sulfuric acid, 464
Sun Salutation (yoga), 240–41
sunflower oil, 132
Superman (exercise), 239, 245
supplements, 57, 86, 227, 259, 436, 442, 487
support system, 13–14, 175, 225, 226. See also buddies
surgeons, weight-loss, 492–93
surgery. See weight-loss surgery
Sweet Beet and Gorgonzola Salad (recipe), 320
sweeteners, 104–5, 405, 406, 413. See also type of sweetener
Synthroid, 445
syrup, 121, 126, 258, 270, 279, 422, 434, 442, 500

tabbouleh, 288
Taco Bell, 284
tahini, 288
tai chi, 155
tangerines, 278
tape measure
    importance of, 225
    scale watch versus, 416–17
target weight, 222
taste/taste buds, 40, 58, 67, 74, 94, 125, 178, 181, 258, 445–46, 462
tea, 103, 268, 275–77, 279, 395, 396, 406, 413, 428, 441
team, YOU, 13–14, 259, 273
teenagers, 501–2
teeth, 60, 61, 447
teetotaler's cocktail, 268
television, 149, 167, 178, 207, 420, 423, 427, 497, 501
temperature, 41, 42, 44, 96, 138, 234
temptation, 31, 197, 206, 207
testosterone, 47, 141, 142, 143, 144–45, 146, 414–15
thermogenesis, 41
thirst, 20, 24, 53, 151, 461, 483
thyme, 281, 392
thyroid, 80, 140–42, 145, 227, 414, 445, 496
thyroid-stimulating hormone test, 146
Tight Pants Syndrome, 81
tilapia, 402
tofu, 266, 288, 438

Tofu or Turkey Dogs with Sauerkraut (recipe), 344
Tofu Scramble (recipe), 292
tomato
    and digestive system, 68
    FAQs about, 393, 399, 402, 408, 439
    and GERD, 68
    and inflammation, 102
    shopping for, 278, 279, 281
    in soup, 393, 402
    and YOU Diet, 263, 266
Tomato-Avocado Salsamole with pita toasts, 268, 276, 358
Tomato Sauce (recipe), 379
tongue, 58, 59, 74
Topamax, 459
topiramate, 459
tortillas, 278, 288
trans fat
    and children's eating habits, 500
    and digestive system, 63
    and elimination diets, 104
    FAQs about, 445
    and impact of fat on health, 120, 121, 126, 131, 132
    and inflammation, 76, 93, 102
    and labels, 269
    and ready-made meals, 287
    and Rule of 5, 53, 270
    and weight-loss drugs, 460
    and YOU Diet, 258
    and YOU strategies, 225
Triceps Push-Ups (exercise), 505
triglycerides, 70, 93, 109–10, 136, 434, 438, 453
Troubleshooting Guide, YOU Diet, 287–88
trout, 102, 193, 438, 439, 448
tryptophan, 183, 193, 419
tummy tucks, 465, 467–68, 469, 470
tuna, 419
turkey, 193, 266, 276, 277, 280, 419, 425
Turkey Tortilla Wraps with Red Baked Potato (recipe), 274, 277, 336
Turkish Shepherd Salad (recipe), 317
turmeric, 102–3, 227, 263, 400, 432
Twenty-Minute YOU Workout
    additions to, 248–53
    equipment for, 160
    exercises for, 233–43, 244–46
    and impact of fat on health, 126
    overview of, 232
    as part of YOU Activity Plan, 230, 231, 233–43, 244–46
    and YOU Diet, 272, 273, 274
Two-Onion Delight (recipe), 300